MAY

Non-Animal Techniques

in

Biomedical and Behavioral Research and Testing

Non-Animal Techniques

in

Biomedical and Behavioral Research and Testing

Michael B. Kapis
Shayne C. Gad

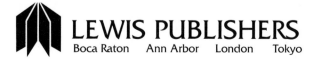

LEWIS PUBLISHERS

Boca Raton   Ann Arbor   London   Tokyo

Library of Congress Cataloging-in-Publication Data

Non-animal techniques in biomedical and behavioral research and
    testing / edited by Michael Kapis and Shayne C. Gad.
        p.   cm.
    Includes bibliographical references and index.
    ISBN 0-87371-504-7
    1. Biology, Experimental.   2. Animal experimentation.   3. Human
experimentation in medicine.   4. Toxicity testing—In vitro.
5. Medicine, Experimental—Data processing.   6. Medicine,
Experimental.   I. Kapis, Michael.   II. Gad, Shayne C., 1948–
R852.N65   1993
619—dc2   92-45746
                                                                            CIP

Direct all inquiries to CRC Press, Inc., 2000 Corporate Blvd., N.W., Boca Raton, Florida 33431.

PRINTED IN THE UNITED STATES OF AMERICA
1 2 3 4 5 6 7 8 9 0
Printed on acid-free paper

Preface

Within the last two decades, there has been a steadily increasing number of researchers, students, and educators investigating and utilizing alternative-to-animal methods in biomedical and psychological research, testing, and education. Some primary incentives for this interest in alternatives are (1) many recent advances in biotechnology, (2) ethical issues involving animal experimentation, (3) accuracy and precision, (4) expedience, and (5) cost effectiveness.

In 1959, Russell and Birch defined alternatives as "Refinement, Reduction, and Replacement", commonly known as the 3 Rs. This volume will focus primarily on two of the 3 Rs — reduction and replacement. Therefore, we define an alternative as any method (primarily non-animal) that either reduces or replaces the need for animal models in biomedical and behavioral research, testing, and education. The exceptions are observational, painless, stress-free, and noninvasive laboratory investigations, as well as the study of animals in their natural environments (ethology).

Alternatives are now involved in every aspect of biomedical and behavioral research, testing, and education. Many of the recent advances in AIDS, heart disease, cancer, stroke, cystic fibrosis, Alzheimer's disease, drug designs, multiple sclerosis, Parkinson's disease, schizophrenia, etc., have benefitted and have been accomplished by the use of alternative methodologies.

In spite of this success, however, many scientists either are unaware or maintain "outdated" views of alternatives, adhering to the traditional practice of using animal models. The purpose of this volume is to inform the reader of the numerous potential applications that alternatives offer to biomedical and behavioral investigations. In order to accomplish this, we invited recognized leading scientists from industry and academia to write on their areas of expertise pertaining to alternatives. Emphasis was placed both on the application and on the strengths and weaknesses of the methods. An exhaustive but unsuccessful effort was made to enlist experts in the areas of physicochemical techniques, medical microbiology, and human autopsies. Since these are important areas of research and testing, we wrote brief chapters on these subjects and included extensive references.

Alternatives have given new meaning to "never say never". What a decade ago was thought to be "impossible" is now often "probable". Only a lack of imagination or ingenuity stands as an impediment to an ever-increasing utilization of alternative methods in biomedical and behavioral investigations.

Michael B. Kapis
Shayne C. Gad

Acknowledgments

I wish to thank everyone involved with supplying information and support for *Non-Animal Techniques in Biomedical and Behavioral Research and Testing.* I wish to extend special appreciation to Rowland Mitchell for proofreading and suggestions, to Kevin Winterfield for inspiration, to the librarians of the San Francisco Bay Area for their assistance, to Jon Lewis and staff at Lewis Publishers for their support and their unbelievable patience, and to Irene, Eleanor, and Cynthia for word processing.

Finally, I owe a special thanks to my wife, Luz, and my son, Christopher, for putting up with me during the lengthy creation of this book.

Michael B. Kapis

To Tine, and a special time. May it somehow and somewhere go on forever. And may the Lord always keep her in the sunshine.

Shayne C. Gad

The Editors

Michael B. Kapis, B.A., B.S., earned his B.A. in Physics from San Jose State University, where he also earned his B.S. and completed his coursework for the M.S. in biological science. He has a wide range of interests in the animal sciences.

During the time he was pursuing his degree in astrophysics, Mike became very interested in techniques and devices that might prevent animal–vehicle collisions. In particular, he is interested in ultrasonic sound and fluorescent markings as possible collision-deterrent mechanisms. His master's thesis involves the effects of alarm signals on deer movements. This interest in animal–vehicle accidents later led

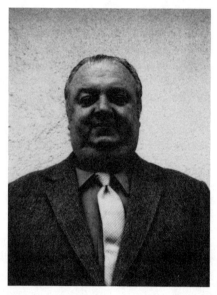

him to change his major from astronomy to biology.

In 1983, while visiting Davao City in the Philippines, Mike became involved with the plight of the endangered Philippine eagle. He later formed a nonprofit organization—Save The Philippine Eagle Fund—and since that time, he has focused his attention on conserving and restoring the rainforest habitat of the Philippine eagle.

Throughout his studies in biology, Mike has had an interest in the use of animals in research, testing, and education. He was concerned about the amount of needless duplication in animal experimentation. Later, he became aware that there were alternative-to-animal methods available. He selected the topic of alternatives for a graduate seminar presentation. He assembled many articles on alternatives while preparing for the seminar, which was well received. In 1986, Mike and a fellow graduate student, Kevin Winterfield, began publishing the quarterly *Alternatives To Animals Newsletter*, geared for the research and academic community.

Shayne C. Gad, Ph.D.,
is Director of Medical Affairs Product Support Services at Becton Dickinson, Research Triangle Park, North Carolina. His interests include neurotoxicology, alternative methods and models, dermal and immune toxicology, and statistics in toxicology. He has published more than 230 abstracts, articles, papers, chapters, and books in the field of toxicology. He is on the editorial boards of the *Journal of Applied Toxicology*, the *Journal of Fire Science*, and the *Journal of Acute Toxicology*; he is also Editor-in-Chief for *Toxicology Methods*. He has served on the National Institute of Standards and Technology Combustion Toxicology

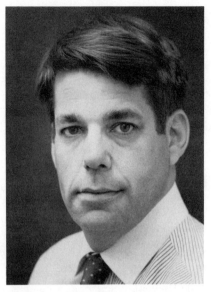

Task Force, the Consumer Product Safety Commission Toxicology Advisory Board, and on the SOT Animals in Research Nominations and Placement Committees; he has also served with trade association groups for Nylon 6, chrome chemicals, cyclohexanone, ketones, and phthalates. He is past president of the American College of Toxicology and is editor of the SOT Reproductive and Developmental Toxicology Newsletter.

Dr. Gad has lectured at Texas, Kansas, Rutgers, Johns Hopkins, and Pittsburgh, has served on several Ph.D. thesis committees, and is a grant reviewer for the Center for Alternatives to Animal Testing at Johns Hopkins University; he also established and taught a bachelor program in toxicology at the College of St. Elizabeth.

Dr. Gad serves on the National Institutes of Health (NIH) Occupational Safety and Health Study Section. He is a member of the Society of Toxicology, the American College of Toxicology, the Teratology Society, the Biometrics Society, and the American Statistical Association, and he is a Diplomate of the American Board of Toxicology.

Contributors

C. L. Alden
Product Safety and Metabolism
Searle
Skokie, Illinois

Sarah Barron
University of Texas System
Center for High Performance
   Computing
Austin, Texas

Charles Bauer, Jr.
NovaScreen®
Nova Pharmaceutical Corporation
Baltimore, Maryland

Maura Charlton
Department of Molecular Psychiatry
Yale University School of Medicine
New Haven, Connecticut

Jesse Driver
University of Texas System
Center for High Performance
   Computing
Austin, Texas

Shayne C. Gad
Medical Affairs Product Support
   Services
Becton Dickinson
Research Triangle Park, North
   Carolina

Alan M. Goldberg
Center for Alternatives to Animal
   Testing
School of Public Health
Johns Hopkins University
Baltimore, Maryland

Virginia C. Gordon
In-Vitro International
Irvine, California

Andrew J. Greenshaw
Department of Psychiatry
University of Alberta
Edmonton, Alberta, Canada

Robert Harkness
University of Texas System
Center for High Performance
   Computing
Austin, Texas

Michael B. Kapis
Alternatives To Animals
San Jose, California

Jennifer L. Kelsey
Division of Epidemiology
Stanford University School of
   Medicine
Stanford, California

Peter H. Klopfer
Department of Zoology
Duke University
Durham, North Carolina

John M. Last
Epidemiology and Community
   Medicine
University of Ottawa
Ottawa, Ontario, Canada

Peter G. Morris
Magnetic Research Center
Department of Physics
University of Nottingham
Nottingham, England

Susan Parker
School of Public Health
Columbia University
New York, New York

Paul S. Prueitt
Neural Network Research Facility
Department of Physics
Georgetown University
Washington, D.C.

Paul M. Sweetnam
Exploratory Medicinal Chemistry
Pfizer Central Research
Groton, Connecticut

Fang Wang
University of Texas System
Center for High Performance
   Computing
Austin, Texas

Frederick Wehr
Consultant
500 Edgevale Road
Baltimore, Maryland

Matthew Witten
University of Texas System
Center for High Performance
   Computing
Austin, Texas

John Yam
Cosmetics & Fragrance Worldwide
The Procter & Gamble Company
Cincinnati, Ohio

Table of Contents

Chapter 8 Ethology and Noninvasive Techniques
Peter H. Klopfer

Chapter 9 Computational Modeling of Biological/Medical Systems
Matthew Witten

Chapter 10 The Human Genome Project: An Overview of Computational Issues in Molecular Biology and Genetics
Sarah Barron, Matthew Witten, Robert Harkness, Fang Wang, and Jesse Driver

CHAPTER 1

Alternatives to Whole Animal Testing

Alan Goldberg and Frederick Wehr

1.0 Introduction

The Center for Alternatives to Animal Testing (CAAT), at the Johns Hopkins University School of Hygiene and Public Health in Baltimore, MD, was founded in 1981. It began as a cooperative venture of the School and the Cosmetic, Toiletry, and Fragrance Association, a body determined to develop ways of testing the safety of their products without having to rely so extensively on expensive, time consuming, and socially sensitive testing on live animals. The School's participation is a natural extension of its ongoing efforts in toxicology—the study of any substance, drug, or product that might be harmful, however mildly—and its intensive and world-wide pursuit of solutions to public health problems.

Today, CAAT is funded by almost 70 companies in the food, drug, cosmetics, consumer products, computer and petrochemical industries, and by individuals that support its mission.

In the years since the founding of the Center, substantial progress has been made toward reducing the number of animals necessary in product testing.[1] It must be recognized at the outset, however, that such institutions as the Food and Drug Administration (FDA) and the Environmental Protection Agency (EPA) are charged with guarding the public from intrusion into the marketplace of potentially

0-87371-504-7/93/$0.00+$.50

harmful chemicals, and *in vivo* (live animal) testing is the proven and accepted method from which these agencies cannot depart without the most positive proof that any *in vitro* alternative testing method proposed is just as good if not superior to *in vivo* testing.[2]

1.1 Why Test?

All testing of any substance to which humans are to be exposed—whether it be a drug, a food preservative or additive, a cosmetic product, one for household use, or whatever—is conducted with two goals. Is the product effective? Can the product be used safely? The investment by American industry in answering these questions is in the billions of dollars annually. Nowhere is the scope and intensity of this research greater than in the drug industry. The reader, we believe, will gain a better understanding of the place and the importance of animal testing if we first review the procedures followed in the development of a new drug and the questions and quandaries posed to researchers as they go about their work.[3]

Scientists in drug research invariably begin with a hypothesis. They assume that a new molecule or a modification of a molecule known to have certain effects on the human body might lead to a medication which would be an improvement over some existing drug or, even more dramatic, provide a cure for a disease to date unaffected by medications. The laws of chemistry limit the extent to which molecular modification is possible. Within those limits, the researchers and their colleagues devise methods to create the molecule envisioned bearing in mind, all along, that the number of potentially helpful molecules—the laws of chemistry notwithstanding—is enormous and that the track they have elected to follow commits the firm to a huge investment. Whether it will be commercially success-ful is unknown. It is estimated that only 1 in about 10,000 compounds formulated turns out to be helpful and that the average cost of developing one new drug may exceed $150 million.

1.2 A New Compound

Once the molecule has been synthesized, several questions arise. Is it more effective than an existing drug? What will be its side effects and are they greater or less than those of an existing drug? Might it prevent the onset of disease? And, more dramatically, might it treat a disease which is now untreatable or cure a disease which is now incurable? Let us suppose that the new molecule has been formulated, that it is stable, and that the rationale for its creation stands up to intellectual examination. Has it already been patented by another firm? If so, did that competitor devise the molecule with the same objective in mind? Maybe their researchers were seeking a cure for a different disease. If so, what are the implications?

After the new compound has been created, it is examined by pharmacologists who must determine whether it has any value. At this point, the testing of the drug on animals and by other methods—more on this later—may begin. Is it harmful and, if so, is there an adequate margin of safety above the therapeutic dose before reaching a toxic dose? Is it beneficial? If so, is it more beneficial than something already in existence? Does it do the unexpected? Usually, the unexpected is a negative and the compound may be retired then and there. If so, a sample or at least a record of the compound will be filed away for possible future use. Occasionally, the unexpected is beneficial or, at least, gives promise of being beneficial. AZT, a drug developed back in the 1960s and then put on the shelf, turned out to be helpful in the treatment of AIDS.

1.3 Looks Promising

Let's move on and assume that the new compound—at least in moderate doses—appears not to be toxic and that it gives promise of being beneficial to humans. Now, how long must we observe the test animals to ascertain that the drug is not having some long-term negative effect, that it will not cause cancer, and that it will not affect the animals' genetic structure. Brilliant men and women with access to astonishingly sophisticated equipment now examined the compound from every conceivable direction, in anticipation that they will be the ones to discover a new miracle drug.

Several years may go by before the initial safety tests are completed. And while the safety tests are underway, other scientists are studying the effectiveness of the compound and exploring the possibility that a further modification might make it better or, for that matter, effective in combating a completely different disease. And if that modification is made, will the drug be safer than the one under test? Questions, questions, questions, all requiring time and money for resolution.

Rarely does a new compound get this far in the testing process. But let us assume that all signs are positive, that the drug continues to hold promise of therapeutic and, equally important, that at therapeutic doses, it appears to be safe for humans. Next, metabolic studies involving *in vitro* human cells and larger mammals are subjected to the compound. The drug passes these tests.

1.4 Clinical Trials

Now it is time for clinical trials, for tests of the medication on healthy people and/or those afflicted with the disease in question. Five or six years may have gone by since the original formulation of the molecule. Volunteers, fully advised of the part they are playing, are given the drug. The typical approach in the clinics is to conduct Phase I studies, with emphasis on safety, in small numbers of healthy volunteers. Since safety is the greatest concern, these studies are not double blind, but are "open" or singly blind, permitting the physician to know as much information as possible. Once a drug is safe in healthy people, small Phase II studies are conducted in patients with the disease for which the drug has been developed. Initially, these are not double blind either, as safety again is the paramount issue. These small studies provide some information about safety, but lack sufficient numbers of patients to draw conclusions about effectiveness. Then, in Phase III, larger numbers of patients are given the drug, with the emphasis on proof of desired activity and to look for unwanted effects. Phase III studies are double-blind tests. That is, neither the patient nor the physician administering the drug knows whether the patient is receiving the drug or a placebo, something that is identical in appearance but totally neutral in medicinal effect. More time passes. The results of the test are studied. The drug is beneficial and not harmful at therapeutic doses.

1.5 Gaining Regulatory Approval

Next begins the long and tedious process of gaining approval for distribution. The U.S. FDA examines and re-examines the data, and questions and re-questions the scientists involved. Ultimately, approval is granted. The marketing of the product begins. After perhaps a decade, the public has a new product and the firm can expect to realize a return on its investment and begin the search for newer and better compounds.

1.6 Animal Testing

Drugs and other substances are usually screened through many tests using animals, including tests for sudden overdose (acute toxicity) and others that can take anywhere from a few days to 2 years to complete.[4] Since every new chemical introduced into the marketplace, every modification of an old chemical that is proposed, and any mixture of chemicals must be tested to understand the risk of exposure and to protect the public from hazard, it is obvious that the extent of *in vivo* testing is substantial. It is also costly and time consuming. The corporations' laboratories in which testing takes place are at the mercy of the animals' metabolism, their life span and/or reproductive cycles, and the variations which exist from one individual to another. Industry and mainstream animal welfare groups seek the common goal—sometimes for different reasons—of finding alternatives wherever possible. Of the many live animal tests, three are often singled out for criticism by animal activists groups—the LD_{50} test (LD stands for lethal dose), and the Draize eye and skin irritation tests. The LD_{50} test is a measure of acute lethality developed in the 1920s. The Draize tests for irritancy requires the chemical in question to be applied to the eye and skin of a rabbit.[5] There will be more about these tests later.

1.7 Alternatives—Refinement, Reduction, Replacement

The principal alternative to animal testing is *in vitro* (literally, "in glass") testing, a broad term which describes testing that does not involve live animals. *In vitro* testing utilizes a battery of living systems—bacteria, cultured animal cells, fertilized chicken eggs, and frog embryos—that can be employed to evaluate the likelihood that a substance might be toxic to humans. In recent years, research has been conducted in which chemicals are tested in cultures of human cells from various organs and tissues so that the question of human toxicity may be answered more directly.[6,7]

Thanks in part to research sponsored by CAAT, a number of *in vitro* techniques have already been developed which have dramatically reduced the number of live animals previously required to determine whether a substance is safe. Such tests, in short, serve to screen substances from consideration or, alternatively, to demonstrate that they are deserving of further evaluation.[8,9]

Several factors have contributed to the increased effectiveness of *in vitro* testing. Among them are advances in procedures dealing with the isolation of cells, improvements in techniques for the culturing of tissue, an enhanced ability to measure extremely small quantities of biologically important materials, and the development of new human specific products. Under the best of circumstances, however, *in vitro* tests, even if thoroughly proven in the laboratory, might well be rejected by manufacturers out of fear of a court case in which the lawyer for the plaintiff argues that the product was not tested in the "standard" way, that is, on live animals. It is a reasonable fear. We hasten to add that legal liability is not the principle issue here. Scientists recognize that no single *in vitro* test can begin to replicate the extremely complex interaction of cells in the human body.[9]

There is another major consideration. Before scientists can expect manufacturers, the regulatory agencies, and the public to accept *in vitro* test results, standards must be established which are not yet in place. At a recent meeting with government officials, representatives of CAAT presented a working plan to standardize the evaluation of *in vitro* testing. Reference laboratories need to be established, methods and techniques must be evaluated, data should be stored in a core repository, and there is clearly the need for a chemical bank which could provide quality control so that tests can be calibrated with standardized chemicals.

Although *in vitro* testing is a young science, it is no longer in its infancy. The *in vitro* literature as applied to toxicology—the study of poisons—contains over 4000 citations in the National Library of Medicine. About half of these articles deal specifically with carcinogenic (cancer causing) or mutagenic (mutation causing) substances. The rest are studies generally identified with eyes, skin, liver, lungs, or other organs. In most of these cases the studies are fundamental in nature and are aimed at understanding the mechanism of the effect that chemicals have on living tissue.

There are numerous *in vitro* testing methods. Almost all, however, are designed to meet one of four goals. Many tests are conducted to determine whether a substance is cytotoxic (destruction of cells) or genotoxic (alteration in genetic material). The results are usually known within hours, at most within a day or two. The material subjected to such tests varies widely (e.g., blood, mucus, and cells from specific organs) and it may come from a variety of sources (e.g., human, animal, plants, insects, and fish, among others).

A second category of tests determines the effect of a substance on the cells of a specific organ, e.g., the liver. Cells from a liver—animal or human—are intended to represent the whole liver. Does the substance inhibit the function of the liver? The researcher might want it to or not, which is to point out in passing that *in vitro* toxicology and drug discovery are two sides of the same coin. Sometimes the results obtained in drug discovery can highlight hazards or in safety testing will provide information that can lead to other uses of chemicals.

There is a third category of *in vitro* testing which mixes two cell types and then adds the substance under examination. The purpose is to determine how any biochemical by-product resulting from the effect of the cell on the chemical might affect the other cell type. For example, a culture consists of cells from both the liver and the kidney. The substance under test is added. The liver cells metabolize (change) the substance. Now, what will be the effect of the substance and/or the by-products of the metabolism on the kidney cells?

A fourth category of *in vitro* testing is very direct. A piece of skin or other tissue, animal or human, is removed and subjected to the substance in question and a specific process or result is measured.

It is important to note that *in vitro* testing does require the use of living cells. What it does not require, as *in vivo* testing does, is the use of whole live animals.

Although *in vitro* alternatives to live animal testing are most often seen as a humane response to the influence of animal activist groups, there are many other societal as well as scientific reasons why *in vitro* methods are highly desirable.[10] We live in a world that produces thousands of new and important chemical entities annually, and there is no realistic way we can test the safety and potential uses of these compounds with the methods or resources (people, money, time) currently available to us. In addition, we are developing new classes of protein drugs—the products of biotechnology—that can not be measured easily by methods or protocols used in the past. To reap the benefits of these new compounds, to separate the few that will prove beneficial from the vast majority that will not, will require the development of procedures or methodologies not yet in existence.

Whatever the substance under scrutiny, it is being tested for both efficacy and toxicity; does it work and work better than an existing compound and what is the risk to using this substance? These latter questions are those which toxicologists address daily, and it will be helpful at this point to devote some time to this science and its use of *in vivo* and *in vitro* technologies.

1.8 Acute Toxicity Testing

In acute toxicity testing, an investigator is observing an immediate response in which an organism's defense mechanisms are rapidly overwhelmed. Where specific endpoints are being determined—e.g., eye irritancy—it may be possible to develop an adequate *in vitro* alternative based on more than one screening system. It must be noted, however, that one of the functions of acute testing is the identification of unexpected toxic effects. The experimental nature of this approach requires that a relatively good model for the whole human being be used. This generally means using a whole mammal because its metabolism and response is at least sufficiently similar to human response to provide an index of hazard.

LD_{50} testing, referred to earlier, determines the median lethal dose. Originally developed to standardize such potent compounds as digitalis, insulin, and diphtheria toxin, the LD_{50} test came to be used as a standard measure by which the toxicity of all chemicals was compared. But as a result of scientific criticism coupled with pressure from animal welfare groups, the LD_{50} test—with a few specific exceptions—appears about to be discounted scientifically. The U.S. FDA, although it never required the LD_{50}, has recently stated explicitly that it does not require LD_{50} tests and that acute toxicity data from alternative tests may be acceptable. However, other countries still do have requirements for the LD_{50}.

The classic method of assessing the potential for eye irritancy of chemicals is the Draize eye-irritancy test—referred to earlier—which in recent years has been criticized by both scientists and animal welfare groups. A principal difficulty with using the test as a regulatory tool is the subjective nature of scoring and evaluating responses. Several *in vitro* replacements of the Draize eye irritancy tests are under study and show promise.[1]

In dermal toxicity testing, some of the same approaches applied to the search for alternatives to eye irritancy will undoubtedly prove successful. Again, there are difficulties in transferring test results from animals to humans. Although very little research into *in vitro* systems for identifying skin irritants has been undertaken to date, there have been increasing numbers of reports of the use of *in vitro* skin cultures to study toxic reactions or mechanisms.

Toxicologists also study phototoxicity, the tendency of a compound to increase the skin's sensitivity to ultraviolet radiation. Phototoxicity studies are currently conducted on animals. Several alternative methods are under investigation at CAAT. These tests are at varying stages of development and some are currently being used.

Another area of acute toxicity in which *in vitro* methods may be expected to contribute to our understanding of potential chemical insult concerns the acute reaction of certain organs or cell cultures to large doses that might occur during unintentional exposures or overdoses. An otherwise helpful and harmless chemical may turn dangerous under certain conditions and dosages. Toxicologists recognize these potential dangers and are examining *in vitro* methods which might give warning of the potential danger. Data derived from such studies could be extremely valuable in the establishment of public emergency limits and in the development of appropriate therapies for acute poisoning cases. A simple example will illustrate: what happens when a child swallows the contents of an entire bottle of a drug which, when taken in prescribed dosages, is beneficial?

In addition to testing for acute toxicity, researchers must be alert to the possibility that a substance may be toxic over the long haul. This is chronic toxicity. Researchers are much more likely to be able to predict the potential dangers here—e.g., the prospects of the substance causing cancer—if they understand the mechanism of the toxic insult than if they rely on empirical testing approaches. In the acute toxicity testing just described, there has been a focused effort to find alternatives to live animal testing following both empirical and mechanistic lines. In chronic toxicity testing, a similar effort is underway to develop short-term tests of substances which might do insidious damage over months or even years, not only one that could alter genetic material but that could affect any organ system.[11]

1.9 The Promise and Potential of *In Vitro* Methods

In vitro testing is both expanding and promising. It is no longer in its infancy and it is nearing adolescence. Clearly, there are reasonable and well-founded hopes that alternatives to testing on live animals will provide a substantial portion of the database necessary for safety assessment. On the other hand, all advances will require the combined use of *in vivo* and *in vitro* testing prior to clinical trials on humans. In any event, animal use in safety testing will be decreased and, as important, a better evaluation of the safety of these products for animal and human use will be established. The development of *in vitro* testing strategies in toxicology affords the opportunity to provide data for risk assessment and for safety evaluation which is more cost effective and rapid, less expensive and will reduce the use of whole animals.

REFERENCES

1. Goldberg, A. M., Ed. *Alternative Methods in Toxicology,* Vols. 1–9 (New York: Mary Ann Liebert, 1983–1993).
2. Flamm, W. G. and R. J. Lorentzen. "The Use of *In Vitro* Methods in Safety Evaluation," in *In Vitro Toxicology—A Journal of Molecular and Cellular Toxicology,* Vol. 1(1) (New York: Mary Ann Liebert, 1986–1987).
3. Schwartz, H. *Breakthrough: The Discovery of Modern Medicines at Janssen* (New Jersey: The Skyline Publishing Group, 1989).
4. U.S. Congress, Office of Technology Assessment, "Neurotoxicity: Identifying and Controlling Poisons of the Nervous System," OTA-3A-436, Washington, D.C. (April, 1990).
5. European Chemical Industry Ecology and Toxicology Center. "Skin Sensitization Testing, Monograph 14," Brussels (March, 1990).
6. Frazier, J. M. and A. M. Goldberg. "Alternatives to Animals in Toxicity Testing," *Sci. Am.* 260(8):24–30 (1989).
7. Rowan, A. and A. M. Goldberg. "Perspectives on Alternatives to Current Animal Testing Techniques in Preclinical Toxicology," *Ann. Rev. Pharm. Toxicol.* 25(1):225–247 (1985).

8. Frazier, J. M. and A. M. Goldberg. "Alternatives to and Reduction of Animal Use in Biomedical Research, Education, and Testing," *Cancer Bull.* 42(4):238–244 (1990).

9. National Research Council. "Use of Laboratory Animals in Biomedical and Behavioral Research," National Academy Press, Washington, D.C. (1988).

10. Zbinden, G. "Animal Experimentation: Are There Practical Answers to an Ethical Dilemma?," in *Medicina E Morale,* chap. 6 (Rome: Universita Cattolica del Sacro Cuore Facolta di Medicina e Chirurgia, 1989) pp 1089–1094.

11. Organization for Economic Co-operation and Development; "Scientific Criteria for Validation of *In Vitro* Toxicity Tests, No. 36," (September, 1990).

CHAPTER 2

Applications of *In Vitro* Methods for the Cosmetic, Household Products, and Pharmaceutical Industries

Virginia C. Gordon

2.0 Introduction

For nearly 80 years, animal tests have been utilized to determine the health and safety risks of chemicals and products to the human population. *In vivo* toxicology assesses these risks in a wide variety of animal tests for irritation to the eyes and skin, penetration into the skin, allergic response to the skin (also called sensitization), photo-irritation, photosensitization, carcinogenicity, mutagenicity, teratogenicity, and lethality.

The events occurring *in vivo* represent a complex series of biochemical and physiological changes. Whole animal tests provide the physiological and metabolic relationships of macromolecules, cells, tissues, and organs necessary to evaluate routes of contact such as ingestion, skin penetration, and inhalation, as well as reversibility of effects. Animal tests often involve subjective assessment of responses and are difficult to standardize.[1-4] Many animals demonstrated insensitivity and poor predictability for human toxicity.[5-10] Animal toxicity tests also were not well validated with respect to human data. The correlation, for instance,

> - Complex Cascade Reactions
>   Difficult to Quantitate
>   Difficult to Interpret
> - Subjective Endpoints
> - Time Consuming
> - Costly

Figure 1.   Discussion of *in vivo* test.

> - Allow for Control of Environmental Conditions
> - Utilize Large Number of Test Organisms or
>   Macromolecules (Cells) per Dose Level
> - Reduce Variability Between Experiments
> - Are Often Quicker and Cheaper
> - Require Smaller Quantities of Test Chemicals
> - Produce Small Quantities of Toxic Waste
> - Reduce Animal Usage

Figure 2.   Advantages of *in vitro* systems.

of rabbit ocular irritation to human ocular irritation was reported as 0.48 in a study by Freeberg.[11] Animal tests are costly and have often involved animal suffering (Figure 1).

Humane considerations have accelerated efforts to find alternative testing methods. The development of these methods may also be a means of improving the accuracy of the original animal tests. *In vitro* methods can provide more insight into mechanisms of damage than evaluation of observable responses in an animal. Many *in vitro* methods are more sensitive, reproducible, rapid, and cost effective than existing animal tests. These advantages greatly increase the applicability of these tests to the cosmetic, household products, and pharmaceutical industries (Figure 2).

In recent years, there has been tremendous growth in the development and utilization of *in vitro* test methods. By eliminating actual testing, many major cosmetics manufacturers have responded to their customers' demands for humane alternatives to traditional test methods.

2.1 Current *In Vitro* Methods

In vitro methods have been based on cell cytotoxicity, inflammatory or immune system response, alterations of cellular, bacterial or fungal physiology, cell morphology, biochemical endpoints, macromolecular targets, and structure activity analysis.[12-17] As public pressure leads more companies away from animal testing, *in vitro* test methods have become a crucial component in comprehensive toxicology programs. To provide additional toxicity checks, many companies have also increased their use of human volunteer studies. General alternatives to *in vivo* test methods are listed in Table 1.

Table 1. **Current *In Vitro* Methods or Methods Used as Alternatives to Animal Testing**

1. Physicochemical Analysis
2. Target macromolecular and biochemical responses
3. Cell culture techniques and methods
4. Microorganism studies
5. Human tissue equivalent methods
6. Isolated tissue assays
7. Computer modeling (structure activity relationships)
8. Human volunteer studies

2.2 Description of Current *In Vitro* Methods

2.2.1 Physicochemical Analysis

Analysis of the physicochemical properties of test substances, including the pH, absorption spectra, partition coefficients, and other parameters, can often indicate potential toxicity. OECD guidelines state that substances with a pH of less than 2 or greater than 11 do not need to be tested *in vivo* for irritancy potential.[18] The UV absorption spectra has been used to suggest the potential for photo-irritant.[19] Physicochemical tests are rapid, cost-effective, easily standardized, and transferable to outside laboratories. They are valuable screens but cannot be used alone to predict *in vivo* toxicity.

2.2.2 Target Macromolecular and Biochemical Responses

Test methods which utilize the analysis of biochemical reactions or changes in organized macromolecules evaluate toxicity at a subcellular level. Due to their simplicity, they can be readily standardized and transferred to outside laboratories, providing yardstick measurements on undiluted and neat chemicals and formulations.

The EYTEX test, developed by Ropak Laboratories,[20,21] has been validated with more than 10,000 substances. The test is based on the measurement of conformational changes in a synthetic biomacromolecular matrix solution called the EYTEX Reagent.[22] Changes in macromolecular conformation and hydration is a prime cause of corneal *in vivo* opacity in response to eye irritants. The test features a complete system of reagents, calibrators, and controls as well as an instrument used to quantitate the turbidity that develops in response to the irritancy levels of a specific formulation. Results are expressed in terms of absolute scores. EYTEX can screen insoluble, opaque and colored chemicals, as well as final formulations. Numerous validation studies have shown that EYTEX produces results comparable to those generated by animal testing.

Many validations of this method have demonstrated a high compatibility, high sensitivity, and good predictive value.[23-29] The method is also readily transferable and is utilized by more than 150 laboratories worldwide. Some of the cosmetic laboratories have used this method with other *in vitro* methods to replace the Draize rabbit eye test. EYTEX alone will not totally supplant the rabbit eye test because there is a small number of substances which cannot be tested with the method. EYTEX only measures chemical irritancy and not other factors such as abrasion, allergy, or recovery from irritation. However, it obviously has a major role to play as part of a battery of *in vitro* alternatives to the rabbit eye test.

SKINTEX™, developed by Ropak Laboratories, is an *in vitro* test for predicting the skin irritation of chemicals and formulations, and is based on a two-compartment physicochemical model.[30] The process of skin irritation has been viewed as consisting mainly of absorption onto or permeation through an external surface, the stratum corneum, to an internal (surface of detection) such as the epidermis. Further diffusion into the dermis is not modeled by SKINTEX. Several studies have demonstrated the value of this method.[31-33]

2.2.3 Cell-Culture Techniques

In vitro cytotoxicity tests indicate basic cell toxicity by measuring different endpoints such as cell viability, proliferation, membrane integrity, DNA or RNA synthesis, or metabolic effects and energy regulation.

The most commonly used approaches are the Neutral Red Release Assay cell viability and membrane damage, the Lowry method, and the Coomassie Blue and Kenacid Blue assays (for cell proliferation and total cell protein).[34-36] A newer method, the MTT or tetrazolium assay, measures mitochondrial function. Another test method quantitates the intracellular lactate dehydrogenase activity test indicative of cell lysis.[37]

In the Neutral Red and total protein assays, cells are treated with various concentrations of the test substance in Petri or multiwell dishes. Then, after a period of exposure, the test substance is washed out of the dish and an analytical reagent is added. In the Neutral Red Assay, the dye accumulated in the lysosomes of viable, uninjured cells is quantitated. In the protein test, Kenacid Blue reacts with cellular protein. Healthy control cells are dark blue and dead cells are lighter in color. These tests determine the IC_{50} (the test sample concentration which kills 50% of the cell). These cell-culture test methods are rapid and reproducible. Most test samples must be diluted prior to analysis, which may alter the physical chemistry that was responsible for causing irritation or toxicity.

The MTT test assays mitochondrial function by measuring reduction of the yellow MTT tetrazolium salt to a blue insoluble product. In a study of 28 test substances (including drugs, pesticides, caffeine, and absorbic acid), the MTT test was shown to be comparable to the Neutral Red technique in terms of effective cytotoxicity screening.[16] The two assays ranked the test substances with a correlation coefficient of 0.939. The two assays demonstrated slight differences for a few test agents.

Inhibition of mitogen-stimulated thymidine incorporation in human peripheral blood mononuclear cells has been reported as a screening method for photosensitizers.[19] In this study, cells from at least three human volunteers were used for testing each chemical.

In the microphysiometer, a hydrogen ion sensor will detect subtle responses to the metabolic process of the cell. The toxic effects and cellular recovery are measured within the cell.[38]

2.2.4 Human Tissue Equivalents

Skin equivalents have been developed by several laboratories. TESTSKIN™, a well-known equivalent, seeds human keratinocytes onto a collagen base or a collagen/glycosaminoglycan matrix containing human fibroblasts.[39] In many respects, the epidermis that develops resembles epidermis *in vivo.* The tissue culture system survives for several weeks and may be useful in studying skin penetration. TESTSKIN is a commercially available skin equivalent system marketed by Organogenesis, Inc. (Cambridge, MA, U.S.A.), and is now being assessed for use in skin penetration studies.

Marrow-Tech, Inc. (Elmsford, NY, U.S.A.), has also developed a human skin model.[40] This model develops a dermal layer made of fibroblasts and their own secreted collagen. An epidermal layer of keratinocytes is added by a dermal/ epidermal junction. While TESTSKIN uses bovine collagen, Marrow-Tech's skin equivalent produces human collagen in its dermal layer.

2.2.5 Isolated Tissue Techniques

Several methods using the eyes or skin of animals are used to assess toxic endpoints. In the isolated or enucleated eye test, eyes are removed from humanely killed rabbits and washed with saline in a temperature-controlled chamber. Isolated eyes are equilibrated and then liquid or powder test substances are applied to the cornea for various time periods. After rinsing, the eye can be monitored for a number of endpoints, including ocular opacity, epithelial integrity (assessed by fluorescein penetration), corneal swelling, and histological examination. Results found in a study of 200 chemicals demonstrated a high level of correlation to *in vivo* findings in rabbits diverse irritants.[41]

A screen for corrosive substances that has been well-validated monitors changes in electrical impedance in rat epidermal slices or full thickness human cadaver skin slices. This is done in a specially constructed chamber.[42] Changes in electrical impedance across the skin slice are indicative of changes in the integrity of the stratum corneum and consequent changes in its barrier function. Corrosive substances alter this integrity.

Using rat and rabbit skin slices *in vitro,* a similar technique for assessing irritancy rather than corrosivity was developed by Duffy.[41] Test substances are applied to the upper stratum corneum, while the under surface is supplied with a culture medium. Changes in the number of enzymes are used to separate irritant and nonirritant chemicals.

2.2.6 Human Volunteer Studies

Human volunteer studies are widely used to assess skin irritation, penetration, and sensitization. Many industries conduct repeat patch tests on human volunteers to predict the potential for dermal irritation and sensitization. Cumulative skin irritancy can be measured by re-applying the test sample for 3 weeks. Skin irritation is usually assessed visually. However, quantitative methods such as laser doppler flowmetry can measure blood flow and skin temperature. The thickness of the skin or skin swelling can be measured with calipers or high-frequency pulsed ultrasound.

Human volunteers are also routinely used in tests for allergic sensitization for cosmetic substances and formulations. The repeat patch test includes an induction phase and a 2-week rest period, followed by a challenge phase to see if sensitization has occurred. A pilot study of 20 human volunteers is often followed by an expanded test study of 80 to 100 human volunteers. If a significant number of positive results occur, there is the possibility of a major problem with the formulation. The relevance of positive results to consumer use must then be evaluated. This is sometimes accomplished with a large product-use test which might study 250 to 500 volunteers in 1 year.

2.2.7 Microorganism Studies

One of the most famous *in vitro* tests is the Ames test.[43] The Ames Reverse Mutation Test uses sensitive strains of the bacteria *Salmonella typhimurium* with metabolic activity provided by the rat liver microsomal S9 enzyme fraction. The test has been very extensively validated in intra- and inter-laboratory trials and detects genotoxic carcinogens with a sensitivity of 90%. In their efforts to eliminate mutagenic substances in the early stages of the development process, most chemical companies have used the Ames test as a primary screening method.

Another test method which uses a fungi is Daniel's Yeast Phototoxicity test which utilizes the yeast *Candida albicans* as the test organism.[44] A 1988 study compared favorably the results of this test with the results of photo-patch testing in volunteers for samples from six furocoumarin-containing plants.[44]

A third test method Microtox test, uses a standardized suspension of luminescent bacteria as a test organism. The amount of light emitted by the bacteria is a natural function of a cell's respiration.[45]

2.2.8 Computer Modeling

Health Designs, Inc., has developed a computer simulation based on 400 chemicals for which there is adequate *in vivo* teratogenicity data. *In vivo* data is

• Quality Assurance Raw Materials and Bulk Products
• Safety in the Workplace
• Formulation Tool
• Prioritization—New Chemicals to be Utilized
• Screen for Safety Evaluation Products
• Replacement Animal Test Method for Certain Industries

Figure 3. Applications of *in vitro* methods.

categorized with respect to species, route and frequency of administration, and time of exposure.

Health Designs, Inc., also developed a computer model, this one based on physicochemical characteristics. The computer model for rabbit skin and eye irritation estimates the probability that exposure to a substance would cause one of four possible categories of skin irritation (non, mild, moderate, or severe), similar to those used in the Draize Test.[17] There are four models: two for substances with molecular ring structures and two for compounds without rings. For either structure, one program predicts whether a substance is likely to cause severe skin irritation and the other predicts whether irritation is likely to be mild, moderate, or negative.

2.3 Applications of *In Vitro* Methods

Nonanimal toxicity tests and testing strategies have been developed, validated, and evaluated. These tests are being developed for use in identifying the potential toxicity of chemicals and products to humans during the process of manufacturing as well as when products are manufactured and sold. Since these tests are capable of assessing potential toxicity they can also be used as indicators for minimizing to toxicity during product development. Since they feature an assessment capability, the tests can also be used to evaluate batch-to-batch variability and provide quality control indicators for raw materials and finished products.

The use of *in vitro* tests in comprehensive industry safety programs will contribute greatly to quality and safety assurance in the future (Figure 3).

2.3.1 Quality Assurance

A comprehensive quality assurance program should include the screening of raw materials, monitoring of bulk products, and batch analysis of finished products. The raw materials used in the cosmetic industry are often manufactured chemicals or blends with 50 to 100% purity.

Large lots of these raw materials with acceptable specification ranges are combined to produce finished formulations. These raw materials often contain impurities with significantly different potential for toxicity to humans. Chemical analysis and physicochemical measurements are a first indicator of purity and potential toxicity (Figure 4).

> • Lot-to-Lot Variability Raw Materials
> • Monitor Bulk Products
> • Batched Analysis Finished Products

Figure 4.   Applications of *in vitro* tests to quality assurance raw materials.

> • Employee Safety Primary Concern
> • MSDS Sheets
> • Intermediates of Large and Small Number — Varying Toxicity

Figure 5.   Applications of *in vitro* tests to safety programs in the workplace.

In vitro safety evaluations are sensitive enough to differentiate the changes in toxicity levels of raw materials from different batch lots and different vendors prior to formulation.

2.3.2 Safety in the Workplace

Every laboratory that uses chemicals must ensure the safety of the employees working with these materials. Incoming chemicals and raw materials must have Material Safety Data Sheets (MSDS) delineating the known toxicity of raw materials. Many chemicals in use today have outdated and subjective assessments of safety on their MSDS sheets. *In vitro* methods can rapidly screen these chemicals so MSDS can be updated.

As raw materials are combined during manufacturing, many small quantities of intermediates are produced. These intermediates may have more toxicity than any of the starting materials. *In vitro* testing methods provide cost-effective ways to evaluate the large number of intermediates which may arise during the manu-facturing process. Animal methods are far too costly and time-consuming to be used for this application. Increased tests with reliable methods ensures the safety of workers by permitting comprehensive safety testing (Figure 5).

2.3.3 Formulation Tool

In research and development departments, both new molecules and combina-tions of new and old molecules are developed. When a series of new molecules or formulations is developed, the toxicity and safety of these materials must be considered and then evaluated. Initial screening will permit faster and less expen-sive development of new products. As an integral part of product development, alternative test methods can rapidly and inexpensively identify irritating chemi-cals so that primarily safe materials are evaluated clinically (Figure 6).

In the pharmaceutical industry, an active ingredient could be reformulated in a series of new skin preparations. An *in vitro* test can provide an initial analysis of the safety of the series of skin preparations with respect to skin irritation. The researcher may be trying to increase skin penetration of the active component.

- New Molecule Screens
- New Combinations of Chemicals Evaluated
- Reformulation of Actives in New Preparations
- Plant Extracts and Proteins Prescreened
- Anti-Irritancy Analysis

Figure 6.   In v*itro* tests expand the capabilities of the formulators.

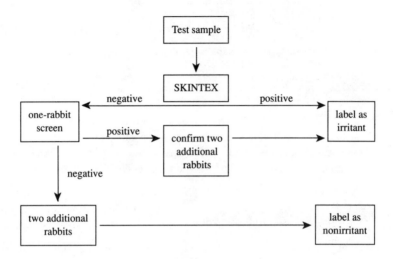

Figure 7.   Tier approach to safety testing.

Once safety is assured by an *in vitro* test then further *in vivo* testing can quantitate increased penetration.

In the cosmetic industry, natural extracts, plant proteins, and low-irritation surfactants can often be added to existing formulations to produce milder formulations. Due to the speed and sensitivity of *in vitro* test methods, many ratios of these protective ingredients in the formulation can be studied to select an optimal ratio of combinations. This application of *in vitro* testing can help manufacturers create new and milder consumer and cosmetic products (Figure 6).

2.3.4 Screen for Safety Evaluation

The use of *in vitro* safety evaluation methods provides an essential function in reduction and refinement of animal tests. Single tests or batteries of tests can screen out severe toxicants so they need not be studied further in animals. The application of *in vitro* tests as prescreens and screens has already substantially reduced the number of animals used in toxicity tests. Many regulatory agencies propose a tier approach to utilization of *in vitro* methods (Figure 7). These proposals suggest that a screening test or combination of tests should be used to eliminate moderate, severe, and corrosive materials from further animal testing.

- Historic *In Vivo* Database
- Validation Test Method(s)
- Utilization Test Batteries
- Raw Materials Well Known and Categorized

Figure 8.   Components in safety programs replacing animal tests. (*M. Balls, 1991*)

- EYTEX
- Neutral Red Release
- Neutral Red Uptake
- Het Cam
- Recovery Test

Figure 9.   One proposed *in vitro* test battery for ocular irritation.

Such proposals recommend only test materials with minimal and mild levels of toxicity be analyzed in animals and then only for substantiation of the *in vitro* result. This substantiation would be performed with one to three animals instead of the six animals required for a standard animal test. The tier approach can reduce animal testing by 50 to 80%.

2.3.5 Replacement of Animal Tests

The Avon Corporation was one of the first major cosmetics manufacturers to eliminate animal testing. Avon's decision to abandon animal testing came after a study of 503 cosmetics and raw materials supported EYTEX as a suitable alternative test method. Using a very large historic Draize database, Avon completed a comparative analysis of *in vitro* and *in vivo* test methods before deciding to eliminate animal testing. Several other cosmetic companies followed Avon's lead and halted Draize rabbit eye testing in 1989 and 1990 (Figure 8).

One test battery (described in Figure 9), which incorporates several scientific methods, has been proposed for ocular irritation. This is only one of several batteries being discussed in the scientific community.[46] This battery combines method with different endpoints, as well as diverse capabilities and endpoints.

Most of the companies that have ceased animal testing or propose replacement utilize combinations of test methods. Test methods can be combined into a battery because the different tests are based on different mechanisms or approaches and have different capabilities and limitations. A comparison of two different approaches used in methods for ocular irritation is presented in Table 2.[46]

2.3.6 Prioritization of New Chemicals

In this world there are more than 8000 chemicals in use. Probably one half lack complete toxicity data. To obtain this toxicity data would utilize many hundreds of thousands of animals at a very substantial cost.

Table 2.   A Comparison of the EYTEX/SKINTEX Approach and the Cell-Culture Approach[46]

The EYTEX/SKINTEX Approach	The Cell-Culture Approach
Narrow mechanistic basis	Wide mechanistic basis
Tight protocols in terms of dosage, exposure, etc.	Infinitely variable protocols in terms of dosage, exposure, etc.
Strong links to regulatory animal tests	Weak links to regulatory animal tests
Results readily classified to match regulatory classifications	Results not readily classified to match regulatory classifications
Able to handle awkward test materials	Not readily able to accommodate awkward test materials
Relatively narrow range of values obtainable	Relatively wide range of values obtainable
Not suitable for repeat-dose studies	Suitable for repeat-dose studies
Not suitable for recovery studies	Suitable for recovery studies

- 6000–8000 Ingredients
  - 3000 No Adequate Toxicity Data
  - $1.2 Billion
- Cost-Effective Screens to Prioritize
- New Molecules Low Toxicity More Quickly Identified
  - Moved Through More Complete Evaluations

Figure 10. Prioritizing new chemicals.

In vitro methods are very important, cost-effective screens to prioritize this list of chemicals. Chemical ingredients with low toxicity *in vitro* would be given top priority for further *in vivo* evaluation. Chemical ingredients with high toxicity *in vitro* tests would be given low priority or would not be utilized.

As new materials are researched and developed, a test battery of *in vitro* methods can provide a preliminary screen of their toxicity. Valuable new molecules and derivatives of these molecules with low toxicity, can more quickly be moved through the toxicological evaluations. More toxic new molecules can be put on a slower development schedule.

2.4 Summary

The importance of *in vitro* assays has increased in recent years. This surge of interest has been fostered by consumer demands to pursue development of alternatives to animal testing with the goal of decreasing the number of animals used for toxicological evaluation of substances. Scientific interest in *in vitro* toxicity methods includes the desire to develop systems which can separate the complex components that occur in the human and thus, define the mechanisms of toxicity. In the future, comprehensive *in vitro* investigational methods may provide more definitive information about the physiological mechanisms caused by a given toxicant than is available with animal studies.

There are many possible applications for *in vitro* systems. *In vitro* tests can be a valuable tool in the assessment of ranking groups of compounds for use as ingredients. *In vitro* methods can be utilized as initial screening methods resulting in the use of a minimum number of animals for toxicity tests and simplifying the process by which new compounds are developed. *In vitro* methods can provide additional safety information too costly to be determined in animal tests. It is very unlikely that an *in vitro* system could ever be developed to mimic the complex cascade of reactions that occur in humans. However, *in vitro* methods can be combined in batteries of tests to mimic diverse mechanisms and complex reactions which occur in humans. Test batteries will be developed and validated to provide as broad databases as possible to assess risk to humans.

In order to protect humans from toxic substances, some *in vivo* animal tests must still be performed. At a minimum, the new *in vitro* tests must be sensitive enough to characterize the potential degree and mechanism of toxicity. The developing *in vitro* systems will provide more information about the mechanism by which a substance causes toxicity. These developments will result in new methods and greater understanding of primary mechanisms in the *in vivo* response. Research, development, validation, and utilization of these alternatives will, however, present important methods to assure human safety with less animal testing. Regulatory agencies will need to evaluate the reliability, reproducibility, and relevance of specific toxicological methods in relationship to the *in vivo* endpoints. With sufficient time, scientific creativity, financial resources, and scientific collaboration, more accurate methods will be developed and utilized which will gradually replace existing animal tests.

REFERENCES

1. Draize, J. H., G. Woodard, and H. O. Calvery. "Method for the Study of Irritation and Toxicity of Substances Applied Topically to the Skin and Mucous Membranes," *J. Pharmocol. Exp. Ther.* 82(1):377–390 (1944).
2. Weil, C. S. and R. A. Scala. "Study of Intra- and Inter-Laboratory Variability in the Results of Rabbit Eye and Skin Irritation Tests," *Toxicol. Appl. Pharmacol.*, 19(1):276–360 (1971).
3. MacDonald, T. O., V. Seabaugh, and H. F. Edelhouser. *Dermatology*, 2nd ed. (New York: McGraw-Hill, 1983), p. 555.
4. Burton, A. B. G. "A Method for Objective Assessment of Eye Irritation," *Food Cosmetic. Toxicol.*, 10(2):209–17 (1972).
5. Zbinden, G. and M. Flury-Roversi. "Significance of the LD50 Test for the Toxicological Evaluation of Chemical Substances," *Arch. Toxicol.* 47(2):77–99 (1981).
6. Schutz, E. "Use of Acute Toxicity Data for Pharmaceuticals," in *The Contribution of Acute Toxicity Testing to the Evaluation of Pharmaceuticals*, D. Schuppan, A. D. Dayan, and F. A. Charlesworth, Eds. (New York: Springer-Verlag, 1986), p. 10–19.
7. Koch, W. H. "Validation Criteria For Ocular Irritation *In Vitro* Alternative Tests," *J. Toxicol. Cut. Ocular Toxicol.* 8(1):17–22 (1989).

8. Griffith, J. F. "Use of Human Experience to Calibrate Draize and *In Vitro* Eye Test Data," *J. Toxicol. Cut. Ocular Toxicol.* 24(1):23–24 (1991).

9. Ennever, F. K., T. J. Noonan, and H. S. Rosenkranz. "The Predictivity of Animal Bioassays and Short-Term Genotoxicity Tests for Carcinogenicity and Non-Carcinogenicity to Humans," *Mutagenesis* 2(2):73–78 (1987).

10. Freeberg, F. E., D. T. Hooker, and G. F. Griffith. "Correlation of Animal Eye Test Data With Human Experience For Household Products: An Update," *J. Toxicol. Cut. Ocular Toxicol.* 5(2):115–123 (1986).

11. Freeberg F. E., et al. "Correlation of Animal Eye Test Data with Human Experience for Household Products," *J. Toxicol. Cut. Ocular Toxicol.* 3:53–64 (1984).

12. Oliver, G. J. A. and M. A. Pemberton. "The Identification of Corrosive Agents for Human Skin *In Vitro*," *Food Chem. Toxicol.* 24(6/7):513–515 (1986).

13. Jackson, E. M., R. D. Hume, and R. F. Wallin. "The Agarose Diffusion Method for Ocular Irritancy Screening: Cosmetic Products, Part II," *J. Toxicol. Cut. Ocular Toxicol.* 7(3):187–194 (1988).

14. Young, J. R., M. J. How, A. P. Walker, and W. M. H. Worth. "Classification as Corrosive or Irritant to Skin of Preparations Containing Acidic or Alkaline Substances, Without Testing on Animals," *Toxicol. In Vitro* 2(1):19–26 (1988).

15. Booman, K. A., J. De Prospo, J. Demetrulias, A. Drieger, J. F. Griffith, G. Grochoski, B. Kong, W. C. McCormick, H. North-Root, M. G. Rozen, and R. I. Sedlak. "The SDA Alternatives Program: Comparison of *In Vitro* Data with Draize Test Data," *J. Toxicol. Cut. Ocular Toxicol.* 8(1):35–49 (1989).

16. Borenfreund, E., H. Babich, and N. Martin-Alguacil. "Comparisons of Two *In Vitro* Cytotoxicity Assays—The Neutral Red (NR) and Tetrazolium MTT Tests," *Toxicol. In Vitro* 2(1):1–6 (1988).

17. Enslein, K. "An Overview of Structure-Activity Relationships as an Alternative to Testing in Animals for Carcinogenicity, Mutagenicity, Dermal and Eye Irritation and Acute Oral Toxicity," *Toxicol. Ind. Health* 4(4):479–497 (1988).

18. OECD. "Acute Eye Irritation/Corrosion," in *OECD Guideline for Testing of Chemicals*, Adopted February 1987.

19. Morrison, W. L., D. J. McAuliffe, J. A. Parrish, and K. J. Bloch. "*In Vitro* Assay for Phototoxic Chemicals," *J. Invest. Dermatol.* 78(6):460–463 (1982).

20. Gordon, V. C. and H. C. Bergman. "EYTEX, an *In Vitro* Method for Evaluation of Ocular Irritancy," in *In Vitro Toxicology: Approaches to Validation,* A. M. Goldberg, Ed. (New York: Mary Ann Liebert, 1987).

21. Gordon, V. C. and H. C. Bergman. "The EYTEX MPA System," in *Progress in In Vitro Toxicology*, A. M. Goldberg, Ed. (New York: Mary Ann Liebert, 1988).

22. Gordon, V. C. and H. C. Bergman. "External Evaluation of the EYTEX System in Six Labs to Determine Intra- and Inter- Lab Accuracy and Precision," in *Progress in In Vitro Toxicology*, A. M. Goldberg, Ed. (New York: Mary Ann Liebert, 1988).

23. Gordon, V. C. and H. C. Bergman. "External Evaluation of the EYTEX System in Twelve Labs to Determine the Correlation of Results with *In Vitro* Results," in *Progress in In Vitro Toxicology*, A. M. Goldberg, Ed. (New York: Mary Ann Liebert, 1988).

24. Gordon, V. C. "The Scientific Basis of the EYTEX® System," *ATLA (Alternatives To Laboratory Animals)* 20:537–548 (1992).

25. Gordon, V. C., C. P. Kelly, and H. C. Bergman. "Applications of the EYTEX Method," presented at the 2nd Int. Conf. Practical *In Vitro* Toxicology, Nottingham, U.K. (1989).

26. Soto, R. J., M. J. Servi, and V. C. Gordon. "Evaluation of an Alternative Method for Ocular Irritation," in *In Vitro Toxicology*, A. M. Goldberg, Ed. (New York: Mary Ann Liebert, 1989).

27. Soto, R. J. and V. C. Gordon. "An *In Vitro* Method for Estimating Ocular Irritation," in EYTEX Users Symposium, Summit, NJ (1990).

28. Dickens, M. S., F. H. Kruszewski, L. H. Heran, K. T. Smith, J. J. Teal, and V. C. Gordon. Application of the EYTEX System to the Evaluation of Cosmetic Products, EYTEX Users Symposium, Summit, NJ (1990).

29. Regnier, J. F. and C. Imbert. "Validation of the EYTEX System as a Screen for Prediction of the Ocular Irritancy Potential of Chemical Products," presentation at ATOCHEM, France (1990).

30. Gordon, V. C. "An *In Vitro* Dermal Safety Test," *J. Drug Cosmet. Ind.* (March, 1990).

31. Gordon, V. C., C. P. Kelly, and H. C. Bergman. "SKINTEX, an *In Vitro* Method for Determining Dermal Irritation," paper presented at the 5th Int. Congr. Toxicology, Brighton, England, July 1989.

32. Gordon, V. C. "Evaluation Of SKINTEX," Ropak Laboratories #51 (1990).

33. Gordon, V. C. "SKINTEX Database," Ropak Laboratories #52 (1991).

34. Borenfreund, E. and J. A. Puerner. "Toxicity Determined *In Vitro* by Morphological Alterations and Neutral Red Absorption," *Toxicol. Lett.* 24(2/3):119–124 (1985).

35. Reader, S. J., V. Blackwell, R. O'Hara, R. H. Clothier, G. Griffin, and M. Balls. "A Vital Dye Release Method for Assessing the Short-Term Cytotoxic Effects of Chemicals and Formulations," *ATLA* 17(1):2837 (1989).

36. Clothier, R. H., L. Hulme, A. B. Ahmed, H. L. Reeves, M. Smith, and M. Balls. "*In Vitro* Cytotoxicity of 150 Chemicals to 3T3-L1 Cells, Assessed by the FRAME Kenacid Blue Method," *ATLA* 16(1):84–95 (1988).

37. Chan, K. Y. "Chemical Injury to an *In Vitro* Ocular System: Differential Release of Plasminogen Activator," *Clin. Eye Res.*, 5(5):357–365 (1986).

38. Gan, C. F. "Microphysiometer Could Open New Avenues in Research," *The Scientist*, 22nd January: 24–26 (1990).

39. Anon., "TESTSKIN: An Analysis," *The Alternatives Report* (4):1–6, Center for Animals and Public Policy, Tufts School of Veterinary Medicine, Massachusetts, (1990).

40. Naughton, G. K. et al. "A Physiological Skin Model for *In Vitro* Toxicity Studies," in *Alternative Methods in Toxicology*, 7th ed., A. M. Goldberg, Ed. (New York: Mary Ann Liebert, 1991).

41. Duffy, P. A. "Irritancy Testing—A Cultured Approach," *Toxicol. In Vitro* 3(2):157–158 (1989).

42. Oliver, G. J. A., M. A. Pemberton, and C. Rhodes. "An *In Vitro* Skin Corrosivity Test—Modifications and Validation," *Food Chem. Toxicol.*, 24(6/7):507–512 (1986).

43. Cooper, J. A., R. Saracci, and P. Cole. "Describing the Validity of Carcinogen Screening Tests," *Br. J. Cancer* 39(1):87–89 (1979).

44. Daniels, F. "A Simple Microbiological Method for Demonstrating Phototoxic Compounds," *J. Invest. Dermatol.* 44(4):259–263 (1965).

45. Bruener, L. H., et al. "Proc. 2nd CTFA Testing Workshop," S. D. Gettings and G. N. McEven, Eds., CTFA Washington D.C. (1990).
46. Balls, M. "Strategic Uses Of EYTEX And SKINTEX," to be published *ATLA* (1991).

CHAPTER 3

In Vitro Testing Program at Procter & Gamble

John Yam and C. L. Alden

3.0 Introduction

Procter & Gamble (P&G) is a leading consumer product company marketing a variety of household cleaning products, beauty and personal care products, foods, beverage, paper products, and pharmaceuticals worldwide. Since so many homes use one or more of P&G's products, P&G places very high regard on product safety. In fact, P&G has a long-standing corporate policy which states that, "P&G products shall be safe for humans and the environment under conditions of intended use and foreseeable misuse." And, "P&G shall meet the requirements of all relevant laws and regulations."

At the same time, P&G is also fully committed to the responsible use of animals. In its Animal Testing Policy, P&G affirms its commitment to:

- Conduct animal testing only when necessary, and only when no acceptable alternative tests exist.
- Maintain the highest ethical and professional standards in animal care and treatment.
- Develop, validate, and adopt new test methods which eliminate the need for animals, reduce the number of animals used, and are less stressful for the animals.

0-87371-504-7/93/$0.00+$.50

This chapter focuses on P&G efforts on the last commitment. Same as many leading scientists working on alternatives, we define alternatives as "Replacement, Reduction, and Refinement," commonly known as the 3 Rs, a definition first proposed by Russell and Birch in 1959. The adoption of this concept is important because it maximizes our ability to bring about actual reduction in the number of animals used.

Some people equate alternatives with only nonanimal or *in vitro* methods. We believe such a view is short sighted. In the near terms, meaningful reduction of animal use and distress will come primarily from reduction and refinement methods that have been or are being developed. We agree that replacement should be the ultimate goal. However, development of methods that lead to replacement of animals is more difficult and therefore requires a longer time to develop.

At P&G, we have taken the mission to search for alternative methods to animal testing seriously. To date, a number of scientists at our Miami Valley Laboratories are devoted to alternative research. Our in-house programs are broad and cover a number of focus areas, including acute oral toxicity, eye irritation, skin irritation, contact sensitization and photoallergy, genetic toxicology, respiratory toxicology, and noninvasive techniques.[1]

In addition to in-house efforts, P&G also supports a number of research programs at universities. In 1989, P&G established a new program, called the University Animal Alternative Research Program, to further encourage development of alternative methods. The program funds up to 50,000 U.S. dollars annually for 3 years per research program, and three new research programs each year. The first three awards were given out in 1990.

DEVELOPMENT AND APPLICATION OF ALTERNATIVES

3.1 Acute Oral Toxicity

The classical LD_{50} test, which for many years has been the standard toxicological test to assess acute oral toxicity, has been criticized for ethical and scientific reasons. While it is now generally accepted that a precise LD_{50} is not essential, the broad scientific community and government agencies agree that acute oral toxicity testing is still necessary to determine the toxic properties of a chemical. At this time, there are no accepted nonanimal alternative methods for acute oral toxicity evaluation. Much work remains to be done before nonanimal tests, such as those based on quantitative structure activity relationships or *in vitro* cell cultures, can be used as substitutes for oral toxicity testing.[2]

P&G does not use the Classical LD_{50} Test, and instead has adopted the Limit Test and the Up-and-Down Method for acute oral toxicity testing. Both tests reduce the use of animals from 40 to 60 used in the Classical LD_{50} Test to 6 to 10 animals per tests.

The Limit Test uses a single "limit dose" which is often 2000 mg/kg body weight. Usually ten animals (five males, five females) are used. The test provides an estimated LD_{50} relative to the selected dose, as well as some information on signs of toxicity. However, the test provides no information on dose response. The Limit Test is most suitable for chemicals that have some information on their acute toxicity from which an appropriate dose can be selected. The test is accepted by most regulatory agencies.

For chemicals for which there is little or no information on acute oral toxicity, the Up-and-Down Method is preferred.[3,4] The method involves the dosing of animals singly, at least 1 d apart, with each successive dose going up or down depending on the effect of the prior dose. If only the female is used, which has been found to be equally or more sensitive than the male, the test requires six to ten animals. In addition to signs of toxicity, the test provides an estimated LD_{50} value which can then be applied to toxicity classification system used by various regulatory agencies. The LD_{50} values obtained from the Up-and-Down Method were found to correlate very well with values obtained from the Classical Test. The Up-and-Down Method is acceptable to the U.S. regulatory agencies, and has been published as a standard test method by the American Society for Testing and Materials (1987).[5]

The British Toxicology Society recently published the results of an international validation study for another approach to evaluate acute oral toxicity, call the Fixed-Dose Procedure, which focuses on toxicity rather than lethality as an end point.[6] The procedure involves dosing ten animals (five males, five females) at a predetermined dose of 5, 50, 500, or 2000 mg/kg body weight, based on the results of a sighting study. Depending on the outcome of the first dose, a second or third dose group may be needed. From the data, the test chemical is classified according to the European Community hazard classification as very toxic, toxic, harmful, or unclassified. The results suggest that the Fixed-Dose Procedure can be used as an alternative test method for ranking test substances for their acute oral toxicity. The procedure is being proposed for adoption by the European Community.

All three alternative methods described above offer advantages in reduction. The choice of which method to use depends on the available information on the toxicity of the chemical, the type of toxicity information required, and certain regulatory requirements which need to be met.[7]

3.2 Eye Irritation

The need for ocular safety testing became clear early in the 1930s when an untested eyelash product caused significant ocular injury and at least one fatality. These injuries prompted Congress to pass federal legislation requiring that materials sold to consumers be safe. In response to the need for methods that assess ocular safety, several animal-based eye irritation tests were developed. In 1942, Draize et al. reported on a procedure that became the standard for assessing ocular irritancy potential. This test, known as the Draize Eye Irritation Test, and its modifications have provided information that has helped assure the ocular safety of products for several decades.

Although the Draize Eye Irritation Test has been used as the standard procedure for making ocular safety assessments, it is not without criticism. One of these is that Draize test results are biased toward overpredicting the degree of human risk.[8-11] Because of these overprediction, P&G researchers initiated studies to find an alternative to the Draize test that was more predictive of human response.

Griffith et al.[8] evaluated the relationship between the volume of test materials applied and the resulting irritation level in the rabbit eye. This study demonstrated that 10 μl of test material applied directly to the cornea allows better differentiation between substances of similar irritancy, and produces an irritation response similar in magnitude and duration to the responses observed in human. This study gave rise to the Low Volume Eye Test (LVET).

In subsequent studies, including studies which directly compared eye irritation response between humans and animals,[10,11] Freeberg et al. confirmed that the LVET more accurately predicts human ocular response than does the standard Draize protocol. The LVET is also less stressful to the test animals. Because of these advantages, P&G has replaced the Draize Eye Irritation Test with the LVET.

In addition to developing alternatives that are modifications of the *in vivo* test, significant effort is being directed toward development of *in vitro* alternatives in the hope the animal tests can some day be replaced. Numerous *in vitro* tests have been proposed as alternatives for *in vivo* eye safety tests.[12] These assays measure endpoints that assess one or more cellular processes that may be linked to eye irritation. Endpoints include cytotoxicity, inflammation, changes in metabolism/physiology, and tissue repair.

In order to minimize the use of animals in the ocular safety assessment process, P&G has proposed a Tier Testing Process (Figure 1).[12] The first step of this process involves obtaining and evaluating all available information on the eye irritation potential and physical/chemical properties of an ingredient or a product that needs to be assessed. Searches include examination of in-house data bases and external data bases such as MEDLINE, TOXLINE, RTECS, trade association data bases, and chemical supplier data. If the information available is sufficient for making a safety assessment, no additional testing is done. When additional information is required, the next step is to evaluate the materials in a battery of *in vitro* tests.

P&G is evaluating a battery of three *in vitro* assays that appear to provide information useful in the ocular safety assessment process. These include the silicon microphysiometer, a device that measures test material-induced changes in basal metabolism in mammalian cells; the microtox test, which measures the ability of test materials to alter bacterial respiratory metabolism; and the neutral red uptake assay, which measures the ability of test materials to inhibit the uptake of the dye neutral red.[13-15]

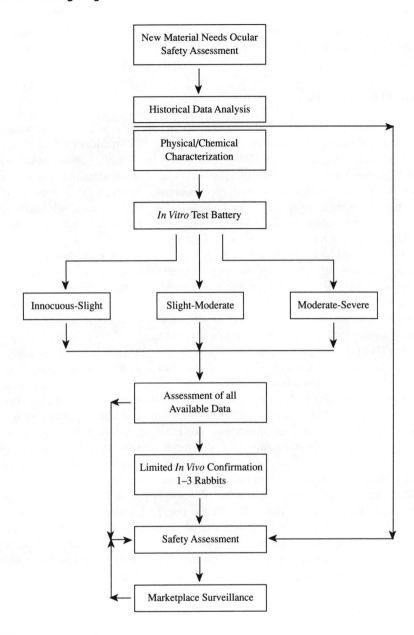

Figure 1. Tier testing process.

When we test chemicals or products for which we have confidence that the *in vitro* assays provide useful data, an eye irritation assessment again may be made without the need for animal testing. For other test materials, such as new chemicals or products where we have little or no previous experience, an *in vivo* test using a limited number of animals (perhaps only one to three) may be necessary. This tiered approach will lead to reduced dependence on animals decreasing our ability to assure the ocular safety of the materials tested.[12]

3.3 Skin Irritation

An evaluation of skin irritancy is an important part of the safety assessment for household cleaning, beauty care, and paper products—products that come into contact with skin. The Draize skin test in rabbits is often the test of choice. At P&G, we have reduced the used of rabbit skin tests to only occasional evaluation of new chemicals which are dissimilar to any known chemicals in our experience, or to meeting strict regulatory requirements for which there are no alternatives. P&G uses a modified protocol which reduces the number of animals used and which minimizes pain.[16]

For most consumer products, our prior experience on the formulations allows us to go directly to humans. Questions associated with animal to human extrapolations are thereby avoided. Here we can do a variety of tests, including single or repeated skin patch tests, clinical mildness tests, and actual product use tests. Excessive irritation can be avoided by conducting pilot range-finding studies using shorter exposure periods or diluted solutions.

For those few situations where *in vitro* testing is still necessary, *in vitro* assays which use human skin cells and which are based on known mechanisms of primary irritant dermatitis in human skin are being developed and validated. Cultured human skin cells have many of the same characteristics as intact human skin. Endpoints being looked at include cytotoxicity, cell viability, morphology, and inflammatory mediator production. For example, cell viability can be assessed by measuring mitochondrial function through metabolism of a vital dye by electron transport chain enzymes in living cells. Cytotoxicity can be assessed by measuring plasma membrane damage through release of the cytoplasmic enzyme lacate dehydrogenase into the culture. Release of the inflammatory mediator prostaglandin E_2 is an endpoint of particular interest because prostaglandin E_2 is known to be important in the process of skin irritation *in vivo*. Osborne and Perkins[17,18] have reported initial success using this strategy. With the rapid development of cultured human skin equivalents, it is likely that *in vitro* tests may soon replace the use of animals for acute skin irritancy testing.

3.4 Contact Hypersensitivity and Photoallergy

A number of animal test methods, including adjuvant tests (e.g., Maximization Test and Optimization Test) and nonadjuvant tests (e.g., the Buehler Method and the Open Epicutaneous Test) are available to evaluate the contact sensitization potential of chemical substances. For many years, P&G has used the Buehler Method and the Human Repeat Insult Patch Test (HRIPT) to assess the contact sensitization potential of chemicals.[19] Ingredients or formulations with appropriate information derived from prior contact sensitization studies are placed directly in HRIPT, thus reducing the number of animal studies being conducted. We have also developed a guinea pig cutaneous basophil hypersensitivity technique which differentiates sensitization from primary irritant reactions in guinea pigs,[20] a question that often comes up in sensitization testing. This diagnostic technique eliminates the need for multiple animal or clinical studies which were previously needed to make the distinction.

P&G is currently evaluating other alternative assays for contact hypersensitivity.[21-23] One promising assay being evaluated is the Local Lymph Node Assay in mice developed by Kimber et al.[24] A major advantage of this assay is that it requires only 1 week to complete as compared to 5 to 6 weeks for a typical guinea pig test. It also uses approximately 50% fewer animals than the Buehler guinea pig test. In this assay, lymph nodes adjacent to the test substance application site are made into a single cell suspension, and lymphocyte proliferation is determined by measuring ^{3}H-thymidine incorporation. Similar to the observation made by Kimber et al.,[24] we found the assay to be capable of detecting moderate to strong sensitizers and even some weak sensitizers; e.g., citronella and cinnamic aldehyde. On the other hand, nonsensitizing irritants (e.g., SLS, glycerol, and benzoic acid) do not cause significant lymphocyte proliferation. This assay is being validated by several laboratories in Europe and the United States. Other opportunities for the development of alternative methods for contact hypersensitivity were recently reviewed by Kimber.[25]

For photoallergy testing, P&G has recently developed a modified mouse ear swelling test.[26] This reduction method was able to detect moderate to strong photoallergens, including musk ambrette, 6-methylcoumarin, and fentichlor. In addition, to having advantages of being a more objective and quicker test, it also uses only half the animals used in other standard tests and does not require the use of adjuvants.

3.5 Respiratory Toxicology

Assessment of toxic exposures to the lung may be made using both *in vivo* and *in vitro* methods. *In vivo* morphologic responses to respiratory toxins has been the mainstay of hazard identification. The development and or refinement of technologies which allow sampling and analysis of respiratory tract fluids or isolation of lung cell populations have provided the basis for recent advances in our understanding of respiratory tract responses to inhaled materials.[27] Simultaneously, we have exploited this understanding to develop methods that can reduce the number of animals used in safety assessment.

Pathologic changes in acute lung damage which appear predictive of a material's ability to cause chronic interstitial lung disease have been identified by analysis of biochemical and cellular constituents of lung lining fluid sampled by bronchoalveolar lavage of exposed animals and by histopathology.[28-29] Bronchoalveolar lavage is used following a single exposure with multiple sampling times up to 2 months after exposure. Biochemical parameters assessed include lactate dehydrogenase for cytotoxicity, total protein for epithelial/endothelial barrier permeability, N-acetylglucosaminidase and β-glucuronidase for inflammatory cell activity. Cellular parameters analyzed include cell number, differential count, and cytology for assessment of inflammatory response and cytotoxicity. Bronchoalveolar lavage can be used as a screening test, thus reducing the number of subchronic and chronic inhalation toxicity tests that need to be conducted. The number of animals required is reduced by approximately 50% and the number of days on test is reduced with this screen.

Cell culture assays are being developed for use as a preliminary nonanimal screen to rank-order potential respiratory toxicants. Driscoll et al.[30] have demonstrated that fibrogenic dusts such as silica and asbestos can activate alveolar macrophages directly *in vitro* to release a leukotriene (LTB4) and tumor necrosis factor. In contrast, the release of these mediators is not stimulated by aluminum oxide or titanium dioxide; two dusts with a low potential to elicit an inflammatory response *in vivo*. This research provides necessary information for the development of a panel of *in vitro* screening assays to predict *in vivo* toxicity.

3.6 Genotoxicity and Carcinogenicity Testing

Over 150 short-term tests have been described for assessing the genotoxic carcinogenic potential of new chemicals or drugs.[31] Most of these are *in vitro* tests. These assays detect DNA damage caused by chemicals or drugs which is correlated with carcinogenic activity in humans and animals. A lifetime animal bioassay for carcinogenic activity of a new chemical or drug typically requires 400 to 600 animals and over a half-million dollars. Extensive reliance on carefully selected short-term tests as prescreens in product development reduces the need for bioassays.[32] Additionally, short-term genotoxicity tests address the potential of a chemical to induce heritable mutation.

Based on knowledge of the endpoints known to be involved in the carcinogenic process, including mutations and chromosome damage, a tiered battery which detects these endpoints is used for assessing the genotoxic potential of new chemicals or drugs in product development.

In the first tier, Tier I, a battery of three *in vitro* short-term tests is used which measures several types of DNA damage including mutation and chromosome damage. The Tier I test battery consists of the Ames assay which measures mutation in bacteria, the mouse lymphoma assay which measures mutation in mammalian cells, and the *in vitro* cytogenetic assay which measures chromosomes in mammalian cells.

A Tier II test battery is used to evaluate further those chemicals or drugs which give positive responses to the Tier I tests. Tier II tests address a chemical's potential to induce heritable effects as well as somatic effects. The tests in this battery include the Drosophila somatic mutation and recombination test (SMART), and an *in vivo* cytogenetic assay which measures chromosome damage in rat bone marrow cells.

Positive results in the Ames or mouse lymphoma assays will trigger a Tier II Drosophila SMART assay. A positive response in the Tier I *in vitro* cytogenetic assay will trigger a Tier II *in vivo* cytogenetic assay.

Other short-term assays are available to investigate further the genotoxicity of a chemical or drug. These assays include the unscheduled DNA synthesis (USD) assay which measure nonspecific DNA damage in rat hepatocytes, the alkaline elution assay which measures nonspecific DNA damage in rat testes, and the Syrian hamster embryo (SHE) cell transformation assay. The SHE assay can detect carcinogenic potential independent of an understanding of the genetic endpoint affected by the chemical. Therefore, the SHE assay detects chemicals which are genotoxic by inducing direct DNA damage or through indirect mechanisms such as the induction of aneuploidy. Extensive exploration of the SHE assay continues as evidence increases that it can also identify other indirect acting agents such as tumor promoters.[33,34]

Negative results in the short-term tests indicate that the chemical or drug is not likely to be carcinogenic. Positive results in Tier I and II tests suggest that the chemical or drug may be carcinogenic. If interest in this product is sufficient, a bioassay would be required to confirm this.

3.7 Developmental Toxicology

Of the approximately 60,000 chemicals in commerce, developmental toxicity data are available for only about 3,000; thus, there is a need to develop rapid, inexpensive, and reliable alternative test methods for developmental toxicity. At present, no nonanimal tests can totally replace the existing reproductive toxicity tests which use live animals. However, a number of *in vitro* tests are being developed as prescreens.[35]

P&G is evaluating the use of the Chick Embryo Retinal Cell Assay as a potential prescreen for teratogens.[36] In this assay, neural retinal cells are obtained from Day 6 chick embryos and are grown as a cell suspension. During incubation, these cells aggregate into spheroids of a specific diameter, grow, divide, and differentiate. Test agents are added on Day 1 to measure their ability to affect the number and size of aggregates which measure cell-to-cell recognition and adhesion, histology of aggregates and expansion of specific proteins which measure differentiation, and protein content as an index of growth. Thus far, the assay has correctly identified 17 materials as teratogens or nonteratogens. Additional work is being done to expand the developmental work to 45 more chemicals.[37]

3.8 Noninvasive Techniques

Noninvasive techniques can play an important role in reduction and refinement of animal use. One such technology is Magnetic Resonance Imaging and Spectroscopy (MRI/MRS). The MRI/MRS technology has broad applications. It can be used to monitor soft tissue changes., e.g., inflammation, tumor growth, and fetal development.[38] With the availability of appropriate reagents, the technique can be applied to measurement of drug metabolism and distribution in specific organs or tissues, imaging blood flow, and perfusion of organs. It can even measure pH changes in the body. The advantage of using the technology is it is noninvasive and painless, and it allows sequential studies to be performed on intact animals. After exploring this technology with several universities, P&G recently installed an MRI/MRS facility at its Miami Valley Laboratories.

Flow cytometry and image analysis are bioanalytical techniques that can reduce the use of animals by measuring the effect of disease or toxicity at the cellular level.[39] These techniques measure changes in cell morphology and function too subtle to be detected from visual inspection and they use very small biological samples, such as blood or culture cells. Cells with specific characteristics can be identified and separated based on their light-scattering properties and interactions with molecular probes. Examples of parameters that flow cytometry and image analysis can measure include changes in cell morphology (size, shape, cytoskeletal structure, and membrane texture), cell biochemistry (RNA, DNA, proteins, surface markers, and chemical accumulation) and cell functions (viability, ion flux, phagocytosis, bacterial killing, and metabolism). This technology allows multiple analyses to be done simultaneously on a small volume of biological samples, thus reducing the number of animals required.

3.9 Computer Applications

Quantitative structure–activity relationships (QSAR) can be useful in estimating the toxicity profile of compounds.[40-42] Three requirements for successful application of QSAR in predictive toxicology is shown in Table 1. One characteristic of a compound across classes that often seems clearly related to toxic potential is lipophilicity as measured by octanol: water partition coefficient. Otherwise, most characteristics considered in available QSAR systems are correlative within a class but less consistent across classes of compounds.[2] Unfortunately, with product formulations, octanol:water partition coefficient cannot be calculated as a single value.

A more promising use of QSAR is in drug design. This can help to reduce the number of animals used in testing for new drug products. Most software is available commercially and can be adapted for specific use. It is, however, not without limitations. Some of the drawbacks include narrow focus and limited accuracy rates of the currently available software programs.

Before any safety tests are conducted, toxicologists should conduct a thorough search of existing data bases, inside and outside the company. P&G has recently upgraded its computer data base system which was first set up in 1966. The new system, the Worldwide Toxicology Data System (WTDS), contains summaries of over 30,000 nonclinical safety studies conducted by the Company. Its primary purpose is to help Company toxicologists determine what company safety testing has already been done on a material being considered for use in products. The system is accessed via a personal computer with a communications link to the

Table 1.   Requirements for Successful Application of QSAR in Predictive Toxicology

1. There should be a well-defined mode of action for the compound considered.
2. The compounds should form part of a congeneric group.
3. There should be a common site of action for the biological effect.

Table 2.   Examples of Professional Practices Which Promote the 3 Rs

1. Reduce the number of product development candidates
2. Judicious use of human clinical testing
3. Avoid testing for trivial constituents and minor formulation changes
4. Utilize epidemiologic data
5. Publish safety data
6. Thoughtfully design studies to minimize animal use or pain
7. Use common controls for testing multiple products
8. Maintain high standards in animal care

IBM mainframe computer where the WTDS resides. The system also features a thesaurus which relates synonymous terms, allowing the user to use familiar terminology. Today over 75 toxicologists in 17 different divisions around the world use the system. Company actives and ingredients from research over the past decades continue to be re-examined for efficacy in new formulations or in new countries. The WTDS helps avoid duplication of safety studies, thus reducing the number of animals used and the cost of product development. Outside sources, e.g., TOXLINE, MEDLINE, and Cosmetic Ingredient Review (CIR), are also reviewed.

3.10   Other Applications

A multiplicity of diverse concepts can be employed to promote the 3 Rs. Individuals in organizations committed to the concept of alternatives often think of new ways to avoid testing without compromising the quality of the safety assessment. These concepts, when implemented, can be termed professional practices, and some examples are given in Table 2. These practices typically do not involve additional testing but can significantly reduce animal use. In 1989, P&G initiated an in-house newsletter, "Alternatives Alert". The newsletter brings to P&G life scientists updates on alternatives developments, new regulatory developments, upcoming meetings, selected publications, and many other areas of interest. The newsletter provides a vehicle for P&G's life science community to share its collective learnings on alternatives development and to encourage scientists to consciously look for ways that will lead to the 3 Rs.

3.11   Validation of Alternative Methods

The word validation often has different meanings to various people, and attempts have been made to better define what it should mean.[43,44] According to the report of the recently held Center for Alternatives to Animal Testing/European Research Group for Alternatives in Toxicity Testing (CAAT/ERGATT) workshop on the validation of toxicity test procedures, a validation process consists of four main steps: intralaboratory assessment, interlaboratory assessment, test database development, and finally, evaluation.[44] It is at the end of this process that a new method can be considered as scientifically validated. Even then, the validation is for a specific purpose with defined limitations.

An equally important process essential for broadscale use of alternative methods is regulatory acceptance. Here there is no defined process. Because regulatory authorities are given the task of protecting the health of the whole population, they tend to be skeptical of new tests that have not been known to be predictive through inter- or intralaboratory testing and that have not been accepted by the general scientific community.[45] At the same time, major corporations or trade associations are reluctant to commit large sums of money for validation activities that may not be acceptable to regulatory agencies.

One obvious solution for this dilemma is to obtain concurrence from regulatory agencies in the design and execution of interlaboratory validation studies. Another option is to form a distinguished scientific panel, selected or agreed to by regulatory agencies, which will review and concur with the design of the validation studies. If such a process can be established and the performance criteria of the validation study is defined, then there is a good chance that the validation study would produce meaningful data for regulatory review and approval. The key to the whole process is independent scientific review. Otherwise, the process can easily disintegrate into fragmented efforts, with individual researchers or companies peddling their pet assay system.

Internally at P&G, we follow the scheme outlined in Figure 2 for adoption of new test methods. It starts with basic research. When a potentially promising test method is identified, the method is subjected to a preliminary evaluation using standard compounds which are of interest to the Company and which cover a broad range of responses. If the test method continues to look promising, we will then initiate the parallel testing phase. In this phase, any test compounds that are submitted to the original test method will be evaluated also with the new method. This is an important phase whereby toxicologists, other than the researcher, can learn about the new method and its capabilities. This familiarity with the new method paves the way for gaining confidence in the acceptance of the new test method. After a reasonable period of parallel testing, the test method is standardized and it will either take the place of the original test method or will serve as an alternate method.

Whatever the process one uses, it is important that the process and its individual steps are well thought out and are based on good science. Only through sound science can alternative methods be developed, adopted for use and accepted by regulatory agencies.

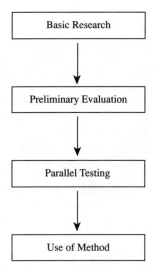

Figure 2. In-company development and adoption of alternatives.

3.12 Conclusions

Much progress has been made on the development of alternative methods for animal testing. Nevertheless, total replacement of animals for safety and efficacy testing is still many years away. At this time, reduction and refinement methods provide the most opportunities for reducing the use of animals and/or relieving pain and distress in animal testing. As alternative technology develops, nonanimal or replacement methods will take on an increasingly important role in further reduction of animal use.[46,47]

At P&G, it is our policy to incorporate new alternative methods into our testing scheme as soon as possible. A number of alternative methods are currently used in both safety and efficacy testing. As a result of the use of these alternative methods, our total use of animals has decreased 45% in the past 6 years, despite major expansion into the health care area and acquisition of new drug companies. More dramatically, over the same period, P&G's use of animals for personal care and household products decreased by 89%. We believe any further reduction in animal use will have to come from breakthrough technology in alternative method development. How does the future look for alternatives development? We believe it is very bright. Over the past few years, alternative methods development has become a respectable science. The science is further fueled by new technology development in bioanalytical techniques and cellular and molecular biology. We believe that in the not-too-distant-future *in vitro* alternative methods will become an integral part of safety and efficacy testing.

REFERENCES

1. Yam, J. and R. E. Winters. "Development of Alternatives in a Consumer Product Company," in *In Vitro Toxicology: New Directions*, A. M. Goldberg, Ed. (New York: Mary Ann Liebert, 1989), pp. 23–31.

2. Phillips, J. C., W. B. Gibson, J. Yam, C. L. Alden, and G. C. Hard. "Survey of the QSAR and *In Vitro* Approaches for Developing Non-Animal Methods to Supersede the *In Vivo* LD_{50} Test," *Food Chem. Toxicol.* 28(5):375–394 (1990).

3. Bruce, R. D. "An Up-and-Down Procedure for Acute Toxicity Testing," *Fund. Appl. Toxicol.* 5(1):151–157 (1985).

4. Bruce, R. D. "A Confirmatory Study of the Up-and-Down Method for Acute Oral Toxicity Testing. *Fund. Appl. Toxicol.* 8(1):97–100 (1987).

5. "Standard Test Methods for Estimating Acute Oral Toxicity in Rats," ASTM Methods, E1162-87, (1987).

6. van den Heuvel, M., D. Clark, R. Fieler, P. Koundaksian, G. Oliver, D. Pelling, N. Tomlinson, and A. Walker. "The International Validation of a Fixed-Dose Procedure as an Alternative to the Classical LD_{50} Test," *Food Chem. Toxicol.* 28(6):469–482 (1990).

7. Yam, J., P. J. Reer, and R. D. Bruce. "Comparison of the Up-and-Down Method and the Fixed-Dose Procedure for Acute Oral Toxicity Testing," *Food Chem. Toxicol.* 29(4):259–263 (1991).

8. Griffith, J. F., G. A. Nixon, R. D. Bruce, P. J. Reer, and E. A. Bannan. "Dose-Response Studies with Chemical Irritants in the Albino Rabbit Eye as a Basis for Selecting Optimum Testing Conditions for Predicting Hazard to the Human Eye," *Toxicol. Appl. Pharmacol.* 55(3):501–513 (1980).

9. Griffith, J. and F. Freeberg. "Empirical and Experimental Basis of Selecting the Low Volume Rabbit Eye Irritation Test as the Validation Standard for *In Vitro* Methods," in *In Vitro Toxicology, Approaches to Validation. Alternative Methods in Toxicology*, Vol. 5, A. Goldberg, Ed. (New York: Mary Ann Liebert, 1987), pp. 303–311.

10. Freeberg, F. E., J. F. Griffith, R. D. Bruce, and P. H. S. Bay. "Correlation of Animal Test Methods with Human Experience for Household Products," *J. Toxicol. Cut. Ocular Toxicol.* 3(1):53–64 (1984).

11. Freeberg, F. E., G. A. Nixon, P. J. Reer, J. E. Weaver, R. D. Bruce, J. F. Griffith, and L. W. Sanders. "Human and Rabbit Eye Responses to Chemical Insult," *Fund. Appl. Toxicol.* 7(4):626–634 (1986).

12. Wilcox, D. K. and L. H. Bruner. "*In vitro* Alternatives: Their Development and Role in Ocular Safety Assessment," *Alternatives Lab. Anim.* 18(1):117–128 (Nov. 1990).

13. Bruner, L. H., K. M. Kercso, J. D. Owicki, J. W. Parce, V. C. Muir. "Testing Ocular Irritancy *in vitro* with the Silicon Microphysiometer," *Toxicol. In Vitro* 5(4):277–284 (1991).

14. Bruner, L. H. and R. D. Parker. "Evaluation of Seven *In Vitro* Alternatives for Ocular Safety Testing," *Fund. Appl. Toxicol.* 17(1):136–149 (1991).

15. Bruner, L. H., Shadduck, J. A., and Essex-Sorlie, D. "Alternative Methods for Assessing the Effects of Chemicals on the Eye," in *Dermal and Ocular Toxicology: Fundamentals and Methods* (Boca Raton, FL: CRC Press, 1991), pp. 585–606.

16. Nixon, G. A., E. A. Bannan, T. W. Gaynor, D. H. Johnston, and J. F. Griffith. "Evaluation of Modified Methods for Determining Skin Irritation in Animals and Humans," *Regul. Toxicol. Pharmacol.* 12(2):127–136 (1990).

17. Osborne, R. and M. A. Perkins. *"In Vitro* Skin Irritancy Testing with Human Skin Cell Cultures," *Toxicol. In Vitro* 5(5/6):563–567 (1990).

18. Osborne, R. and M. A. Perkins. "Evaluation of Human Skin Cell Cultures for *In Vitro* Skin Irritancy Testing," in *In Vitro Toxicology: Mechanisms and New Technology,* Vol. 8, A. Goldberg, Ed. (New York: Mary Ann Liebert, 1991), pp, 317–324.

19. Robinson, M. K., T. L. Nusair, P. H. S. Bay, J. Stotts, and P. J. Danneman. "A Risk Assessment Process for Allergic Contact Sensitization," *Food Chem. Toxicol.* 27(7):479–489 (1989).

20. Robinson, M. K., E. R. Fletcher, G. R. Johnson, W. E. Wyder, and J. K. Maurer. "Value of Cutaneous Basophil Hypersensitivity(CBH) Response for Distinguishing Weak Contact Sensitization from Irritation Reactions in the Guinea Pig," *J. Invest. Dermat.* 94(5):636–643 (1990).

21. Robinson, M. K. and D. L. Sneller. "Use of an Optimized *In Vitro* Lymphocyte Blastogenesis Assay to Detect Contact Sensitivity to Nickel Sulfate in Mice," *Toxicol. Appl. Pharmacol.* 104(1):106–116 (1990).

22. Gerberick, G. F., C. A. Ryan, E. R. Fletcher, D. L. Sneller, and M. K. Robinson. "An Optimized Lymphocyte Blastogenesis Assay for Detecting the Response of Contact Sensitized or Photosensitized Lymphocytes to Hapten or Photohapten Modified Antigen Presenting Cells," *Toxicol. In Vitro* 4(4/5):289–292 (1990).

23. Gerberick, G. F., C. A. Ryan, E. R. Fletcher, A. D. Howard, and M. K. Robinson. "Increased Number of Dentritic Cells in Draining Lymph Nodes Accompanies the Generation of Contact Photosensitivity," *J. Invest. Dermat.* 96(3):355–361 (1991).

24. Kimber, I., J. A. Mitchell, and A. C. Griffith. "Development of a Murine Local Lymph Node Assay for Determination of Sensitizing Potential," *Food Chem. Toxicol.* 24(6–7):585–586 (1986).

25. Kimber, I. "Aspects of the Immune Response to Contact Allergens: Opportunities for the Development and Modification of Predictive Test Methods," *Food Chem. Toxicol.* 27(11):755–762 (1989).

26. Gerberick, G. F. and C. A. Ryan. "A Predictive Mouse Ear-Swelling Model for Investigating Topical Photoallergy," *Food Chem. Toxicol.* 28(5):361–368 (1990).

27. Driscoll, K. E. and R. C. Lindenschmidt. "Symposium on New and Developing Techniques in Respiratory Toxicology," *Toxicology* 60(1/2):1–3 (1990).

28. Driscoll, K. E., R. C. Lindenschmidt, J. K. Maurer, and G. Ridder. "Pulmonary Responses to Silica or Titanium Dioxide: Inflammatory Cells, Alveolar Macrophage-Derived Cytokines and Histopathology," *Am. J. Resp. Cell Molecular Biol.* 2(4):381–390 (1990).

29. Lindenschmidt, R. C., K. E. Driscoll, M. A., Perkins, J. M. Higgins, J. K. Maurer, and K. A. Belfiore. "The Comparison of a Fibrogenic and Two Nonfibrogenic Dusts by Bronchoalveolar Lavage," *Toxicol. Appl. Pharmacol.* 102(2):268–281 (1990).

30. Driscoll, K. E., J. M. Higgins, M. Laytart, and L. L. Crosby. "Differential Effects of Mineral Dusts on the *In Vitro* Activation of Alveolar Macrophage Eicosanoid and Cytokine Release," *Toxicol. In Vitro* 4(4/5):284–288 (1990).

31. Waters, M. D., H. F. Stack, J. R. Rabinowitz, and N. E. Garrett. "Genetic Activity Profiles and Pattern Recognition in Test Battery Selection," *Mutatation Res. (Netherlands)* 205:(1–4):119–138 (1988).

32. International Commission for Protection Against Environmental Mutagens and Carcinogens. "Testing for Mutagens and Carcinogens; the Role of Short-Term Genotoxicity Assays," *Mutatation Res. (Netherlands)* 205(1–4):3–12 (1988).

33. LeBoeuf, R. A. and G. A. Kerckaert. "The Induction of Transformed-Like Morphology and Enhanced Growth in Syrian Hamster Embryo Cells Grown at Acidic pH," *Carcinogenesis* 7(9):1431–1440 (1986).

34. LeBoeuf, R. A., G. A. Kerckaert, J. A. Poiley, and R. Raineri. "An Interlaboratory Comparison of Enhanced Morphological Transformation of Syrian Hamster Embryo Cells Cultured Under Conditions of Reduced Bicarbonate Concentration and pH is not Carcinogen Specific," *Mutatation Res. (Netherlands)* 222(3):205–218 (1989).

35. Daston, G. P. and R. A. D'Amato. "*In Vitro* Techniques in Teratology," in *Benchmarks: Alternative Methods in Toxicology*, M. A. Mehlman, Ed. (New Jersey: Princeton Scientific Publishing, 1989), pp. 79–109.

36. Daston, G. P., D. Baines, and J. E. Yonker. "Chick Embryo Neural Retinal Cell Culture as a Screen for Development Toxicity," *Toxicol. Appl. Pharmacol.* 109(2):352–366 (1991).

37. Fitzgerald, M. P., G. P. Daston, and E. Elmore. "Optimization of the Chick Embryo Retinal Cell Assay for Teratogens," *Teratology* 41(5):557 (1990).

38. Daston, G. P., T. A. Neubecker, Y. E. Yonker, L. J. Busse, R. G. Pratt, R. C. Samaratunga, and S. R. Thomas. "Magnetic Resonance Imaging of Congenital Hydrocephalus in the Rat," *Fund. Appl. Toxicol.* 9(3):415–422 (1987).

39. Melamed, M. R., T. Lindmo, and J. L. Mendelsohn, Eds., *Flow Cytometry and Sorting*, 2nd ed. (New York: Wiley-Liss, 1990).

40. Purchase, R., J. Phillips, and B. Labe. "Structure-Activity Techniques in Toxicology," *BIBRA Bull.* 29:5–9 (1990).

41. Enslein, K. "An Overview of Structure-Activity Relationships as an Alternate to Testing in Animals for Carcinogenicity, Mutagenicity, Dermal and Eye Irritation, and Acute Oral Toxicity," in *Benchmarks: Alternative Methods in Toxicology*, M. A. Mehlman, Ed. (New Jersey: Princeton Scientific Publishing, 1989), pp. 59–78.

42. Rosenkranz, H. and S. G. Klopman. "CASE, the Computer-Automated Structure Evaluation System, as an Alternative to Extensive Animal Testing," in *Benchmarks: Alternative Methods in Toxicology*, M. A. Mehlman, Ed. (New Jersey: Princeton Scientific Publishing, 1989), pp. 29–36.

43. Frazier, J. M. "Scientific Criteria for Validation of *In Vitro* Toxicity Tests," *OECD Environ. Monog.* No. 36, (Sept 1990).

44. Balls, M., P. Blaauboer, D. Brusick, J. Frazier, D. Lamb, M. Pemberton, C. Reinhardt, M. Roberfroid, H. Rosenkranz, B. Schmid, H. Spielmann, A-L. Stammati, and E. Walum. "Report and Recommendations of the CAAT/ERGATT Workshop on the Validation of Toxicity Test Procedures," *ATLA* 18(1):313–337, (Nov 1990).

45. van den Heuvel, M. J. and R. J. Fielder. "Acceptance of *In Vitro* Testing by Regulatory Authorities," *Toxicol. In Vitro* 4(4/5):675–79 (1990).

46. Gad, S. C. "Recent Developments in Replacing, Reducing, and Refining Animal Use in Toxicology Research and Testing," *Fund. Appl. Toxicol.* 15(1):8–16 (1990).

47. Spira, H. "Alternatives: Moving into the Nineties," *Bull. Int. Council Lab. Sci .* 67:19–23 (1990).

CHAPTER 4

In Vitro Techniques for Use in Drug Discovery

Paul Sweetnam, Charles Bauer, Jr., and Maura Charlton

4.0 Introduction

The pharmaceutical industry's role in drug discovery has expanded over the past several decades. Along with increased technical and financial commitment to this effort, the industry has developed more rational methods to identify novel therapeutic agents. This chapter was designed to provide an overview of the integration of two well-established technologies, radioligand binding and cell culture, into an effective research tool for drug discovery. Before describing this integration it is appropriate to briefly review the scientific principles on which each technology is founded.

4.1 Radioligand Binding

4.1.1 General Considerations

Cellular communication by means of chemical messengers and membrane bound receptors is the biological foundation of radioligand binding. While the role of chemical messengers in biological systems was first proposed early in this century,[1] it was not until 1956 that the attachment of a drug to a specific receptor

Table 1.   Protocol for Screening Test Agents for Activity at Nerve Growth Factor Receptor Binding Sites

1. Membrane Suspension Preparation
    PC12 cells are cultured to confluency in T150 flasks (Dulbecco's Modified Eagle's Medium [DMEM] + 5% Horse Serum + 5% Fetal Bovine Serum + 200 mM L-glutamine). *Note:* cells harvested into a 50 ml conical centrifuge tube. The cells are washed with 50 ml of DMEM and centrifuged at 1000 rpm for 10 min at 25°C in a table-top centrifuge. The pellet is resuspended in 50 ml of DMEM and passed through a syringe with an 18G11/2 needle to prevent clumping of cells. Wash cells an additional time as described above. The cells are resuspended to a concentration of 2.5×10^6 cells/ml in DMEM/0.1% BSA (pH 7.7 at 25°C) such that each well will receive 5×10^5 cells. Keep cell suspension on ice until ready for use (no longer than 10 min).

2. Radioligand Stock Solution
    ^{125}I-NGF is obtained from Dupont-New England Nuclear (Cat. #NEX-215) and is diluted to a concentration of 3.0 nM in DMEM/0.1% BSA (pH 7.7 at 25°C), such that the final radioligand concentration in the assay is 0.3 nM.

3. Unlabeled Ligand Stock Solution
    A stock solution of 0.1 μM 2.5S Nerve Growth Factor (NGF) is prepared in 4% DMSO just prior to starting the experiment. 2.5S NGF is available from Biomedical Technologies Inc. (Cat. #BT-206).

4. Test Compound Stock Solution
    A stock solution for each test compound of 1 mM in 4% DMSO if possible. Addition of other vehicles may be necessary.

5. Content for Total Wells
    Prepare wells (.65-μM Multiscreen filtration plates) in triplicate for measuring total binding by pipetting 25 μl of 4% DMSO, 25 μl of radioligand stock, and 200 μl of cell suspension. A separate set of total wells should be prepared per plate.

6. Content for Nonspecific Wells
    Prepare wells (.65-μM Multiscreen filtration plates) in triplicate for measuring nonspecific binding by pipetting 25 μl of unlabeled ligand stock solution, 25 μl of radioligand stock, and 200 μl of cell suspension. A separate set of nonspecific wells should be prepared per plate.

7. Content for Test Compound Wells
    Prepare wells (.65-μM Multiscreen filtration plates) in triplicate for measuring test substance binding by pipetting 25 μl of test substance stock, 25 μl radioligand stock, and 200 μl of cell suspension.

8. Incubation Conditions
    Each 96-well filtration plate is placed in a 37°C incubator for 45 min.

9. Termination
    At the end of the incubation period, the plate is removed from the oven and the contents are removed using the Millipore Multiscreen Filtration system. The wells are rinsed five times with cold phospate buffered saline (PBS).

10. Quantitation of Radioactivity
    Each filter is placed in separate 12 × 55 mm Rohren tubes from Sarsted (Cat. #55.484) and radioligand bound is assessed via gamma scintillation counting.

11. Results (In dpm)
Total binding:	14,000
Nonspecific binding:	4,700
Test compound 1 binding:	13,950
Test compound 2 binding:	14,000
Test compound 3 binding:	4,750
Test compound 4 binding:	4,900

The nonspecific dpm are subtracted from total dpm, leaving what is defined as specific binding. Generally these are further expressed as percent inhibition of binding when no test substance was present—i.e., total binding tube (14,000 dpm) − nonspecific binding tube (4,700 dpm) = specific binding (9,300 dpm) is defined as 0% inhibition; whereas test compound 4 binding (4,900 dpm) − nonspecific binding (4,700 dpm) = specific test compound binding (200 dpm) when expressed as percent inhibition: (9,300 − 200)/9300 × 100 = 97.8% inhibition.

was linked to the efficacy of that drug.[2] This attachment, or binding, allows the use of radioisotope-labeled chemicals (radioligands) to study the interaction of select drugs at specific receptors and to identify potential drug candidates from the screening of libraries of synthetic and natural chemicals (Table 1).

The radioligand binding assay, as inferred by its name, is based on the binding of the radioligand to a specific receptor. The kinetics of this binding must be saturable, competitive, specific, and reversible.[3] The endpoint of a receptor binding assay is the quantification of the radioligand bound to the receptor as measured by the disintegration of the radioisotope, i.e., disintegrations per minute (dpm). In most assays the radioligand has the potential to interact nonselectively with other membrane proteins present in the assay or possibly the glass fiber filters used to terminate the binding reaction. For this reason the specific binding to the receptor of interest must be determined. This is accomplished by quantifying the nonspecific binding component, the amount of radioligand bound in the presence of an unlabeled drug at a concentration which fully blocks the receptor of interest. The specific dpm bound is determined by subtracting the nonspecific dpm from total dpm bound (specific binding = total binding − nonspecific binding). The greater the ratio of total binding as compared to nonspecific binding, the more dependable an assay will be as a drug discovery tool. Specific binding is normally reported as the percent of total binding, with values >70% the criteria required for a dependable assay. (The reader is referred elsewhere for a more detailed description of the concepts and theory of radioligand binding.[4,5])

A dose–response study is one experimental approach used to predict the relative potency of a drug or test compound at a receptor site. This information is generated by holding the receptor concentration, radioligand concentration, and all other experimental conditions constant, while varying the concentration of the inhibiting or unlabeled drug (Figure 1). Drug discovery efforts routinely use modified dose–response formats to screen thousands of compounds for their ability to inhibit binding at a targeted receptor.

Radioligand binding is a sensitive, reliable, and reproducible *in vitro* technique capable of generating a large amount of analytical/quantitative information rapidly. Used as a screening tool, the radioligand binding assay can generate information on thousands of test compounds in a short period of time while utilizing a very limited number of laboratory animals. This provides a cost effective, ethical approach when compared to many of the *in vivo* or whole animal approaches used by drug companies in the past.

4.1.2 Radioligand

The development of radiolabeled drugs with high specific activity and affinity were technical advances essential in establishing radioligand binding as a standard method used to determine the details and dynamics of drug–receptor interactions. The small concentration of any given receptor type in a specific tissue, typically

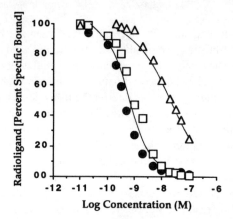

Figure 1.   Dose–response curve. The competition of [^{125}I] endothelin-1 by increasing concentrations of three different endothelin peptides, (□) ET-1, (●) ET-2, (△) ET-3.
In this experiment, the relative inhibitory potencies of each peptide were determined using a thoracic smooth muscle cell line (A10) receptor source.[15] In this
study, ET-1 and ET-2 were equipotent in displacing [^{125}I]ET-1, while ET-3 was
a magnitude less potent. Endothelin is a potent vasoconstricting peptide which
regulates smooth muscle contraction. The development of an endothelin antagonist could be useful in the treatment of cardiovascular disorders, including
coronary angina, cerebral vasospasm, and hypertension.

in the fmol/mg membrane protein range, dictated the need for an extremely
sensitive assay. The ability of a binding assay to detect bound radiolabel to such
a small number of receptors could only reliably be achieved by radioligands with
specific activities >20 Ci/mmol.[6] Radioligands of higher affinity result in "tighter"
binding to a receptor, reducing concerns surrounding the binding kinetics of the
assay, i.e., dissociation/association rates and lowering the concentration of
radioligand needed, thus simplifying technical aspects of the assay. In general,
higher affinity radioligands, dissociation constants (K_d) under 10 nM, contribute
to lowering of the nonspecific binding component.

   The degree of selectivity of a radioligand for a targeted receptor is an important
issue when developing an assay to be used in a drug discovery screening effort.
The more selective the drug for the target receptor, the less the possibility of that
drug binding to other receptor types. If other receptors in the tissue used in the
assay have K_ds for the radioligand similar to the receptor targeted, they will
contribute to the specific binding component in that assay. Therefore, it is
important that the selectivity of a radioligand is well-established so as to correct
for any unwanted receptor interaction in the assay. Selectivity can be determined by employing dose–response studies using a wide variety of reference
drugs which target other receptor types. For example, spiperone, a nonselective
dopamine ligand interacts with alpha 1, alpha 2, beta, dopamine 1, dopamine 2,
serotonin 1, serotonin 2, histamine 1, and muscarinic 1 at submicromolar concentrations.

4.1.3 Tissue/Receptor

Dissected animal tissue, mainly rodent, is the major source of receptor used in binding assays. In many instances the use of such tissue is based on the vast literature which exists concerning the development and characterization of assays targeting over 100 different receptor types.[7] There are, however, technical limitations to the use of dissected animal tissue. First, radioligand binding assays have defined limits on the tissue concentrations which can be utilized without compromising the validity of the results obtained. In most instances as tissue concentration increases there is a corresponding increase in nonspecific binding of the radioligand (Figure 2). Consequently, if the desired receptor population is small and only associated with one cell type in a tissue, the other cell types, which play no role in specific receptor binding, can function to increase the nonspecific binding component of the assay. Therefore, the use of a tissue source composed of only one cell type, i.e., a cell line, might have an advantage over dissected animal tissue in certain assays. However, the use of a clonal line does not guarantee an increase in receptor density as compared to dissected animal tissue. Second, animal tissues routinely used in the assays display a great deal of receptor heterogeneity. This heterogeneity is a direct reflection of the number of different cell types, each expressing a unique complement of receptors. As stated previously, many of the available radioligands bind to more than one type of receptor. It is possible that the receptor heterogeneity found in most tissues could compromise specific binding in certain radioligand binding assays. Therefore, any assay using a ligand of limited selectivity and dissected animal tissues must be rigorously examined before use in a targeted drug discovery effort. The inappropriate identification of a potential lead therapeutic agent could result in time consuming and costly delay. Once again, the use of a tissue source composed of only one cell type could decrease the number of different receptor types in the assay and increase the selective nature of that assay.

In addition to the technical problems which arise from the use of animal tissue, there are a number of ethical/financial issues scientists must continually address. These issues may limit the availability of laboratory animals for biomedical research purposes in the future, so it becomes the responsibility of the scientific community to discover alternate methods which will not compromise the contributions being made by the pharmaceutical industry in the area of human health care.

4.2 Cell Culture

4.2.1 General Considerations

Since its inception in 1907,[8] the ability to maintain viable animal and insect cells *in vitro* has improved dramatically, expanding the utility of cell culture in biomedical research. There are now several excellent books detailing the various

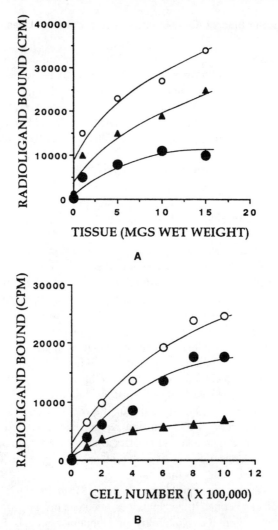

Figure 2.   Tissue/cell linearity. The determination of the tissue concentration or cell number necessary for optimum specific binding in the Nerve Growth Factor (NGF) assay [(○) total binding, (▲) nonspecific binding, and (●) specific binding]. The greatest difference between the total and nonspecific binding is the tissue concentration or cell number at which optimum specific binding occurs. The specific binding of [125I]NGF determined against increasing concentration of homogenized PC12 cell membrane preparation (A) and intact "viable" PC12 cells (B). The nonspecific binding component using intact PC12 cells increases at a gradual rate as compared to the membrane preparations resulting in better specific binding in the intact cell assay than for the tissue preparation. This difference may be the result of the inherent stickiness of [125I]NGF, a large peptide, for homogenized membranes preparation. NGF stimulates the growth of certain types of neurons in the central and peripheral nervous system.[21] The development of an NGF agonist may be useful in the treatment of certain traumatic or biochemically induced neurodegenerative conditions.

Table 2. Receptor Binding Assays Utilizing Established Cell Lines

Cell Line	Receptor Binding	Radioligand	Ref.
A10	Atrial Natriuretic Peptide$_2$	[^{125}I] ANP	14
	Endothelin$_A$	[^{125}I] Endothelin	15
C6 glioma	Benzodiazepine	[^{3}H] Flunitrazepam	16
	Beta Adrenergic	[^{125}I] Dihydroalprenolol	17
Fibroblast (3T3)	Platelet Derived Growth Factor	[^{125}I] PDGF	18
HL60	Histamine$_2$	[^{3}H] Tiotidine	19
	Tumor Necrosis Factor	[^{125}I] TNF	20
L929	Tumor Necrosis Factor	[^{125}I] TNF	20
HCN-1A	Chloride channel	[^{3}H] TBOB	31
	Endothelin$_A$	[^{125}I] Endothelin	31
	NMDA ion channel	[^{3}H] MK801	31
PC12	Nerve Growth Factor	[^{125}I] NGF	21
	Purinergic$_{2Y}$	[^{35}S] ADPBS	22
NIE-115	Bradykinin	[^{3}H] Bradykinin	23
	Muscarinic	[^{3}H] QNB	24
	Neurotensin	[^{3}H] Neurotensin	25
	Serotonin$_3$	[^{3}H] GR-65630	26
SK-N-SH	Muscarinic$_3$	[^{3}H] N-Methylscopolamine	27
SK-N-MC	Neuropeptide Y$_1$	[^{125}I] NPY	28

techniques currently available in the area of cell culture.[9,10] Cultured cells are an accepted alternative to animal tissue as a receptor source for radioligand binding studies and have been used for over 20 years in the study of drug–receptor interactions. However, the widespread use of cultured cells in drug discovery screening efforts is still in its infancy. NovaScreen®, the drug discovery arm of Nova Pharmaceutical Corporation, now has over 20 assays utilizing cultured cells and is continually looking to convert other assays from animal tissue to cells (Table 2).

Established cell lines, homogeneous populations (clones) of animal or insect cells, can be cultured in precisely controlled environments, lessening the problem of cellular and receptor heterogeneity commonly associated with animal tissues and some primary cell culture models. Selectivity of the radioligand used may not be an issue due to the limited receptor heterogeneity. Cultured cells also provide the distinct advantage of allowing scientists to use the same *in vitro* model for receptor binding as well as other pharmacological (functional) assays targeting the same receptor. The use of intact or living cells, which better mimic the *in vivo* situation, is particularly advantageous compared to the extensively washed and homogenized tissue preparations routinely used in binding assays. With any biological model, one must be careful to understand its limitations when interpreting results, and a cell culture model is no exception. It should be noted that cells grown in culture may not function as their *in vivo* counterparts for several reasons: (1) anatomically, cells develop and are maintained in a 2-D not a 3-D array; (2) cells are maintained in an artificial growth medium; (3) a clonal cell line is removed from the influence of other cells; and (4) "continuous" cell lines are functionally different from their normal cell counterparts. For the purpose of receptor binding these differences may not be as critical, given the ability of the researcher to completely characterize a drug–receptor interaction of interest. At the molecular level, the ability of the receptor to interact with a drug should be similar for whole cells and *in vivo* models (although an altered biologic response to receptor occupancy is possible).

4.2.2 Primary Cell Culture

Cultured cells are routinely categorized as either "primary" or "continuous/immortal" cells based on their *in vitro* growth characteristics. Primary cell cultures are started from freshly dissected normal animal tissue which has been mechanically or enzymatically dissociated to a suspension of individual cells. These cells are then allowed to adhere to an artificial substrate and developed in a defined environment. This type of culturing has several disadvantages when used for drug discovery. These cells have a limited capacity to undergo cell division and can be maintained for only a finite period of time in culture, consequently, new starter cultures must be prepared on a regular basis. Cells which cannot divide in culture, i.e., neurons, must be cultured before differentiation is complete; this requires the use of embryonic tissue. These cultures also have a limited life span in culture, in addition to the technical and ethical problems in using embryonic tissue. Further, the ability to generate a homogeneous population of primary neuronal cells is difficult, and in most instances impossible (Figure 3).

4.2.3 Continuous/Immortal Cell Culture

One of the biggest advances in cell culture technique was the discovery of "continuous/immortal" cell lines. These lines were initially established from various tumors, neoplastic cell growths,[11] although primary cells can now be immortalized by virally induced transformation.[10,12] "Continuous" cells in culture divide indefinitely and lend themselves readily to cloning, the establishment of a cell line from a single cell. Thus, "continuous" cell lines can provide ready access to a homogeneous population of cells, increasing the reproducibility of an assay by standardizing the model system.

There are problems associated with the use of continuous cell lines in the field of drug discovery. In particular is the limited number of different receptor types that have been identified and characterized on established cell lines (Table 2). However, the growing number of cell lines available increases the probability of finding a line suitable for any drug discovery effort. For example, a human cortical neuronal cell line (HCN-1A) established from a cortical biopsy of a patient with unilateral megaencephaly has many of the properties of a developing cortical neuron.[11] For this reason, HCN-1A is being used in neurochemical studies targeting neuronal development and differentiation (see Figure 4). The American Type

Culture Collection in Rockville, MD is an excellent source of continuous cell lines, with over 1800 different lines now available, however, receptor identification and characterization is needed.

4.2.4 Molecular Biology/Cloned Receptors

Recent advances in the field of molecular biology are expanding the uses of cell culture and its role in drug discovery. Cell lines can now be genetically engineered to express high levels of a particular receptor (Figure 5).[13] The ability of a cell to express millions of one receptor type on its surface greatly enhances a radioligand binding assay's specific binding component and selectivity. High level expression systems may also enhance the development of nonradiolabeled ligands, i.e., fluorescent ligands. These ligands will have lower sensitivity but the large increases in receptor number will be more than adequate to establish a workable specific binding signal. Molecular biology will also allow for expression systems based on the use of human receptors. This could potentially enhance its scientific relevance as compared to nonhuman *in vitro* models now being used.

4.3 Radioligand Binding and Drug Discovery

The implementation of a drug discovery and development effort tends to be somewhat generic throughout the pharmaceutical industry. This scheme is outlined in Figure 6. Radioligand binding and cell culture technologies can make significant contributions in the early stages of this effort. A more detailed description of these contributions follows.

4.3.1 Phase I Drug Discovery

In this phase of drug discovery the radioligand binding assay is used as a rapid way to identify compounds, from synthetic chemical or natural product libraries, which inhibit binding to the receptor of interest. With a synthetic chemical library, all compounds can be screened in a random manner because thousands of samples can be tested in a period of several days. This serendipitous approach to drug discovery has been used successfully by many pharmaceutical companies. Conversely, a semirandom approach can be used where portions of the library are screened. Compounds are preselected to represent the various structural groups in that library. The preselection of compounds is an important consideration if the receptor binding assay being utilized as a screening tool is technically difficult; an example of this would be an assay designed around the use of a peptide growth factor whose availability is limited.

The purpose of the initial screen is to give the researcher a structural starting point, or template, for further drug development. Rarely, if ever, do structures identified in Phase I screening represent the final structure of a marketed drug. Many development efforts start with a compound of potency and selectivity which

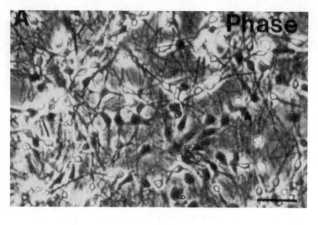

A

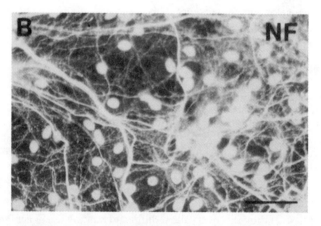

B

Figure 3.   Primary dissociated spinal cord culture. Cell cultures obtained from embryonic central nervous system tissue are an excellent example of the cellular heterogeneity associated with primary culture models. The heterogeneity is demonstrated by using antibodies which label cell-type specific markers. (A) Phase micrograph of spinal cord culture (unlabeled), (B) neurons are identified by the presence of neurofilament-like immunoreactivity; (C) astrocytes are identified by GFAP, glial fibrillary acidic protein; and (D) oligodendrocytes by GalC, galactoside cerebroside-like immunoreactivity.[29] Homogeneous or nearly homogeneous primary cell cultures from embryonic central nervous system tissue can be obtained by utilizing various mechanical and biochemical manipulations, however, these are time consuming and difficult.[9]

are not useful from a pharmacological standpoint and must be structurally modified. The ideal screening assay must identify not only strong but also weak inhibitors of binding. Therefore, the concentration of compounds tested is a relatively high one, between 1 and 10 μM. However, as with other components of

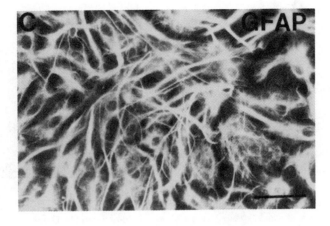

C

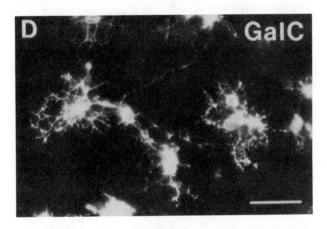

D

the binding assay, the concentration of test samples must also be carefully selected because high concentrations can nonspecifically inhibit radioligand binding in certain assays.

In the case of a natural product library, individual samples or extracts are composed of numerous unidentified chemical structures. Here receptor binding identifies inhibitory activity, and chemists must isolate and purify the appropriate structure. Receptor binding is used to monitor this progress. Natural products, because of their heterogeneous nature, tend to increase the variability of an assay which functions well when used for screening of synthetics. It may therefore be necessary to redesign the assay to correct for this variation.

Following the initial identification of a compound which possesses inhibitory activity, it is important to verify that activity on a fresh disbursement of the sample in order to eliminate the possibility of a false positive in the initial screen. False

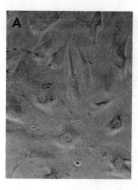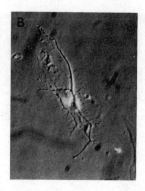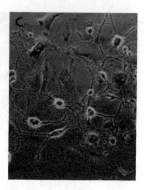

Figure 4.   Human cortical neuronal cell line. The first established neuronal cell line displays an epithelioid-like morphology when undifferentiated (A). Under the appropriate conditions, i.e., the presence of NGF, HCN-1A cells differentiate into morphologically mature neuron (B, C). The nontransformed and homogeneous (clonal) nature of the cells in culture make them an excellent *in vitro* model in drug discovery/development.

positives can occur for a number of reasons, ranging from the inherent variability of a specific assay, to a technical mistake such as the improper dispensing of tissue into a test tube. Conversely, the potential for false negatives, the inability to detect inhibitory activity, can be determined by the addition of hidden positive controls throughout the assay.

4.3.2 Phase II Drug Discovery/Development

The binding characteristics of the lead compound, once confirmed in Phase I, need to be determined in more detail. Two important characteristics, the potency and the selectivity of the binding, can be generated from dose–response studies (Figure 1). This information will serve as the reference point for monitoring lead compound improvements made through structural modification. As implied earlier, the ideal drug candidate would not only be of high affinity, but also selective in nature. Obviously, a compound which lacks binding selectivity may not be a good lead drug candidate. The selective nature of the candidate can be determined by profiling its activity against related and nonrelated receptor binding assays. It is often difficult for a drug discovery group, due to limited technical resources, to determine a broad receptor binding profile for a lead compound. To assist Phase II drug discovery efforts, NovaScreen®, a receptor binding service, has developed a profiling system to determine the activity of a drug candidate against 38 different receptor binding assays (Table 3).

Phase II and III drug discovery and development are time consuming and costly stages requiring significant receptor biochemistry and chemistry expertise and effort. It should be made clear that these stages normally function in tandem, with Phase III functional assays performed on the most potent and selective compound(s) identified.

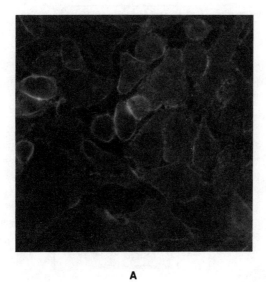

A

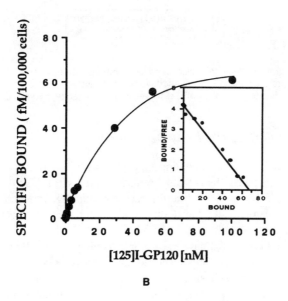

^{125}I-GP120 [nM]

B

Figure 5. Characterization of the cloned human CD4 receptor. The ability of the HIV-1 viral envelope glycoprotein, gp120, to interact with the CD4 receptor is one of the first steps in viral infectivity. A gp120/CD4 binding assay was developed with a cloned CD4 receptor for use as a drug discovery tool.[13] (A) The immunohistochemical identification of the human CD4 receptor on the surface of Chinese hamster ovary cells (CHO). (B) The characterization of the gp120/CD4 interaction using radioligand binding saturation/scatchard analysis to determine the affinity of the receptor ($K_d = 5$ nM) and the amount of receptor protein expressed (6.8 pM/100,000 cells).

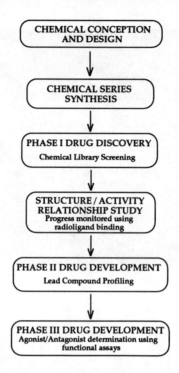

Figure 6.   Pharmaceutical drug discovery/development strategy. This schematic represents a simplified discovery/development strategy where receptor binding is
used as the primary tool to discover and characterize potential drug candidates.

4.3.3 Phase III Drug Discovery/Development

Drugs function by either activating a receptor (agonist activity) or blocking the
ability of that receptor to be activated (antagonist activity).[13] Using the lock and
key model typically used to describe receptor binding, one can see that the
probability of identifying a key (compound) which can fit into the lock (the
receptor) is more probable than identifying a key which can turn the lock. As
predicted from this model, Phase I receptor screening historically identifies compounds which function as antagonists and not agonists. However, binding assays
alone can not accurately determine the agonist or antagonist potential of a lead
compound. Phase III assays are designed to make agonist/antagonist determina-
tions. These *in vitro* assays measure the actions initiated through the occupancy
of a receptor by an appropriate agonist. In the past, these tests were designed
around isolated tissue preparations or whole animal models. As stated previously,
one of the advantages of using an intact cell culture preparation for binding studies
is the ability of the researcher to use the identical culture system in Phase III work.
A number of functional assays are now routinely studied in such systems, including biochemical, electrophysiological, and morphological assays (Figure 7). These

Table 3.   Receptor Selectivity *PROFILE®* for Imipramine

Receptor/Selectivity	Radioligand	Percent inhibition (Average; N = 2)		
		$10^{-9}M$	$10^{-7}M$	$10^{-5}M$
Adenosine				
Adenosine 1	[3H] CP	−3.7	7.6	9.6
Adenosine 2	[3H] CGS 21680	−0.9	6.9	1.1
Adrenergic				
Alpha 1	[3H] Prazosin	0.7	16.1	96.4
Alpha 2	[3H] RX 781094	−12.5	−2.5	68.8
Beta	[125I] Dihydroalprenolol	−10.1	4.4	9.4
Amino Acids				
Excitatory				
NMDA	[3H] CGS 19755	12.8	−5.1	3.9
Quisqualate	[3H] AMPA	−3.7	−7.9	−3.8
Kainate	[3H] Kainic Acid	−5.1	−6.8	−9.4
Glycine	[3H] Glycine	−1.0	−6.0	−12.5
PCP	[3H] TCP	−7.8	−8.4	31.7
Sigma	[3H] DTG	6.7	37.2	97.5
Inhibitory				
Benzodiazepine	[3H] Flunitrazepam	0.6	3.1	8.0
$GABA_A$	[3H] GABA	−1.9	4.6	3.5
$GABA_B$	[3H] GABA + Isoguvacine	−6.4	−5.0	−4.7
Glycine	[3H] Strychnine	−7.4	−9.0	6.0
Biogenic amines				
Dopamine 1	[3H] SCH 23390	−2.8	2.1	12.4
Dopamine 2	[3H] Sulpiride	−0.1	5.9	88.1
Histamine 1	[3H] Pyrilamine	7.3	66.0	109.8
Serotonin 1	[3H] 5–HT	9.1	11.7	25.9
Serotonin 2	[3H] Ketanserin	−0.6	22.0	96.2
Channel proteins				
Calcium, T&L	[3H] Nitrendipine	8.5	4.4	2.0
Calcium, N	[125I] Omega–Conotoxin	−3.2	5.0	4.6
Chloride	[3H] TBOB	−2.9	2.8	−2.3
Potassium, low cond.	[125I] Apamin	−1.8	0.7	3.3
Cholinergics				
Muscarinic 1	[3H] Pirenzepine	−2.7	49.5	101.1
Muscarinic 2	[3H] AF–DX 384	5.2	22.6	95.9
Nicotinic	[3H] NMCl	1.5	14.1	5.7
Opiate				
Mu [3H]DAGo	−0.9	−0.7	13.7	
Delta	[3H] DPDPE	−0.7	0.3	9.0
Kappa	[3H] U–69593	−8.1	−2.8	17.1
Prostanoids				
Leukotriene B_4	[3H] LTB_4	0.6	0.2	−5.1
Leukotriene D_4	[3H] LTD_4	1.5	−3.0	−0.4
Thromboxane A_2	[3H] SQ 29548	−4.1	0.8	0.6
Reuptake Sites				
Norepinephrine	[3H] Desmethylimipramine	−11.0	9.4	24.3
Serotonin	[3H] Citalopram	−1.9	81.5	95.4
Dopamine,cocaine site	[3H] WIN 35428	−6.4	26.5	62.0
Second Messenger Systems				
Adenylate cyclase				
Forskolin	[3H] Forskolin	2.7	4.7	8.1
Protein kinase C				
Phorbol ester	[3H] PDBU	−5.8	7.2	19.9

Note: Values are expressed as the percent inhibition of total specific binding and represent the average of duplicate tubes at each of the three concentrations tested.

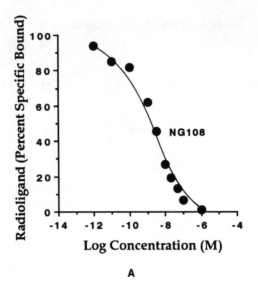

A

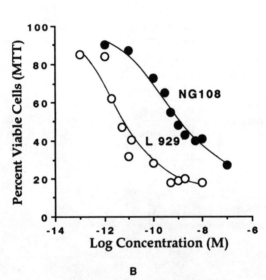

B

Figure 7.   Cytotoxicity assay. (A) Concentration–response curve generated for the binding of [^{125}I] tumor necrosis factor alpha (TNFα) to a viable neuroblastoma cell line (NG108). (B) The functional activity of TNFα has also been determined using the NG108 cell line.[30] Using NG108 cells it should be possible to identify compounds which inhibit TNFα binding and subsequently determine if those compounds are either agonists or antagonists. TNFα is a cytokine which has numerous actions which modulate the immune response.

assays can be as simple as determining if a cell shape is altered by drug administration, to determining the effect of a drug on the electric potential of that cell's membrane.

4.4 Conclusions

The objective of pharmaceutical drug discovery is: "The identification of new potential therapeutic agents in a rapid, reliable, and efficient manner." To this end, the simplicity of the radioligand binding assay makes it an outstanding resource to identify and monitor subsequent stages of a drug's development. The integration of radioligand binding and cell culture is serving to expand and simplify many of the approaches used by the pharmaceutical industry over the past century. Cultured cells can provide an *in vitro* system which can be used in all three phases of drug discovery, thereby significantly reducing the need to use more complicated isolated tissue or whole animal models. In addition, standardizing the *in vitro* system used by the biochemical and functional research units involved in the discovery effort aids in the interpretation of data between the various groups. As a result, development of radioligand cell culture models could have a significant impact on the many ethical and scientific issues facing the pharmaceutical industry in the next decade.

REFERENCES

1. Parascandola, J. "Origins of the Receptor Theory," in *Towards Understanding Receptors*, J. W. Lamble, Ed. (Amsterdam: Elsevier North-Holland, 1981), pp. 1–7.
2. Clark, A. J. *The Mode of Action of Drugs on Cells* (London: Edward Arnold, 1933).
3. Burt, D. R. "Criteria for Receptor Identification," in *Neurotransmitter Receptor Binding*, H. I. Yamamura, S. J. Enna, and M. J. Kuhar, Eds. (New York: Raven Press, 1978), pp. 41–55.
4. Bennett, J. P. "Methods in Binding Studies," *Neurotransmitter Receptor Binding*, H. I. Yamaura, S. J. Enna, and M. J. Kuhar, Eds. (New York: Raven Press, 1978).
5. Ferkany, J. W. "Radio-Receptor Assays for Amino Acids and Related Compounds," in *Neuromethods*, Vol. 3, A. Bolton, G. Baker, and J. Wood, Eds. (Clifton, NJ: Humana Press, 1985), pp. 117–153.
6. *Receptor Binding Techniques*, 1980 Short Course Syllabus (Bethesda, MD: Society for Neuroscience, 1980).
7. Kinnier, W. J. "Receptor Binding as a Method for Drug Discovery," in *Methods in Neurotransmitter Receptor Analysis*, H. I. Yamamura, S. J. Enna, and M. J. Kuhar, Eds. (New York: Raven Press, 1990), pp. 245–258.
8. Harrison, R. G. "Observations on the Living Developing Nerve Fiber," *Proc. Soc. Exp. Biol. Med.* 4(1):140–143 (1907).
9. Shahar, A., J. de Vellis, A. Vernadakis, and B. Haber, Eds. *A Dissection and Culture Manual of the Nervous System* (New York: Alan R. Liss, 1989).

10. Jakoby, W. B. and I. H. Pastan, Eds. *Methods in Enzymology*, Vol. 58, *Cell Culture* (New York: Academic Press, 1979).

11. Ronnett, G. V., L. D. Hester, J. S. Nye, K. Connors, and S. H. Snyder. "Human Cortical Neuronal Cell Line: Establishment from a Patient with Unilateral Megalencephaly," *Science* 248(4955):603–605 (1990).

12. Hartley, J. W. and W. P. Rowe. "Production of Altered Cell FOCI in Tissue Culture by Defective Moloney Sarcoma Virus Particles," *Proc. Natl. Acad. Sci. U.S.A.* 55(4):780–786 (1966).

13. To, L. P., V. Balasubramanian, M. E. Charlton, T. A. Francis, C. Doyle, and P. M. Sweetnam. "Development and Characterization of a Whole-Cell Radioligand Binding Assay for [^{125}I]gp120 of HIV-1," *J. Immunoassay* 13(1):61–83 (1992).

14. Neuser, D. and P. Bellemann. "Receptor Binding, cGMP Stimulation and Receptor Desensitization by Atrial Natriuretic Peptides in Cultured A_{10} Vascular Smooth Muscle Cells," *FEBS Lett.* 209(2):347–351 (1986).

15. Cain, M. J., R. K. Garlick, and P. M. Sweetnam. "Endothelin-1 Receptor Binding Assay for High Throughput Chemical Screening," *J. Cardiovasc. Pharmacol.* 17(Suppl. 7):S150–S151 (1991).

16. Syapin, P. J. and P. Skolnick. "Characterization of Benzodiazepine Binding Sites in Cultured Cells of Neural Origin," *J. Neurochem.* 32(3):1047–1051 (1979).

17. Fishman, P. H. and J. P. Finberg. "Effect of the Tricyclic Antidepressant Desipramine on β-Adrenergic Receptors in Cultured Rat Gliomoa C_6 Cells," *J. Neurochem.* 49(1):282–289 (1987).

18. Huang, J. S., S. S. Huang, B. Kennedy, and T. F. Deuel. "Platelet Derived Growth Factor -Specific Binding to Target Cells," *J. Biol. Chem.* 257(14):8130–8136 (1982).

19. Sawutz, D. B., K. Kalinyak, J. A. Whitsett, and C. L. Johnson. "Histamine H_2 Receptor Desensitization in HL-60 Human Promyelocytic Leukemia Cells," *J. Pharmacol. Exp. Ther.* 231(1):1–7 (1984).

20. Tsujimoto, M., Y. K. Yip, and J. Vilcek. "Tumor Necrosis Factor: Specific Binding and Internalization in Sensitive and Resistant Cells," *Proc. Natl. Acad. Sci. U.S.A.* 82(22):7626–7630 (1985).

21. Landreth, G. E. and E. M. Shooter. "Nerve Growth Factor Receptors on PC_{12} Cells: Ligand-Induced Conversion from Low- to High-Affinity States," *Proc. Natl. Acad. Sci. U.S.A.* 77(8):4751–4755 (1980).

22. Powell, J. A., R. A. Zeppetello, M. A. Connolly, P. M. Sweetnam, and W. J. Kinnier. "The Identification and the Pharmacological Characterization of the P_{2Y} Receptor on PC-12 Cell Line", *IBRO* Abstract (1991).

23. Snider, R. M. and E. Richelson. "Bradykinin Receptor-Mediated Cyclic GMP Formation in a Nerve Cell Population (Murine Neuroblastoma Clone N1E-115)," *J. Neurochem.* 43(6): 1749–1754 (1984).

24. Burgermeister, W., W. L. Klein, M. Nirenberg, and B. Witkop. "Comparative Binding Studies with Cholinergic Ligands and Histronicotoxin at Muscarinic Receptors of Neural Cell Lines," *Mol. Pharmacol.* 14(5):751–767 (1978).

25. Gilbert, J. A., C. J. Moses, M. A. Pfenning, and E. Richelson. "Neurotensin and its Analogs-Correlation of Specific Binding with Stimulation of Cyclic GMP Formation in Neuroblastoma clone N1E-115," *Biochem. Pharmacol.* 35(3):391–397 (1986).

26. Lummis, S. C. R., G. J. Kilpatrick, and I. L. Martin. "Characterization of $5HT_3$ Receptors in Intact N1E-115 Neuroblastoma Cells," *Eur. J. Pharmacol. Mol. Pharmacol. Sect.* 189(2/3):223–227 (1990).

27. Fisher, S. K. and A. M. Heacock. "A Putative M_3 Muscarinic Cholinergic Receptor of High Molecular Weight Couples to Phosphoinositide Hydrolysis in Human SK-N-SH Neuroblastoma Cells," *J. Neurochem.* 50(3):984–987 (1988).

28. Gordon, E. A., T. A. Kalhout, and P. H. Fishman. "Characterization of Functional Neuropeptide Y Receptors in a Human Neuroblastoma Cell Line," *J. Neurochem.* 55(2):506–513 (1990).

29. Sweetnam, P. M., H. R. Sanon, L. A. White, B. J. Brass, M. Jaye, and S. R. Whittemore. "Differential Effects of Acidic and Basic Fibroblast Growth Factors on Spinal Cord Cholinergic, GABAergic, and Glutamatergic Neurons," *J. Neurochem.* 57(1):237–249 (1991).

30. Blake, D., I. Baker, M. Connolly, J. Ferkany, and P. Sweetnam. "TNF-α Induced Cytotoxicity in NCB20 and NG-108 Neuroblastomas," *Soc. Neurosci.* Abstract 15:437 (1989).

31. Charlton, M., M. Connolly, J. Lancaster, A. Snowman, L. Williams, and P. Sweetnam. "Biochemical, Immunological, and Molecular Characterization of HCN-1A Cells," *Soc. Neurosci.* Abstract 18:31 (1992).

CHAPTER 5

Structure–Activity Approaches as an Alternative to Animal Testing for Predicting Toxicity in Man

Shayne C. Gad

5.0 Introduction

There are currently believed to be approximately 70,000 synthetic chemicals in common use. Some 5,000 additional structures are added to this total each year. Clearly not all of these can (or should) be evaluated for adverse health and environmental effects by traditional animal testing; structure–activity relationship (SAR) methods are an approach for reducing animal usage in testing by identifying those compounds which may require it.

SAR methods have become a legitimate and useful part of toxicology over the last 15 years or so. These methods are various forms of mathematical or statistical models which seek to predict the adverse biological effects of chemicals based on their structure. It should be noted that, as discussed below, SAR approaches have a long and successful history of use in pharmacology and medicinal chemistry. In these cases, however, the mechanisms of biological activity tend to be considerably better defined and simple (such as activity at a single biochemical receptor) than in toxicology. The use of SAR in pharmacology and drug design has significantly reduced the number of animals used in screening for new therapeutics. The prediction may be of either a qualitative (mutagen/nonmutagen) or quantitative (median lethal dose) nature, with the second group usually being denoted as QSAR (quantitative structure–activity relationship) models. The basic mathematical techniques utilized to construct such models are mathematical modeling and reduction of dimensionality methods, as discussed elsewhere by this author.[1]

The concept that the biological activity of a compound is a direct function of its chemical structure is now at least a century old.[2] During most of this century, the development and use of SARs were the domain of pharmacology and medicinal chemistry. These two fields are responsible for the beginnings of all the basic approaches in SAR work, usually with the effort being called drug design. An introductory medicinal chemistry text[3] is strongly recommended as a starting place for SAR. Additionally, *Burger's Medicinal Chemistry*,[4] with its excellent overview of drug structures and activities, should enhance at least the initial stages of identifying the potential biological actions of *de novo* compounds using a pattern recognition approach.

Having already classified SAR methods (based on their predictive objectives) into qualitative and quantitative, it should also be pointed out that both of these can be approached on two different levels. The first is on a local level, where prediction of activity (or lack of activity) is limited to other members of a congeneric series of structural near neighbors. The accuracy of predictions via this approach is generally greater, but is of value only if one has sufficient information on some of the structures within a series of interest.

The second approach is prediction of activity over a wide range, generally based on the presence or absence of particular structural features (functional groups). Particularly in this form of use, SAR approaches are utilized as initial screens to identify those compounds that some form of secondary screen (testing with an *in vitro* model) or confirmatory test (whole animal test) must be carried out.[5]

This means that for toxicology, SARs have a small but significant and growing number of uses at present. These can all be generalized as identifying potentially toxic effects, or restated as three main functions:

1. For the selection and design of toxicity tests to address end points of possible concern.
2. If a comprehensive or large testing program is to be conducted, SAR predictions can be used to prioritize the tests, so that outlined questions (the answers to which might preclude the need to do further testing) may be addressed first.
3. As an alternative to testing at all. Though in general it is not believed that the state-of-the-art for SAR methods allows such usage, in certain special cases (such as selecting which of several alternative candidate compounds to develop further and then test) this use may be valid and valuable.

5.1 Basic Assumptions

Starting with the initial assumption that there is a relationship between structure and biological activity, we can proceed to more readily testable assumptions.

First, the dose of chemical is subject to a number of modifying factors (such as membrane selectivities and selective metabolic actions) which are each related in some manner to chemical structure. Indeed, absorption, metabolism, pharmacologic activity, and excretion are each subject to not just structurally determined actions, but also to (in many cases) stereospecific differential handlings.

Given these assumptions, actual elucidation of SARs requires the following:

1. Knowledge of the biological activities of existing structures
2. Knowledge of structural features which serve to predict activity (also called molecular parameters of interest)
3. One or more models which relate item 2 to item 1 with some degree or reliability

There are now extensive sources of information as to both toxic properties of chemicals and, indeed, biological activities. These includes books, journals, manuals, and computerized data bases. The reader is directed to Wexler's book[6] as a guide to accessing the different sources of toxicology information, but is cautioned to remember that there is also extensive applicable information in the realms of medicinal chemistry and pharmacology, as exemplified by Burger's.[4]

5.2 Molecular Parameters of Interest

Which structural and physicochemical properties of a chemical are important in predicting its toxicologic activity are both open to considerable debate.[7-9] Table 1 presents a partial list of such parameters. The reader is referred to a biologically oriented physical chemistry text (such as Reference 10) both for explanations of these parameters and for references to sources from which specific values may be obtained.

There are now several systems available to study the three dimensional structural aspects of molecules and their interactions. The first are the various molecular modeling sets, which can actually be very useful for some simpler problems. The second are the molecular design and analysis packages which are available for main frame computers. Last, molecular graphics software packages have become available recently for such microcomputers as the Apple IIe, Macintosh, and IBM. Use of such forms of graphics structural examination as tool or method in SAR analysis has been discussed.[11-13] Such methods are generally called topological methods.

5.3 SAR Modeling Methods

A detailed review of even the major methodologies available for SAR/QSAR modeling in toxicology is beyond the scope of this chapter or book. Though we will briefly discuss the major approaches, the reader is directed to one of the several very readable introductory articles[14-17] for somewhat detailed presentations.

Table 1.   Molecular Parameters of Interest

Electronic effects
    Ionization constants
        Sigma substituent constant
    Distribution constant
    Resonance effect
    Field effect
    Molecular orbital indices[a]
        Atomic/electron net charge
        Nucleophilic superdelocalizability
        Electrophilic superdelocalizability
        Free radical superdelocalizability
        Energy of the lowest empty molecular orbital
        Energy of the highest occupied molecular orbital
        Frontier self-atom polarizability
        Frontier atom-atom polarizability
        Intermolecular coulombic interaction energy
        Electric field created at point [A] by a set of charges
          on a molecule

Hyprophobic parameters
    Partition coefficients
    P_i substituent constants
    R_M value in liquid-liquid chromatography
    Elution time in high-pressure liquid chromatography [HPLC]
    Solubility
    Solvent partition coefficients
    pKa

Steric effects
    Intramolecular steric effects
        Steric substituent constant
        Hyperconjugation correction
    Molar volume
    Molar refractivity, MR substituent constants
    Molecular weight
    Van der Waals radii
    Interatomic distances

Substructural effects
    Three dimensional geometry
    Fragment and molecular properties (see Chu 1980 for
      substituent effects)
    Chain lengths

[a]   Calculated or theoretical parameters

To begin with, it should be made clear that all the actual techniques involved in the performance or SAR analysis have already been presented in the text. It is only their actual application to data which sets such analysis apart from the forms of modeling at which we have previously looked.

All the current major SAR methods used in toxicology (see Purchase et al.[18] for an overview) can be classified based on what kinds of compound-related or structural data they use and what method is used to correlate this structural data with the existing biological data.

The more classical approaches use physicochemical data (such as molecular weight, free energies, etc.) as a starting point. The major approaches to this are by manual pattern recognition methods, cluster analysis, or by regression analysis. It is this last, in the form of Hansch or linear–free energy relationship (LFER) which actually launched all SAR work (other than that on limited congeneric cases) into the realm of being a useful approach. Indeed, still foremost among the QSAR methods is the model proposed by Hansch and his co-workers.[19] It was the major contribution of this group to propose the incorporation of earlier observations of the importance of the relative lipophilicity, to biologic activity into the formal LFER approach to provide a general QSAR model for biological effects. As a suitable measure of lipophilicity, the partition coefficient (log P) between 1-octanol and water was proposed, and it was demonstrated that this was an approximately additive and constitutive property and that it was therefore calculable, in principle, from molecular structure. Using a probabilistic model for the Hansch equation, which can be expressed as:

$$\log(1/C) = k\pi^2 = k'\pi + \rho\sigma + k''$$

$$\log(1/C) = -k(\log p)^2 + k'(\log p) + \rho\sigma + k''$$

where
$$C = \text{the dose that elicits a constant biological response (e.g., } ED_{50}, LD_{50})$$
$$\pi = \text{the substituent lipophilicity}$$
$$\log p = \text{the partition coefficient}$$
$$\sigma = \text{the substituent electronic effect of Hammet}$$
$$k, k', \rho, \text{ and } k'' = \text{the regression coefficients derived from the statistical curve fitting}$$

The reciprocal of the concentration reflects the fact that higher potency is associated with lower dose, and the negative sign for the π^2 or $(\log p)^2$ term reflects the expectation of an optimum lipophilicity, designated π_0 or log p_0.

The statistical method used to determine the coefficients above is multiple linear regression. A number of statistics are derived in conjunction with such a calculation, which allow the statistical significance of the resulting correlation to be assessed. The most important of these are s, the standard deviation, r^2, the coefficient of determination or percentage of data variance accounted for by the model (r, the correlation coefficient is also commonly cited), and F, a statistic for assessing the overall significance of the derived equation, values, and confidence intervals (usually 95%) for the individual regression coefficients in the equation. Also very important in multiparameter equations are the cross-correlation coefficients between the independent variables in the equation. These must be low to assure true "independence" or orthogonality of the variables, a necessary condition for meaningful results.

In a like manner, there are a number of approaches for using structural and substructural data and correlating these to biological activities. Such approaches are generally classified as regression analysis methods, pattern recognition methods, and miscellaneous others (such as factor analysis, principal components, and probalistic analysis).

The regression analysis methods which use structural data have been, as we will see when we survey the state of the art in toxicology, the most productive and useful. "Keys"—or fragments or structure—are assigned weights as predictors of an activity, usually in some form of the Free-Wilson model,[20] which was developed at virtually the same time as the Hansch. According to this method, the molecules of a chemical series are structurally decomposed into a common moiety (or core) that may be substituted in multiple positions. A series of linear equations of the form are constructed

$$BA_i = \sum_j a_j x_{ij} + \mu$$

where BA = the biological activity
x_j = the jth substituent with a value of a 1 if present and 0 if not
a_j = the contribution of the jth substituent to BA
μ = the overall average activity

All activity contributions at each position of substitution must sum to zero. The series of linear equations thus generated is solved by the method of least squares for the aj and μ. There must be several more equations than unknowns and each substituent should appear more than once at a position in different combinations with substituents at other positions. The favorable aspects of this model are

1. Any set of quantitative biological data may be employed as the dependent variable.
2. No independently determined substituent constants are required.
3. The molecules comprising a sample of interest may be structurally dismembered in any desired or convenient manner.
4. Multiple sites of variable substitution are readily handled by the model.

There are also several limitations: a substantial number of compounds with varying substituent combinations is required for a meaningful analysis; the derived substituent contributions give no reasonable basis for extrapolating predictions from the substituent matrix analyzed; and the model will break down if nonlinear dependence on substituent properties is important or if there are interactions between the substituents.

Pattern recognition methods comprise yet another approach to examining structural features and/or chemical properties for underlying patterns that are associated with differing biological effects. Accurate classification of untested molecules is again the primary goal. This is carried out in two stages. First, a set of compounds, designated the training set, is chosen for which the correct classification is known.

A set of molecular property descriptors (features) is generated for each compound. A suitable classification algorithm is then applied to find some combination and weight of the descriptors that allow perfect classification. Many different statistical and geometric techniques for this purpose have been used and were presented in earlier chapters. The derived classification function is then applied in the second step to compounds not included in the training set to test predictability. In published work these have generally been other compounds of known classification also. Performance is judged by the percentage of correct predictions. Stability of the classification function is usually tested by repeating the procedure several times with slightly altered, but randomly varied, sets or samples.

The main difficulty with these methods is in "decoding" the QSAR in order to identify particular structural fragments responsible for the expression of a particular activity. And even if identified as "responsible" for activity, far harder questions for the model to answer are whether the structural fragment so identified is "sufficient" for activity, whether it is always "necessary" for activity, and to what extent its expression is modified by its molecular environment. Most pattern recognition methods use as weighting factors either the presence or absence of a particular fragment or feature (coded 1 or 0), or the frequency of occurrence of a feature. They may be made more sophisticated by coding the spatial relationship between features.

Enslein[21] has published a good concise description of the problems involved in applying these methods in toxicology.

5.4 Applications in Toxicology

SAR methods have been developed to predict a number of toxicological end points (mutagenesis, carcinogenesis, dermal sensitization, lethality [LD_{50} values], biological oxygen demands, and teratogenicity) with varying degrees of accuracy, and models for the prediction of other end points are under development. Some of these existing models are presented by category of use in Table 2. Additionally, both the Environmental Protection Agency and the Food & Drug Administration (FDA) have models for mutagenicity/carcinogenicity that they utilize to "flag" possible problem compounds. FDA is currently accepting some SAR "data" for use in characterizing the potential environmental risks of new drugs and pharmaceutical process intermediates.

It should be expected that qualitative models are more "accurate" than quantitative ones, and that the more possible mechanisms associated with an endpoint, the less accurate (or more difficult) a prediction. Personal experience in the use of such models has certainly shown this to be the case. However, if a commercial organization modifies one of the existing models by adding data about proprietary structures in their realm of interest, accuracy (predictive value) can be significantly improved.

Table 2.   Existing SAR Models for Toxicology End Points

Endpoint	Prediction		Ref.
	Quantitative	Qualitative	
Mutagenicity	X		22
		X	23
	X		24
Carcinogenicity	X		25
	X		22
		X	23
	X		26
Sensitization	X		27
LD_{50}		X	24
Teratogenicity	X		24
Biological oxygen demand		X	28
Ocular irritation	X		28

REFERENCES

1. Gad, S. C. and C. S. Weil. *Structure and Experimental Design for the Toxicologist* (Caldwell, NJ: Telford Press, 1988).
2. Crum-Brown, A. and T. Fraser. "The Relationship of Chemical Structure and Biological Activity," *Trans. Roy. Soc. Edinburgh* 25:693 (1869).
3. Foye, W. O. *Principles of Medicinal Chemistry* (Philadelphia: Lea & Febiger, 1974).
4. Wolff, M. E. *Burger's Medicinal Chemistry* (New York: John Wiley, 1980).
5. Gad, S. C. "A Tier Testing Strategy Incorporating *In Vitro* Testing Methods for Pharmaceutical Safety Assessment," *Hum. Innovations Alternatives Anim. Exp.* 3:75–79 (1989).
6. Wexler, P. *Information Resources in Toxicology* (New York: Elsevier/North Holland, 1982).
7. Kaufman, J. J., V. Lewchenko, P. C. Hariharan, and W. S. Kuski. "Theoretical Predictions of Toxicity," in *Product Safety Evaluation*, A. M. Goldberg, Ed. (New York: Mary Ann Liebert, 1983) pp. 333–355.
8. Tamura, R. M. "A Model for Toxicologic Prediction," in *Product Safety Evaluation*, A. M. Goldberg, Ed. (New York: Mary Ann Liebert, 1983) pp. 317–330.
9. Tute, M. S. "Mathematical Modeling," in *Animals and Alternatives to Toxicity Testing*, M. Balls, R. J. Riddel, and A. N. Worden, Eds. (New York: Academic Press, 1983) pp. 137–166.
10. Chang, R. *Physical Chemistry with Application to Biological Systems* (New York: MacMillan, 1981).
11. Cohen, J. L., W. Lee, and E. J. Lien. "Dependence of Toxicity on Molecular Structures: Group Theory Analysis," *J. Pharm. Sci* 63(7):1068–1072 (1974).
12. Gund, P., J. D. Andosf, J. B. Rhodes, and G. M. Smith. "Three-Dimensional Molecular Modeling and Drug Design," *Science* 208(4451):1425–1431 (1980).
13. Hansch, C., D. Kim, A. J. Leo, E. Novellino, C. Silipo, and A. Victtoria. "Toward a Quantitative Comparative Toxicology of Organic Compounds," *CRC Crit. Rev. Toxicol.* 19(3):185–226 (1989).

14. Chu, K. C. "The Quantitative Analysis of Structure-Activity Relationships," in *Burger's Medicinal Chemistry*, Vol. 1, M. E. Wolff, Ed. (New York: John Wiley, 1980) pp. 393–418.

15. Olson, E. C. and R. E. Cristoffersen. *Computer Assisted Drug Design* (Washington:ACS 1979).

16. Topliss, J. G. *Quantitative Structure-Activity Relationships of Drugs* (New York: Academic Press, 1983).

17. Goldberg, L. *Structure-Activity Correlations as a Predictive Tool in Toxicology* (New York: Hemisphere, 1983).

18. Purchase, R., J. Phillips, and B. Lake. "Structure-Activity Techniques in Toxicology," *Food Chem. Toxic.* 28(6):459–462 (1990).

19. Hansch, C. in *Drug Design*, Vol .1, E. J. Ariens, Ed. (New York: Academic Press 1971) chap. 2.

20. Free, S. M. and J. W. Wilson. "A Mathematical Contribution to Structure-Activity Studies," *J. Med. Chem.* 7(4):395–399 (1964).

21. Enslein, K., M. E. Tomb, and T. R. Laner. "Structure-Activity Models of Biological Oxygen Demand," in *QSAR in Environmental Toxicology*, K. L. E. Kaiser, Ed. (Dordrecht: Reidel, 1984).

22. Asher, I. M. and C. Zervos. "Structural Correlates of Carcinogenesis and Mutagenesis," Office of Science, FDA, Washington, (1977).

23. Niculescu-Duvaz, I., T. Craescu, M. Tugulea, A. Croisy, and P. C. Jacquignon. "A Quantitative Structure-Activity Analysis of the Mutagenic and Carcinogenic Action of 43 Structurally Related Heterocyclic Compounds," *Carcinogenesis* 2(4):269–275 (1981).

24. Enslein, K., T. R. Lander, M. E. Tomb, and W. G. Landis. "Mutagenicity (Ames): A Structure-Activity Model," *J. Teratogenesis, Carcinogenesis Mutagenesis* 3(6):503–514 (1983).

25. Franke, R. "Structure-Activity Relationships in Polycyclic Aromatic Hydrocarbons: Induction of Microsomal Aryl Hydrocarbon Hydroxylase and Its Possible Importance in Chemical Carcinogenesis," *Chem.-Biol. Inter.* 6(1):1–17 (1973).

26. Enslein, K. and P. N. Craig. "Carcinogenesis: A Predictive Structure Activity Model," *J. Toxicol. Envir. Hlth.* 10(4–5):521–530 (1982).

27. Dupuis, G. and C. Benezra. *Allergic Contact Dermatitis to Simple Chemicals: A Molecular Approach* (New York: Marcel Dekker, 1982).

28. Enslein, K. "Estimation of Toxicological Endpoints by Structure-Activity Relationships," *Pharmacol. Rev.* 36(2):131–134 (1984).

CHAPTER 6

Biological Studies in Psychiatry: Neurochemical Measurements with Human Subjects

A. J. Greenshaw

6.0 Introduction

Chemotherapy in psychiatry has been formally established since the middle of this century. Initial progress, although relying heavily on traditional pharmacological laboratory methods, was also the result of fortuitous and careful clinical observation. The extent to which the analysis of drug action in humans can be assessed neurochemically is discussed in relation to recent advances in neuropharmacology and the use of indirect measures of brain activity such as receptor changes on blood cells, alterations in hormone concentrations or drug-induced physiological responses. The advent of positron emission tomography as a window on brain receptors is also discussed. The possibilities for using these approaches to improve our understanding of and treatments for mood disorders and schizophrenia are considered. The limitations of these approaches are contrasted with the limitations of experiments with nonhuman species and possibilities for future human research are briefly discussed.

0-87371-504-7/93/$0.00+$.50
© 1993 by Lewis Publishers

6.1 The Advent of Chemotherapy in Psychiatry

The middle of this century yielded great advances in the treatment of mental disorders, principally through the discovery of effective drug treatments for schizophrenia and depression. In the 1940s Charpentier[1] synthesized phenothiazines in an attempt to discover new antihistamine drugs. Chlorpromazine was identified as a sedative compound and, based on the clinical observations of Laborit,[2] was identified as a major tranquilizer in human patients. These properties of chlorpromazine were successfully applied to the treatment of agitated psychiatric patients and led to the establishment of a class of compounds which are now widely used in the treatment of psychiatric disorders, particularly schizophrenia.

In the same period drugs were developed that had clear efficacy in the treatment of tuberculosis. One such compound iproniazid, a monoalkyl derivative of isoniazid, was observed to induce euphoria and psychostimulant effects in patients. This serendipitous observation led to the use of iproniazid in an attempt to improve the mood of depressed patients with a variety of medical diseases.[3] By the late 1950s iproniazid was established as an effective antidepressant drug. In addition to iproniazid, the effects of imipramine (originally developed as a potential antihistamine), were reassessed following the discovery of chlorpromazine as an antipsychotic. This drug, although structurally very similar to chlorpromazine, was ineffective as an antipsychotic. Nevertheless, Kuhn[4] observed the beneficial effects of imipramine in the treatment of mental depression. The discovery of these three drugs gave rise to the widespread and effective development of chemotherapy in psychiatry.

In assessing the rise of drug treatment in psychiatry it is important to recognize that these developments were the result of basic and clinical research involving both the testing of new compounds in classical pharmacological tests with laboratory animals and careful clinical observation leading to serendipitous conclusions with human patients. The careful evaluation of controlled clinical trials followed on from this initial work.[3]

6.2 Approaches to Neurochemical Measurements in Human Subjects

At the present time both basic and clinical research into the causes and effective treatment of psychiatric disorders have generated a very complex body of information concerning brain chemistry. Fundamental to this area of investigation is the underlying assumption that changes in processes of communication between nerve cells (neurons) in the brain form the basis of psychiatric disorders. Inherent to this assumption is an understanding of the basic process by which each neuron secretes a chemical messenger (neurotransmitter) across the intervening space (synaptic cleft) to the next neuron. This neurotransmitter then interacts with a specialized protein (receptor) on the surface (membrane) of the neuron which results in transduction of this chemical event, through a series of biophysical events, to a change in the activity of that neighboring neuron. Alterations of neuronal communication may obviously be manifest at several levels, e.g., changes in the availability of the neurotransmitter through altered processes of formation (synthesis) or breakdown (catabolism); altered receptor protein structure or altered number of receptors; and changes in the transduction of receptor activity to alterations in neural excitation. The interested reader is referred to the text by Cooper, Bloom, and Roth[5] for further information concerning these topics. Research with laboratory animals has played an important role in increasing our understanding of the bases of psychiatric disorders and improving treatment strategies. To a large extent such studies have relied on the development of "models" of illness and of drug action in tests with tissues from laboratory animals or behavioral tests with whole laboratory animals.[6] This dependence on nonhuman species as test subjects is primarily due to the difficulties of assessing changes in brain chemistry in human patients and to problems associated with collecting and interpreting information from postmortem human brain samples. The development of laboratory animal "models" and an analysis of their suitability in this context is beyond the scope of this discourse (the reader is referred to References 6 and 7). A question which is less frequently raised concerns the extent to which humans may be used in this endeavor and addresses the types and limitations of approaches to analysis of brain chemistry in live patients.

The literature concerning neurochemical changes in psychiatric disorders is vast. It is the purpose of this chapter to provide an overview of approaches to the assessment of some biological changes in psychiatric disorders in humans. It is, therefore, not possible to describe the state of the art, but merely to indicate some illustrative aspects—hopefully to reveal future possibilities. It is important to understand at the outset that this is not yet an area full of "hard facts" relating biochemical dysfunction clearly to disease. Nevertheless, with the advent of the 90s as the "decade of the brain", it is apparent that substantial progress is being made even if we are faced with a particularly difficult nut to crack! For an overview of biological theories of psychiatric disorder, the reader is referred to Baker and Dewhurst[8] and Seeman,[9] for useful summaries. Far more detailed accounts are available in an extensive text edited by Meltzer.[10]

There are principally three approaches to the assessment of neuronal function in studies of psychiatric disorders and mechanisms of psychotherapeutic drug action.

1. Measurement of the relationship between psychiatric symptoms and circulating levels of substances relating to brain chemistry in peripheral body fluids (i.e., blood and urine) or in cerebrospinal fluid (CSF); attempt to correlate levels of such substances with symptom changes, and relate these changes to drug treatment or other forms of effective therapy.

2. Measurement of receptors for brain chemicals involved in neural processing either in brain (by means of some noninvasive imaging technique, e.g., Positron Emission Tomography) or homologues of these receptors which may be present on cells in the peripheral circulation (e.g., receptors for the neurotransmitter norepinephrine which are present on blood platelets such as α_2-adrenoceptors). Here again, attempts are made to correlate changes in the properties or abundance of these receptors with the occurrence of psychiatric symptoms and to assess the effects of therapeutic intervention with drugs or other treatments.

3. The use of single test administrations of drugs which are used to probe receptor-mediated responses. In this case a drug will be administered to a patient and its effect will be measured in terms of altered levels of circulating hormones or changes in a physiological response such as heart rate, blood pressure, or body temperature.

6.3 The Measurement of Neuroactive Compounds in Human Body Fluids

With respect to the measurement of circulating substances related to brain chemistry, in peripheral body fluids, most work has focused on the biogenic amines (principally dopamine, noradrenaline, 5-hydroxytryptamine [5-HT]; and to a lesser extent noncatecholic phenyl alkyl amines such as 2-phenylethylamine and tryptamine) and their metabolites. This research area has generated a vast database with hundreds of studies reported in recent decades. As has recently been pointed out,[11] it was originally hoped that clear patterns of biochemical disturbances would emerge from these studies which could serve as reliable "state" or "trait" markers. Nevertheless, over the past 40 to 50 years few such markers have emerged as unambiguous indicators of disease states in psychiatry.

Numerous factors have contributed to the problems encountered in interpreting the results of these studies.[11] Foremost, and a particular problem for psychiatry, has perhaps been the issue of the heterogeneity of psychiatric disorders.[12] It is a fact that progress in understanding the biological basis of psychopathology is inextricably tied to the clear diagnostic evaluation of mental abnormality. This is a striking point when considering our attempts to develop new and more effective drug treatments—whether basic (i.e., laboratory animal studies) or clinical (i.e., human studies) research is evaluated. With "classical medical illness" typically there is a clearly defined physiological system which may be finely dissected and analyzed in purely mechanistic terms (consider cardiology). In the case of psychiatric and certain neurological disorders this is simply not the case. The same marvelous variety of experience that the human brain affords us also, not surprisingly, renders the task of assessing mental dysfunction an extremely subtle and complex affair. This consideration alone suggests that research in biological psychiatry is currently an heuristic process. Effective psychiatric treatments have emerged and are continually being improved upon; this is reassuring evidence that significant progress is being made. At our present stage of understanding, however, we still cannot clearly predict the clinical efficacy of psychotherapeutic drugs from basic research studies.

Apart from this issue of diagnostic heterogeneity and the ongoing attempts to refine the classification of psychiatric disorders, there are numerous other factors that have obfuscated the interpretation of human biochemical measurements. These factors, which are more directly amenable to our scientific methods, are represented by: biochemical individuality, environmental influences, and analytical limitations. Individual differences in sex, age, weight, height, ethnic origin, and circadian rhythms all have influences on the measure of the metabolism of chemicals related to brain function. Additional environmental concerns include diet, history of drug use (including cigarette smoking and alcohol ingestion), physical and mental stress, and even body posture at the time of sampling. Finally, the quality of analytical techniques is highly significant especially when comparing earlier studies to the findings of recent research (this is particularly true for compounds such as the trace amines which exist at very low concentrations and require high resolution chemistry[13] although it is clearly important to have highly accurate and reliable quantitation of all compounds both within and between studies). This issue of accuracy is particularly critical for human studies in which interindividual variability of sample values is typically high, although it is also an important concern for basic research. It will be evident to the reader that these sources of interpretative difficulty (for they may not simply be regarded as sources of error in measurement) apply to all of the approaches adopted to assess neuronal function in studies of psychiatric disorders and mechanisms of psychotherapeutic drug action.

6.4 Measurements of Receptor-Related Mechanisms—a Possible Key to Understanding Actions of Psychotherapeutic Drugs

The most useful studies have been those in which biochemical concentrations have been monitored in an attempt to predict drug responses or in which such concentrations have responded to drug treatment in a manner which parallels the clinical response. It is, in fact, this kind of study which has also been most successful in furnishing useful data with the other approaches alluded to earlier — i.e., measurement of receptors for neurotransmitters in the brain (e.g., by positron emission tomography [PET]) or on cells in the peripheral circulation (e.g., α_2-adrenoceptors on platelets); or pharmacological assessment of receptor mediated responses (e.g., measurement of differences in clonidine-induced changes in blood pressure and heart rate which may reflect α_2-adrenoceptor responses).

The current focus of interest in investigating the biological bases of psychopathology is the neurotransmitter receptor. The reason for this is to be found in the time/course of clinical responses to drug treatment. Psychiatric symptoms such as depressed mood, suicidal ideation, and thought disorder typically fade into remission only after prolonged exposure to drug therapy for what may be a period of several weeks.[14] This delay in clinical improvement is somewhat enigmatic as the primary biochemical effects of these drugs emerge within minutes or, at most, within hours of administration.[15] One key factor that may tie drug action to clinical improvement is that of plasticity at the level of the receptor. A classical response of a receptor population to drug stimulation is a gradual decrease in the number of receptors. Conversely, blockade of stimulation will classically result in increases in the number of receptors for a given target population.[16] It has been claimed that such adaptive responses may underlie the emergence of therapeutic responses to biological treatments in psychiatry.[17] The study of receptor changes is important in the evaluation of the emergence of adverse psychopathology. An example of this may be seen in the manifestation of movement disorders such as tardive dyskinesia in the context of antipsychotic drug treatment and withdrawal. In addition to ethical concerns and ongoing related attempts to reduce laboratory animal use, the assessment of receptor function in humans is of obvious importance, particularly considering the limitations of "animal models" that are currently available.[18]

6.5 Studies Related to Antidepressant Drug Action

Most of the human work concerning antidepressant drugs has focused on the *in vivo* assessment of receptor function. Strategies for assessing noradrenergic receptor function have been described in detail.[15,19] Seiver and colleagues[20] have also recently discussed strategies for assessing 5-HT receptors in humans. In the case of dopamine receptors, circulating levels of the hormones prolactin and growth hormone have been extensively measured to functionally assess receptor activity.[21,22]

The investigation of peripheral homologues of central nervous system receptors is, with the exception of the usual practical difficulties of clinical studies, largely equivalent in procedure to basic research protocols. Peripheral tissue receptor sources such as blood platelets (for α_2 adrenoceptors, 5-HT$_2$ receptors, and imipramine binding sites[23-28]) and lymphocytes and lymphoblasts (for β-adrenoceptors[29-31]) are readily available. Leukocytes, fibroblasts, and adipose tissue also have adrenergic receptor sites.[32-35] The analyses of these homologous sites entail two fundamental assumptions. The first is that they are truly homologous and may be used as a convenient window for assessing central receptor changes. The second assumption is that drug action is equivalent in the brain and in the periphery. In terms of functional studies, peripherally active pharmacological challenges have been used to assess cardiac responses[15,19] changes in body temperature[36] and hormonal responses (for recent reviews see References 11, 37, and 38).

A useful summary of results obtained with this approach in relation to depression has been compiled by Heninger and Charney.[15] The focus on receptor changes in this context really began in the mid 1970s.[39] For this reason, and in contrast to the measurement of biogenic amines and their metabolites,[11] there is a limited number of studies in the literature. Nevertheless, it is encouraging that these limited data describing the effects of antidepressant drug treatments on measures of human receptor function generally parallel those of basic studies involving nonhuman species. α_2-Adrenergic (platelet) binding is reduced by some chronic treatments with antidepressants although conflicting reports have appeared.[27] Fewer data are available for β-adrenoceptor (lymphocyte) function. Measurements of plasma levels of the receptor-related compound cyclic adenosine monophosphate (cAMP) do, however, indicate reduced responses to β-adrenergic stimulation following administration of salbutamol (which acts to stimulate β_2-adrenoceptors[40]—see Reference 41 for a discussion of this approach). Nevertheless, some laboratory animal studies indicate that the lymphocyte model may be inappropriate as long-term administration of antidepressants does not invariably decrease β-adrenergic receptors on lymphocytes under conditions whereby brain β-adrenoceptor density is reduced.[30] This issue of equivalence is also questioned by a report of increased β-adrenoceptor binding on human leukocytes following treatment with antidepressants or antipsychotics.[42] The effects of antidepressant treatment on platelet imipramine binding sites are also a focus of controversy at this time.[43]

At the present time insufficient data are available to provide a clear view of emergent antidepressant induced changes in receptors in humans. Most human studies have characterized receptor states in depressed patients versus control subjects. A useful summary of comparisons between results of receptor studies from laboratory animal experiments and from human studies has been provided by Pinder.[44] Many receptor changes that emerge with chronic antidepressant treatment may be predicted from an analysis of direct drug-receptor interactions in radiochemical binding studies. Nevertheless, there are drugs which may induce receptor changes similar to those observed following antidepressant treatment *without* inducing any therapeutic effect.[45] Such observations clearly indicate the need for caution in interpreting clinical improvement in terms of receptor adaptation. In addition, the issue of diagnostic complexity must be considered,[12] as described earlier. Thus, in the case of antidepressants, it is probably unreasonable to expect all clinically effective drugs to exhibit equivalent potency in the clinic and in terms of specific receptor measurements. A clearer distinction between subtypes of affective disorder and related pharmacological responses may yield a more meaningful analysis of the emergent human receptor database in the next few years.

6.6 Antipsychotic Drug Action—the Advent of PET Analysis

Antidepressant drugs and the affective disorders represent the most complex case in assessing biological correlates of psychiatric disorder. An extremely challenging and yet apparently simpler area is that of antipsychotic drug action and the treatment of schizophrenia. In this disorder, the therapeutic effects of drugs have been quite clearly related to the blockade of brain receptors for dopamine (see Reference 9 for a review). These antipsychotic effects of drugs are widely accepted to be mediated by the D_2 subtype of the dopamine-receptor family. This picture is currently in a state of potential upheaval as three receptors

(D_3, D_4, and D_5) have been further identified by molecular techniques[46,47,48] and have yet to be evaluated. Nevertheless, the available literature concerning D_1 and D_2 dopamine-receptor function illustrates the possibilities for and applications of receptor analysis in the context of antipsychotic drug action.

No useful peripheral receptor homologues of brain dopamine receptors exist in accessible tissues. Fortunately, recent work has been conducted using PET in this context.[49] This technique enables researchers to track the location and relative concentration of radioactively labeled drugs and other molecules *in vivo*. Although first applied to assess receptors in nonhuman primate brain, this technique was sufficiently refined in the last 5 years to permit quantitation of receptors in the living human brain.[50] In the first studies [^{11}C] methylspiperone was used to label D_2 receptors in the brain but recent studies with [^{11}C] raclopride and [^{11}C] piquindone have provided the advantage of increased specificity.[51,52] The labeled drug [^{11}C]SCH23390 has also been used to assess the density of D_1 receptors in human brain.[53] By application of these PET techniques it has become possible to measure the location and density of these receptors in the brains of live patients. There are clear advantages of this approach relative to that of postmortem brain analysis. The data generated indicate an increase in D_2 dopamine receptor density but no change in that of D_1 receptors in the brains of schizophrenic patients. One issue that is unresolved, however, concerns the cause of the D_2 receptor elevation. As with postmortem analysis of brain dopamine receptors, there is some controversy concerning the density of dopamine receptors in brains of schizophrenic patients who were *not* on drug treatment. Farde and colleagues[51] reported that elevated D_2 receptor density in schizophrenics is simply a function of drug treatment, and not the disease process. Such an interpretation is well supported by a careful recent postmortem study by Kornhuber et al.[54] The debate continues with some groups contending that the receptor elevation is disease-related. The results of the PET studies available to date are complicated by various pharmacokinetic and pharmacodynamic factors which influence the rapid establishment of a pseudoequilibrium between the free circulating labeled drug and that bound to the receptors. One recent study successfully incorporated PET, diagnostic assessment of symptoms, and a hormonal measure of dopamine receptor activity.[55] This is clearly the best possible approach, in which different forms of evidence may be integrated to obtain a comprehensive analysis. Nevertheless, at this stage the controversy continues.

In terms of hormonal indices of dopamine activity, both prolactin and growth hormone have been used to measure the functional state of dopamine receptors *in vivo*.[21,22,56] Growth hormone release is stimulated by dopamine, whereas this neurotransmitter inhibits the release of the hormone prolactin. Despite the advantage and the ease of accessibility of such measurements, such procedures suffer from problems of specificity. Hormonal responses are almost invariably governed by multiple neural receptor systems, inferences from changes in these measures are therefore less specific (see References 56 and 57 for recent reviews).

Again, despite limited availability of data the effects of drug treatments on these measures of human receptor function generally parallel those of preclinical studies involving nonhuman species. Such analyses relate particularly to D_2 dopamine receptor function.[9,21] Particular emphasis has been placed on prolactin which is increased by administration of dopamine receptor-blocking antipsychotic drugs.[21,57]

6.7 Conclusion

The purpose of this chapter is to provide a general overview and an introduction to the analysis of neurochemical changes in psychiatric patients and control subjects. The measurement of indices of neurochemical activity in humans has historically been fraught with technical difficulties. Many earlier studies suffered from a failure to recognize sources of interpretative difficulty in terms of diagnostic grouping or general procedural issues. Contemporary research suffers from these flaws to a lesser extent but apparent progress is tempered by a growing understanding of the complexity of this research area. Traditional pharmacological methods have been invaluable in revealing directions for human studies, and will undoubtedly continue to provide a major input until our understanding of brain function is greatly increased. Nevertheless, there will be continued growth and refinement of neurochemical research with human subjects which will exploit the possibilities afforded by PET analysis and future technological advances. To attempt to finally unravel the mysteries of biological events that lead to psychiatric disorders, human measurements are absolutely necessary, for these are disorders of human thought, affect, and behavior.

REFERENCES

1. Charpentier, P. "Sur la Constitution d'us Dimethylamino-*N*-Phenothiazine," *C.r. hebd. Seanc. Acad. Sci.* 225(5):306–308 (1947).
2. Laborit, H. "Therapeutique Neuroplegique et Hibernation Artificielle: Essai d'eclairissement d'une Equivoque," *Presse Medicale* 62(17):359–362 (1954).
3. Pletscher, A. "The Discovery of Antidepressants: Winding Path," *Experientia*, 47(1):4–8 (1991).
4. Kuhn, R. "The Imipramine Story," in *Discoveries in Biological Psychiatry*, F. J. Ayd and B. Blackwell, Eds. (Philadelphia: J. B. Lippincott, 1970).
5. Cooper, J. R., F. E. Bloom, and R. H. Roth. *The Biochemical Basis of Neuropharmacology*, 4th ed. (New York: Oxford University Press, 1982).
6. Boulton, A. A., G. B. Baker, and R. T. Coutts, Eds. *Neuromethods*, Vol. 10, *Analysis of Psychiatric Drugs* (Clifton, NJ: Humana Press, 1988).
7. Carlton, P. L. *Behavioural Pharmacology*, (New York: McGraw Hill, 1983).
8. Baker, G. B. and W. G. Dewhurst. "Biochemical Theories of Affective Disorders," in *Pharmacotherapy of Affective Disorders*, W. G. Dewhurst and G. B. Baker, Eds. (New York: New York University Press, 1985).

9. Seeman, P. "Dopamine Receptors and the Dopamine Hypothesis of Schizophrenia," *Synapse* 1(2):133–152 (1987).
10. Meltzer, H. Y., Ed. *Psychopharmacology: The Third Generation of Progress* (New York: Raven Press, 1987).
11. Davis, B. A. "Biogenic Amines and Their Metabolites in Body Fluids of Normal, Psychiatric and Neurological Subjects," *J. Chromatogr.* 466(1):89–218 (1989).
12. Bland, R. C. "Clinical Features of Affective Disorders. I. Diagnosis, Classification, Rating Scales, Outcome and Epidemiology," in *Pharmacotherapy of Affective Disorders*, W. G. Dewhurst and G. B. Baker, Eds. (London: Croom Helm, 1985).
13. Boulton, A. A. and A. V. Juorio. "Brain Trace Amines," in *Handbook of Neurochemistry*, A. Lajtha, Ed. (New York: Plenum Press, 1982).
14. Lapierre, Y. D. "Course of Clinical Response to Antidepressants," *Prog. Neuro-Psychopharmacol. Biol. Psychiat.* 9(5/6):503–507 (1985).
15. Heninger, G. R. and D. S. Charney. "Mechanism of Action of Antidepressant Treatments: Implications for the Etiology and Treatment of Depressive Disorders," in *Psychopharmacology: The Third Generation of Progress*, H. Y. Meltzer, Ed. (New York: Raven Press, 1987).
16. Cannon, W. G. and A. Rosenblueth. *The Supersensitivity of Denervated Structures* (New York: Macmillan, 1949).
17. Ackenheil, M. "The Mechanism of Action of Antidepressants Revised," *J. Neural Transm.*, 32(Suppl):29–37 (1990).
18. Greenshaw, A. J., D. J. Sanger, and T. V. Nguyen. "Animal Models for Assessing Antidepressant, Neuroleptic and Anxiolytic Drug Action," in *Neuromethods*, Vol. 10, *Analysis of Psychiatric Drugs*, A. A. Boulton, G. B. Baker, and R. T. Coutts, Eds. (Clifton, NJ: Humana Press, 1988).
19. Siever, L. J., T. W. Uhde, and D. L. Murphy. "Strategies for Assessment of Noradrenergic Function in Patients with Affective Disorders," in *Neurobiology of Mood Disorders*, R. M. Post and J. C. Ballenger, Eds. (Baltimore: Williams & Wilkins, 1984b)
20. Siever, L. J., L. B. Guttmacher, and D. L. Murphy. "Serotonin Receptors: Evaluation of Their Possible Role in Affective Disorders," in *Neurobiology of Mood Disorders*, R. M. Post and J. C. Ballenger, Eds. (Baltimore: Williams & Wilkins, 1984a).
21. Meltzer H. Y., D. J. Goode, and V. S. Fang. "The Effect of Psychotropic Drugs on Endocrine Function. I. Neuroleptics, Precursors and Agonists," in *Psychopharmacology: A Generation of Progress*, M. A. Lipton, A. DiMascio, and K. F. Killam, Eds. (New York: Raven Press, 1978).
22. Sachar, E. J. "Neuroendocrine Response to Psychotropic Drugs," in *Psychopharmacology: A Generation of Progress*, M. A. Lipton, A. DiMascio, and K. F. Killam, Eds. (New York: Raven Press, 1978).
23. Carstens, M. E., A. H. Engelbrecht, V. A. Russell, C. Aalbers, C. A. Gagiano, D. O. Chalton, and J. J. F. Taljaard. "Alpha$_2$-Adrenoceptor Levels of Platelets of Patients with Major Depressive Disorders," *Psychiatr. Res.* 18(4):321–331 (1986a).
24. Carstens, M. E., A. H. Engelbrecht, V. A. Russell, C. Aalbers, C. A. Gagiano, D. O. Chalton, and J. J. F. Taljaard. "Imipramine Binding Sites on Platelets of Patients with Major Depressive Disorder," *Psychiatr. Res.* 18(4):333–342 (1986b).
25. Garcia-Sevilla, J. A., C. Udina, M. J. Fuster, E. Alvarez, and M. Casas. "Enhanced Binding of [^{3}H](-) Adrenaline to Platelets of Depressed Patients with Melancholia: Effects of Long-Term Clomipramine Treatment," *Acta Psychiatr. Scand.* 75(2):150–157 (1987).

26. Kafka, M. S., J. I. Nurnberger, L. Siever, S. Targum, T. W. Uhde, and E. S. Gershon. "Alpha$_2$-Adrenergic-Receptor Function in Patients with Unipolar and Bipolar Affective Disorders," *J. Affect. Dis.* 10(2):163–169 (1986).

27. Kafka, M. S. and S. M. Paul. "Platelet α-Adrenergic Receptors in Depression," *Arch. Gen. Psychiatr.* 43(1):91–95 (1986).

28. Piletz, J. E., D. S. P. Schubert, and A. Halaris. "Evaluation of Studies on Platelet Alpha$_2$ Adrenoreceptors in Depressive Illness," *Life Sci.* 39(18):1589–1616 (1986).

29. Berrettini, W. H., C. B. Cappellari, J. I. Nurnberger, and E. S. Gershon, "Beta-Adrenergic Receptors on Lymphoblasts," *Neuropsychobiol.* 17(1/2):15–18 (1987).

30. Chalecka-Franaszek, E. and J. Vetulani. "Lack of Effect of Chronic Imipramine Administration of β-Adrenoceptor Density on Rat Lymphocytes," *Pol. J. Pharmacol. Pharm.* 38(4):385–390 (1986).

31. Wood, K., K. Whiting, and A. Coppen. "Lymphocyte Beta-Adrenergic Receptor Density of Patients with Recurrent Affective Illness," *J. Affect. Dis.* 10(1):3–8 (1986).

32. Galant, S. P., L. Doniseti, S. Underwood, and P. A. Iusel. "Leukocyte β-Adrenergic Receptor Assay in Normals and Asthmatics," *N. Engl. J. Med.* 299(17):933–936 (1978).

33. Maguire, M. E., R. A. Wiklund, H. J. Anderson, and A. G. Gilman. "Binding of [^{125}I] Iodohydroxybenzylpindolol to Putative β-Adrenergic Receptors of Rat Glioma Cells and Other Cell Clones," *J. Biol. Chem.* 251(5):1221–1231 (1976).

34. Tharp, M. D., B. B. Hoffmann, and R. J. Lefkovitz. "α-Adrenergic Receptors in Human Adipocyte Membranes: Direct Determination by [^{3}H] Yohimbine Binding," *J. Clin. Endocrinol. Metab.* 52(4):709–714 (1981).

35. Williams, L. T., R. Snyderman, and R. J. Leftowitz. "Identification of β-Adrenergic Receptors in Human Lymphocytes by [^{3}H] Alprenolol Binding," *J. Clin. Invest.* 57(1):149–155 (1976).

36. Lesch, K. P., S. Mayer, J. Disselkamp-Tietze, A. Hoh, G. Schoellnhammer, and H. M. Schulte. "Subsensitivity of 5-hydroxytryptamine$_{1A}$ (5-HT$_{1A}$) Receptor-mediated Hypothermic Response to Ipsapirone in Unipolar Depression," *Life Sci.* 46(18):1271–1277 (1990).

37. Muller, E. E. "The Neuroendocrine Approach to Psychiatric Disorders: A Critical Appraisal," *J. Neural Transm.* 81(1):1–15 (1990).

38. Deakin J. F. W., I. Pennell, A. J. Upadhyaya, and R. Lofthouse. "A Neuroendocrine Study of 5HT Function in Depression: Evidence for Biological Mechanisms of Endogenous and Psychosocial Causation," *Psychopharmacology* 101(1):85–92 (1990).

39. Vetulani, J., J. V. Dingall, and F. Sulser. "A Possible Common Mechanism of Action of Antidepressant Treatments," *Naunyn-Schmied. Arch. Pharmacol.* 293(2):109–114 (1976).

40. Lerer, B., R. B. Epstein, and R. H. Belmaker. "Subsensitivity of Human β-Adrenergic Adenylate Cyclase after Salbutamol Treatment of Depression," *Psychopharmacology* 75(2):169–172 (1981).

41. Palmer, G. C. "Clinical Considerations of the Cyclic Nucleotides in Psychiatry and Neurology," *Integr. Psychiat.* 3(2):99–111 (1985).

42. Pandey, G. N., P. G. Janicak, S. C. Pandey, and J. M. Davis. "Effect of Treatment with Antidepressants and Neuroleptics on Human Leukocyte Beta-Adrenergic Receptors," *Psychopharmacol. Bull.* 25(2):257–262 (1989).

43. Wagner, A., A. Anberg-Wistedt, M. Asberg, L. Bertilsson, B. Martensson, and D. Montero. "Effects of Antidepressant Treatments on Platelet Tritiated Imipramine Binding in Major Depressive Disorder," *Arch. Gen. Psychiat.* 44(10):870–877 (1987).

44. Pinder, R. M. "Antidepressant Drugs of the Future," in *Psychopharmacology: Recent Advances and Future Prospects*, S. D. Iversen, Ed. (Oxford: Oxford University Press, 1986).

45. Uhde, T. W., L. J. Siever, and R. M. Post. "Clonidine: Acute Challenge and Clinical Trial Paradigms for the Investigation and Treatment of Anxiety Disorders, Affective Illness and Pain Syndromes," in *Neurobiology of Mood Disorders*, R. M. Post and J. C. Ballenger, Eds. (Baltimore: Williams & Wilkins, 1984).

46. Giros, B., M-P. Martres, P. Sokoloff, and J-C. Schwartz. "Clonage du Gene du Receptor Dopaminergique D_3 Humain et Identification de son Chromosome," *C. R. Acad. Sci. Paris* 311(13):501–508 (1990).

47. Sunahara, R. K., H-C. Guan, B. F. O'Dowd, P. Seeman, L. G. Laurier, G. Ng, S. R. George, J. Torchia, H. H. M. Van Tol, and H. B. Niznik. "Cloning of the Gene for a Human Dopamine D_5 Receptor With Higher Affinity for Dopamine Than D_1," *Nature* 350(6319):614–619 (1991).

48. Van Tol, H. H. M., J. R. Bunzow, H-C. Guan, R. K. Sunahara, P. Seeman, H. B. Niznik, and O. Civelli. "Cloning of the Gene for Human Dopamine D_4 Receptor With High Affinity For the Antipsychotic Clozapine," *Nature* 350(6319):610–614 (1991).

49. Sedvall, G. "PET Imaging of Dopamine Receptors in Human Basal Ganglia: Relevance to Mental Illness," *TINS* 13(7):302–308 (1990).

50. Farde, L., E. Ehrin, L. Eriksson, T. Greitz, H. Hall, C. Hedstrom, J-E. Litton, and G. Sedvall. "Substituted Benzamides as Ligands for Visualization of Dopamine Receptor Binding in the Human Brain by Positron Emission Tomography," *Proc. Natl. Acad. Sci. U.S.A.* 82(11):3863–3867 (1985).

51. Farde, L., H. Hall, E. Ehrin, and G. Sedvall. Quantitative Analysis of D_2 Dopamine Binding in the Living Human Brain by PET," *Science* 231(4735):258–261 (1986).

52. Sedvall, G., E. Ehrin, and L. Farde. "Stereoselective Binding of ^{11}C-Labelled Piquindone (Ro22-1319) to Dopamine-D_2 Receptors in the Living Human Brain," *Human Psychopharmacol.* 2(1):23–30 (1986).

53. Sedvall, G., L. Farde, S. Stone-Elander, and C. Halldin. "Dopamine D_1-Receptor Binding in the Living Human Brain," in *Neurobiology of Central D-1-Dopamine Receptors*, G. R. Breese and I. Creese, Eds. (New York: Plenum, 1986).

54. Kornhuber, J., P. Riederer, G. P. Reynolds, H. Beckmann, K. Jellinger, and E. Gabriel. "[^{3}H]-Spiperone Binding Sites in Postmortem Brains from Schizophrenic Patients. Relationship to Neuroleptic Drug Treatment, Abnormal Movements and Positive Symptoms," *J. Neural Transm.* 75(1):1–10 (1989).

55. Farde, L., F-A. Wiesel, P. Jansson, G. Uppfeldt, and G. Sedvall. "An Open Label Trial of Raclopride in Acute Schizophrenia. Confirmation of D_2-Dopamine Receptor Occupancy by PET," *Psychopharmacol.* 94(1):1–7 (1988).

56. Lal, S. "Growth Hormone and Schizophrenia," in *Psychopharmacology: The Third Generation of Progress*, H. Y. Meltzer, Ed. (New York: Raven Press, 1987).

57. Rubin, R. T. "Prolactin and Schizophrenia," in *Psychopharmacology: The Third Generation of Progress*, H. Y. Meltzer, Ed. (New York: Raven Press, 1987).

ADDITIONAL READING

Brown, G. M., S. H. Doslow, and S. Reichlin, Eds. *Neuroendocrinology and Psychiatric Disorders* (New York: Raven Press, 1984).

Cooper, J. R., F. E. Bloom, and R. H. Roth. *The Biochemical Basis of Neuropharmacology*, 4th ed. (New York: Oxford University Press, 1982).

Gregory, R. L. and O. L. Zangwill. *The Oxford Companion to the Mind* (Oxford: Oxford University Press, 1987).

Iversen, S. D. Ed. *Psychopharmacology: Recent Advances and Future Prospects* (Oxford: Oxford University Press, 1986).

Meltzer, H. Y. Ed. *Psychopharmacology: The Third Generation of Progress* (New York: Raven Press, 1987).

CHAPTER 7

Network Models in Behavioral and Computational Neuroscience

Paul S. Prueitt

7.0 A Brief History of Neural Networks—The Early Epoch

The advocates of new approaches toward modeling cognitive and behavioral processes have struggled over the last 50 years to define how insights derived from newly discovered facts could be unified with existing theoretical preferences within the intellectual communities that collectively form the academy. To understand the modern developments in cognitive and behavioral sciences one should be aware of some of this early history, and to gain an oversight on the reoccurring themes in neural network and artificial intelligence research, and to make a judgment on the value of some of the themes that act as control parameters. A comprehensive history is available from a number of sources.[1,2] An examination of this history demonstrates the existence of belief constraints that have shaped, and continue to shape, the investigation of the brain–behavior interface.

The history of neural networks takes form in the 1940s with two papers by Warren McCulloch and Walter Pitts.[3] The first paper develops a logical calculus in which all or no "neurons" receive excitatory and or inhibitory inputs from other all or no neurons. Five physical assumptions are given (see below).

0-87371-504-7/93/$0.00+$.50
© 1993 by Lewis Publishers

1. The activity of the neuron is an "all-or-none" process.
2. A certain fixed number of synapses must be excited within the period of latent activity in order to excite a neuron at any time, and this number is independent of previous activity and position on the neuron.
3. The only significant delay within the nervous system is synaptic delay.
4. The activity of any inhibitory synapse absolutely prevents excitation of the neuron at that time.
5. The structure of the net does not change with time.[3]

An important underlying premise of the 1943 paper was that the fundamental relations of psychology are determined by two-valued logic and expressible in the formal logic of Russell and Whitehead's *Principa Mathematica*. In addition to a formal analysis of both feed forward and recurrent nets, the 1943 McCulloch and Pitts paper contained a number of figures representing examples of nets that conform to their five assumptions. The second paper[4] was more accommodating to neurophysiology and contained the rudimentary concept of a back propagated error term.

It was Rosenblatt's judgment[5] that boolean logic was not suitable for discussing either the processes of the human brain or the behavioral substrate to higher order cognitive function. His networks were formulated, in the early 1950s, in the language of probability, although the interpretation of this language as continuous dynamics expressed as concentration is in contrast to the recent interest in fuzzy logics.[6] In this interpretation, the Rosenblatt perceptron is similar to the modern theory embedding fields of Grossberg[7,8] as well as to the linear association models[1] of cognitive science.

An emphasis on a continuum representational space for modeling process activity leads us to the second theme constraining the evolution of modern neural network theory, i.e., population dynamics defined as interacting populations is sufficient for a comprehensive theory of brain function. In such a theory, system evolution can be defined by deterministic differential equations. This tradition should be traced back to Rashevsky's attempts in the 1950s to establish the principles of relational biology.[9] The approach, seen only from the perspective of Rashevsky, appears to not account for the apparent indeterminism that we observe in human exercise of choice or that is observed in the exercise of control by a more general class of intentional systems.

I underscore the word "appears" because the full story is not told without dealing directly with the formal reality of deterministic chaos, a reality that is only just beginning to be examined.[10] Rashevsky's attempt to formulate a widely acceptable set of foundation principles for relational biology was largely unsuccessful due to the prevailing scientific sentiment, and thus the deeper questions involving control of system evolution through intersystem modulation did not fully mature. Indeed the continuous, and analytic, approach towards the brain–behavior interface has only marginally endured the pressure of unfavorable sentiment from the psychological community in particular. The stage was not set for a serious attack on the problem of determining origin of control and other related issues. The technical difficulty of the theory of deterministic chaos, as well as other deep physical processes theory and the present clutter of neuroscience and psychological theory provides a barrier for all but a few.

The cognitive and behavioral theories of the 1950s and 1960s were not followed by the development of a mathematical formalism adequate to embody higher order cognitive function. The prevailing view was, and still is, that cognitive processes are simply not amenable to formal understanding. Given this view, the research community felt constrained to treat the human brain as though it were a computational device not very different from the von Neuman computer. The constraint also derived a legitimacy from a hard nosed, and misplaced, scientific materialism.

The constraints placed by a narrowly defined scientific materialism has had both a positive and a negative effect on the general nature of the inquiry about brain and behavior. The positive effect is that scientific materialism has outlawed the re-introduction of scientific vitalism. The negative effect has been the denial of the very characteristic of the brain–behavior interface that makes it so interesting, i.e., the origin of willful control.

The relationship between discrete symbolic analysis, boolean formalisms, and scientific materialism is an interesting one but cannot be fully treated here. Several points are important to note, however. The artificial neural network (ANN) research published in the early 1960s was occupied with state vectors, more boolean logic, statistics, and Turing machines. We feel that this research has been overly influenced by the symbolic analysis of data as a means of information management. Most of the early ANN research, Grossberg's work is an important exception, was concerned with constructing a general theory of computation, from which it was assumed that biological computation would follow as a special instance. This research developed in parallel with early artificial intelligence and cognitive science.

Today, artificial intelligence and cognitive science enjoy considerable success in generating research support from federal agencies, particularly the Department of Defense. There is, moreover, considerable perceived scientific correctness in relating global theories of brain function back to the belief in a universal computational grammar. However, relatively little, in terms of understanding natural intelligence, has been advanced by this program. With a diminishing return from basic research in artificial intelligence and cognitive science, a distinct possibility should be considered. Discrete symbolic analysis and boolean formalism, when taken as the only valid scientific paradigm, has obscured important questions that can only be answered elsewhere.

Time and space are continuums, whereas logical symbols are, to some extent, a discrete packet. To the extent that semantics is stripped away from these discrete packets during the formalization of a model, the discretization of a state space into symbols formally eliminates the possibility of deterministic chaos. A continuum has many properties that (nonesoteric) discrete spaces do not have, such as uncountability. Of importance in considering the nature of deterministic chaos, a major difference has to do with point neighborhoods, i.e., for points in a continuum given any two points there exists a point between these two points. The discrete spaces do not have this property. This condition, expressed as having neighborhoods of positive radius without neighbors, restricts the possibility of modeling the phenomena of choice, since the sensitivity to initial condition of future possible trajectories provides nonrule-based branching. Interestingly, the issue of informational uncertainty is a factor in modeling the origin of control. A perception–action cycle has a duration, or event window, over which choice must be exercised, and clearly this is a discretization of experience into temporal chunks. Thus, while discretization eliminates nonhomogenous features within an event window, choice requires the ability to preferentially treat substructures in order to shape the dynamics at the end of the event.

The only way out is if a single symbol could have more than one meaning *without regard to context*. This situation is difficult to imagine and this leads to a Gödel[11] type conclusion:

> Symbolic reasoning has formal limitations that have not and perhaps can not be overcome by simply improving computational technology;[12] and, thus building faster (digital) computers will not identify the origin of control within biological systems.

If this type of Gödel statement is correct, then where does this leave our inquiry into the brain and behavior? The answer lies with integration of discrete *and* continuous processes acting in temporal hierarchies. The discrete event is then seen as an emergent property of microprocesses acting collectively under the constraint of macroprocesses, and thus the property of being discrete is very much dependent on the object's environment and constituents. In this case, the origin of control is deterministically constrained by the nature and condition of constituent microprocesses. This statement of ontology about the implicit nature of the world[13] is not fully reflected in any discrete formalism.

With continuum spaces, the choice of a specific evolutionary path within the critical regions of a dynamic may occur via random fluctuation of processes occurring at faster time scales. Control in biological systems, however, may occur via intersystem modulation directed by intercomponent language.[14,15] In this view, the origin of observed control, while the dynamic is in a critical region, can be clarified by reference to the existence of natural languages. Natural and synthetic languages then becomes of special interest. The central implication of intercomponent languages is that the nonlocality of some constraints are not expressed in a local syntax — thus giving rise to what are called semantic and pragmatic axes that cannot be (easily) reduced to syntax. These intercomponent languages may be responsible for interaction dynamics at all levels of physical organization. The role of deterministic chaos in intercomponent modulation and the emergence of natural language is still speculative and digresses from our short historical account of network theories of cognitive and behavioral science.

7.1 Neural Networks—The Middle Epoch

During the 1970s and 1980s, programs were developed[16-29] that continued the network research that found continuous dynamics and biology significant. Hopfield's work,[23] based upon a simplified field equation for fully connected summative neurons, found wide support in the physical science communities. As is pointed out in Anderson and Rosenfeld's[1] introduction to a reprint of Hopfield,[23] neural-network theory became respectable within the scientific community in his hands. The information storage algorithm that he developed has a biological interpretation and exploited well-understood mathematical theories involving energy functions. This led to the successful modeling of a general class of optimization problems including the traveling salesman problem. Hopfield's work, along with the work of others,[16,19,24] showed the feasibility of content-addressable memory. The potential for content addressable memory and information processing provides a fundamental challenge to symbolic analysis and the computer metaphor.

It is important, however, to establish an overview of the historical facts and recognize that the respectability provided by Hopfield's 1982 and 1984 papers[1] was established not due to a theory of biological interaction but due to a formalization of an optimization principle in terms familiar to the electronic engineering, physics, and mathematics communities. In spite of the introduction of a new principle, the origin-of-control issue was not raised within the literature associated with the early formulation of a distributed theory of computation. The challenge presented by Hopfield's papers was not sufficient to induce a major paradigm shift in cognitive or behavioral science, but rather led to a slight modification of an existing paradigm in physics and electrical engineering. The central issue of the origin of intentional control could not yet be addressed.

The general notion of a dynamic system, with attractor regions and energy functions, has been very productive for engineering applications, but neither the Hopfield model, nor any of its contemporaries, admit to the storage of stable limit cycles and the degree of variability required of more profound models of neurobiology. The stable limit cycle would be one way in which a behavioral program could be expressed. Neither is there a notion of deterministic chaos. In the Hopfield system, random noise is important as a mechanism for seeking global rather than local minimum, but the notion of a system's behavioral intent was not linked to the existence of indeterminism in certain critical regions. This is a severe limitation.

In biological systems we observe the temporary emergence of cognitive and sensory processes that appear to be created from stimuli interaction with neurosubstrata. Once these synergisms are formed they have a stable existence for some finite period of time, during which they will manifest an influence on other

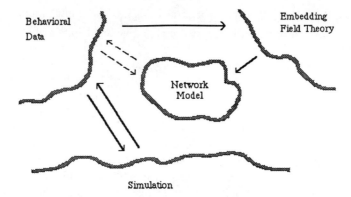

Figure 1.   A schematic interpretation of the role of embedding field theory. Large data bases of behavioral data have accumulated over the last 50 years. Much of this data exists as clusters that have little theoretical connections with each other. Embedding field theory is designed to embody the salient features of individual clusters of behavioral data, resulting in network models of the underlying simulation. The broken line represents a feedback loop to behavioral science from the predictive quality of the network model.

processes. Specific biological constraints on the creation, annihilation, and control of such synergisms must exist in the neurosubstrata and in the more global constraints associated with electromagnetic field potentials.[39]

The theory of embedding fields[7,8] was defined, in part, by the restriction of model instantiation equations to first order differential equations and defined in part by a methodology that selects a body of behavioral studies to be analyzed. The published literature is identified by Grossberg as the source of data sets representing these behavioral studies. Through the application of modeling principles, the theory of embedding fields seeks a system of first order differential equations reflecting a firm grounding in the behavioral research. The result has been the development of a small set of design principles for modeling the behavioral data. Five such design principles were identified in Prueitt and Levine[14] as:

1. Associative learning—to enable strengthening or weakening of connections between events based on contiguity or probable causality
2. Lateral inhibition—to enable choices between competing percepts, drives, categorizations, plans, or behaviors
3. Opponent processing—to enable selective enhancement of events that change over time
4. Neuromodulation—to enable contextual refinement of attention
5. Interlevel resonant feedback—to enable reality testing of tentative classifications

The analysis of existing research literature in specialized behavioral science has resulted in predictive models as demonstrated in Grossberg's work on visional illusions,[18] in work on adaptive motor control,[30] in work on attentionally modulated conditioning,[25,28] and in perceptual chunking.[27] In the continuous versions of

Adaptive Resonance Theory (ART II and ART III)[3] stimulus input is played across an ensemble of interaction populations.[28] The esemble, called the input field, processes the input and interacts with a number of re-entrant systems, resulting in learning, memory retrieval, and classification. These processes are occurring within a model that is defined by differential equations and evolved through the use of a computer (no closed-form solution exists). The theory of embedding fields can also be utilized in the modeling of specific experimental research that has been produced from lesion studies or neuroinhibitors.[29,31]

7.2 Discrete and Continuous ANNs

Network models have been used in neuromodeling as well as in theoretical immunology. For an extensive review see References 1, 2, 20, and 32 for neural networks and References 33 and 34 for immune networks. Both neural and immune networks share the common feature of being a realization of the promise implicit in the application of population dynamics to modeling biological processes. Neural network algorithms generally suppose physical nodes, representing neurons, ensembles of neurons, or sometimes subcellular units, and physical connections between nodes. Sometimes the notions of nodes and connections take the form of an analogy rather than a representation of physical processes and the term "connectionism" is often used as a general rubric for the theoretical context of such algorithms. In such cases, the dynamics often are described as next-step functions and some important features of continuous dynamics are lost.

It is in this twilight zone of discrete versus continuous formalism that the field of ANN is torn into two very different camps, the first one (continuous ANNs) very concerned about the description of deterministic trajectories in a continuum and the second (discrete ANNs) insistent on computability using the closure and reversible properties of a formal ring of numbers.[35] These differences are exploited in the push and pull of various communities who often use ANN theory to show consistency of their model with a specific ANN paradigm.

The loss of continuous dynamics is a feature of numerical integration, which results in an approximate solution for systems of differential equations. This loss is acceptable to some because of the existence of theorems that prove various properties such as convergence, completeness, or closure. It is reasoned that numerical integration evolves the description of the system dynamics in the future in such a way as to continue a closed correspondence to the underlying substrate processes that are being modeled. Thus the approximation is sometimes not so important.

From the other quarter, difference equations and related symbolic analyses may in fact not be approximating a continuous dynamic. A purely symbolic analysis of language, for example, is acceptable to some because their interest is in modeling very high level cognitive or sensory processes in which symbolic processes are dominate features. However, the discretization of the basic elements of the formalism modeling these processes is critically important. This often amounts to a selection of a finite basis of elements upon which the real world must be mapped. The issue is not so much a question of feasibility if we consider a representation of a static world by a finite bases, but a challenge is placed on that representation by the nonstationarity of the real world.

The network principle of artificial neural systems makes the assumption that static networks, with a fixed number of variables, are sufficient to model higher order cognitive functions. The introduction of continuous variables, by embedding field theory, for example, provides the formal tools needed to address the complexities of choice, but these tools have been largely ignored with deference to systems that are conservative and asymptotically stable, i.e., without limit cycles. Neither has there been a wide acceptance of the notion of the variable selection of basis elements. Formal systems having a variable number of variables have been called piece-wise formal[14] because the *a priori* selection of a set of observables, and the measurement of these observables with variables corresponds to the development of an episodic event in behavioral space.

The completion of an episode corresponds with the collapse of a set of observables, e.g., measured by the system's variables, as these observables begin to fail in their role as useful measurement devices for the animal.[12] At the time of this collapse, the set of rules governing the animal's behavior also (partially or completely) collapses; leading to a restructuring of the behavioral space. This phenomena occurs, for example, when an animal's appetite is satiated after eating a large meal. As a methodology for modeling episodic dynamics, it is suggested that piece-wise formal models of the organization, duration, and collapse of behavioral episodes should be used. These models will undergo nonstationary forcings, i.e., small alterations, on the model's axiomatic foundations. The small alterations will result, when the episode ends, in a nonlinear restructuring of the dynamics. The greatest open questions center around the task of specifying the dynamics of the transition period.

7.3 The Impending Paradigm Shift

To develop a scientific approach towards understanding biologically feasible models of the brain–behavior interface, we require both a greater exploitation of the network principle to provide a model of willful intent, and the appreciation of its limitations to provide a model of episodic transitions. Thus we conceive a future possibility, rather than a present one, when we talk about biologically feasible computational models of the sensory and cognitive processes that act through this interface. The development of biologically feasible models of sensory and cognitive processes must be facilitated in the present by thoughtful development of basic research. The rate of development of high quality computational models is dependent on:

1. Acceptance and cooperation within the medical community
2. High funding levels for basic research on new computational paradigms that deal squarely with the distributed and nonlocal nature of sensory and cognitive processes

3. Overcoming a strongly felt bias imposed by the network principle and reinforced by engineering type ANN research

The evaluation of better computational models of brain and behavior is assisted by two factors. First, many have made the observation that, throughout history, psychology has used analogy to compare the workings of the human brain with the most complex system currently understood by prevailing scientific and social views. Recent advances in quantum theory[36] and molecular computing provide a new metaphor which has a nonlocal nature and is nonboolean. Second, a fundamental change in description is underway in which analogies to nonbrain processes are being replaced with a direct analysis of the subprocesses of the brain.

However, as is to be expected, we move in the direction at different speeds. In a recent article in *Behavioral Research Methods, Instruments, and Computers*, Walter Schneider[37] writes about a possible paradigm shift in psychology that is framed by "connectionism". Schneider, however, defines connectionism in terms that do not represent, for us, a real shift in cognitive science or artificial intelligence, since for Schneider connectionism "does not incorporate either the microstructure (e.g., differential polarization, depending on whether the synapse contacts the cell body or the dendrite) or macrostructure (e.g., very specific neuroanatomical connections between regions of the cortex) of neurophysiology" (p. 73).[37] If this is a paradigm shift within cognitive science then we believe that cognitive science will continue to not address the full range of issues required of 21st century behavioral science. The two areas will continue to be separated by foundational inconsistencies.

Schneider's view is similar to the view of many, but not all, who work in the neural network paradigm, thus pointing out an important nonhomogeneity within the community. Another group sees this viewpoint as "shallow" and would extend the meaning of connectionism to a richer definition by generalizing the term to include weakly coupled locally defined dynamic systems as models of neurophysical processes. This approach provides the potential for modeling willful intent and, when arranged in a temporal hierarchy, the potential for modeling emergent episodes. This is not, however, a small shift in formal technique but rather a radical departure from a narrow scientific materialism that cannot make the connection between symbolic processes and biological ones. Models of neurophysical processes can provide an understanding of psychological processes and vice versa, while retaining the distinction that models of neurophysical processes cannot always be identified exactly as a model of psychological processes.[38]

The problem of language becomes apparent when a term such as connectionism (or "parallel distributed processing") is used in a shallow fashion. A richer semantics is excluded by the analysis of those who would have us believe that the brain's computational ability can be understood by developing a general theory of computation based on present day computers. Historically, it has been difficult to counter the "rationality" of this view, particularly since research and development funding has been traditionally applied to a specific set of short-term goals that are easily defined. In this sense we have developed science into 30-s sound bites and have failed to define long-term objectives that address central questions, such as the questions of the origin of willful intent or the origin of control. Once the shallow view became dominate, then those who were biologically or behaviorally oriented found themselves on the outside of a rigid paradigm and confronted with the pressure of scientific correctness. "Good theories rarely develop outside the context of a background of well-understood real problems and special cases".[40]

Clearly, medical science cannot be happy, and should not be, with a type of neural network research that is narrowly concerned with engineering. A preoccupation with engineering applications has disguised a large body of neural network research that is concerned with neurological function and neuropsychology and is willing to discuss biological feasibility. The dominance of shallow connectionism within the neural network community has shaped a judgment by many in the medical field that neural network research is without value to medical research. This is not an informed judgment. Moreover, the medical community has not acted in a cooperative fashion with the modeling community and thus has helped create an artificial barrier to the development of a richer modeling paradigm capable of producing great value to medical research and practice.

To build valid nonanimal models for behavioral science, something we are just beginning to do, we need not only better mathematical and computational tools but also a mature theory of the biological basis of psychological processes such as cognition and sensation. The general methodology for developing an algorithm and then implementing this algorithm in neuroscience involves awareness of neuroscience, behavioral science, and mathematical theory. This methodology involves at least a five level process, within numerous iterations between the levels (Figure 2).

Behavioral or experimental models are often described as flow charts having unknown internal dynamics (e.g., Skinner). The specification of a transfer function that conceivably produces qualitative matches to data can only be biologically feasible if the underlying substrate processes are well understood. Unfortunately, biological substrate processes are not generally understood in a context that allows behavioral researchers a basis for speculation. Thus we need a boot strapping method to allow known substrate dynamics to develop in behavioral context. To begin this method, a dynamical system and a corresponding algorithm is specified that conceivably could provide qualitative matches to the behavioral model and a correspondence between known neuroprocesses and the dynamical system's variables.

Once a dynamical system, preferably with continuous evolution rules, has been specified then a computational instantiation of the refined algorithm is developed. Qualitative matching between the model and computer simulations are then used to provide evidence for or against the model. At this point, methodology requires starting over by modifying and giving detail to the original flow chart.

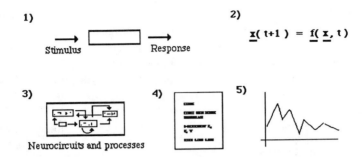

Figure 2. (1) Behavioral or experimental models are described as flow charts having unknown internal dynamics. (2) A dynamical system, and algorithm, is designed that conceivably could provide qualitative matches to the model. (3) A correspondence between known neuroprocesses and the dynamical system's variables are identified. (4) A computational instantiation of the refined algorithm is developed. (5) Qualitative matching between the model and computer simulations are used to provide evidence for or against the model.

Although a complete specification of the identity of the major players involved in neuroprocesses and corresponding system variables eludes basic sciences, a partial list of fundamental players in the network modeling of neural and immune response processes has been developed. For example, we now have clear evidence that processes within neurons, and even within membranes, involve complex information processing. It is also well known that synaptic transmission induces changes in receptor sensitivity that induce specific messenger RNA transcription of proteins. The resulting protein production involves diffuse gene expression and this expression involves global variations of synaptic behavior. A dominant problem is to specify how behavioral and experimental theory can be modeled as interactions between subsystem models that are rich enough to embody neurophysical process at this level of detail.

7.4 Does Neural Network Research Require a New Notion of Scientific Inquiry?

There is a general concern by the neural network research community that advanced investigation in neuropsychology, psychophysics, and computational neuroscience is inhibited by problems in communicating underlying principles between scientific disciplines and to the American public. We note that a lack of information about neural network research presents, to government and business communities, fundamental difficulties in making optimal decisions about funding and resource allocation. As a further indication of the seriousness of the problem, valuable contributions from the neural network community to other disciplines are often lost due to the wide scope of knowledge needed to read the neural network research literature. To accept this condition as status quo is to underestimate the significance of this scientific inquiry to medicine and behavioral science.

Scientific inquiry necessitates a cooperative hearing of philosophical notions, the common use of language, and a purpose derived from our search for individual meaning. Without a wide dissemination of our fundamental notions and without adherence to the principles of scientific methodology, the neural network community faces the prospect of working within an artificially restricted marketplace of ideas. The methodology must, however, be one that constantly examines our assumptions and the natural limitations of formal language.[11] Thus an iterative refinement of science is directed by both theoretical and phenomenological considerations.

It is the principle of iterative refinement that leads us around some of the fundamental difficulties involved in a modern scientific inquiry about biological and cognitive processes. For example, iterative refinement allows us to utilize conceptual form and theory as illusionary processes that must undergo adaptive change. The principle of iterative refinement implies that a structurally stable paradigm should not necessarily be taken as proof of a particular set of views but rather as a possible sign that theorists have lost contact with the real world. Not all of the difficulties facing behavioral and computational neuroscience are circumvented by iterative refinement, however, and thus we are again brought to the question of new language development and of cooperative research.

Another very important dimension to the future of ANN research defines an opportunity to develop a science of education from neural network and computation neuroscience research. The next steps require a vision of the eventual application of behavioral and computational neuroscience research to educational theory and suggests computational theory adequate to begin the long journey. The younger generation is excited about the prospect of contributing to the emerging information-age-based technology. This interest is particularly true about object oriented programming and neural networks. Thus behavioral and computational neuroscience can provide a motivational input into the educational processes as well as provide a greater understanding of natural intelligence.

Research on the nature of motivation, intelligence, memory, and selective attention hints at a science of education that can select from concepts of traditional educational theories having value and delegitimize those concepts that are founded on speculation or mythology. In addition to increasing student motivation, a direct application of computational models of behavior promises to increase our understanding of human learning behaviors and thus improve the institutional insight available to teachers and professors.

7.5 Summary

This chapter provides an overview of five decades of research on network models of neural systems. The discussion points to the existence of strongly held viewpoints about the proper approach towards integrating medical science and behavioral science databases into a unified science complete with mathematical expression. Discrete versus continuous modeling approaches are contrasted in order to bring into focus the role each must play in modeling sensory and cognitive processes. A challenge is presented to the medical and artificial neural network communities to seek a unification of computational neuroscience, behavioral science, and neural networks.

REFERENCES

1. Anderson, J. A. and E. Rosenfeld. Eds. *Neurocomputing, Foundations of Research* (Cambridge, MA: MIT Press, 1988).
2. Levine, D. S. *Introduction to Neural and Cognitive Modeling* (Hillsdale, NJ: Erlbaum Press, 1991).
3. McCulloch, W. S. and W. Pitts. "A Logical Calculus of the Ideas Immanent in Nervous Activity," *Bull. Math. Biophys.* 5(4):115–133 (1943).
4. Pitts, W. and W. S. McCulloch. "How We Know Universals: the Perception of Auditory and Visual Forms," *Bull. Math. Biophys.* 9(3):127–147 (1947).
5. Rosenblatt, F. "The Perceptron: A Probabilistic Model for Information Storage and Organization in the Brain," *Psychol. Rev.* 65(6):386–408 (1958).
6. White, D. and D. Sofge. *Handbook of Intelligent Control: Neural, Adaptive and Fuzzy Approaches* (New York: Van Nostrand, 1992).
7. Grossberg, S. "A Neural Theory of Punishment and Avoidance. I. Qualitative Theory," *Math. Biosci.* 15(1/2):39–67, (1972).
8. Grossberg, S. "A Neural Theory of Punishment and Avoidance. II. Quantitative Theory," *Math. Biosci.* 15(3/4):253–285, (1972).
9. Rashevsky, N. *Mathematical Biophysics*, Vols. 1 and 2 (New York: Dover, 1960).
10. Berge, P., Y. Pomeau, and C. Vidal. *Order Within Chaos: Towards A Deterministic Approach To Turbulence* (New York: J. Wiley, 1984).
11. Nagel, E. and J. R. Newman. *Gödel's Proof* (New York: New York University Press, 1958).
12. Kugler, P. N. and M. T. Turvey. *Information, Natural Law, and the Self-Assemble of Rhythmic Movements* (Hillsdale, NJ: Lawrence Erlbaum Associates, 1987).
13. Bohm, D. *Wholeness and the Implicate Order* (New York: Routledge & Kegan Paul, 1980).
14. Prueitt, P. S. and D. S. Levine. "Specifying a Theory of Sensory and Cognitive Processes," in progress. Also available as NNRF #31, Physics Dept., Georgetown University, Washington, D.C.
15. Pattee, H. "The Nature of Hierarchial Control in Living Matter," in *Foundations of Mathematical Biology*, Vol. 1, *Subcellular Systems* (New York: Academic Press, 1972).
16. Amari, S. I. "Neural Theory of Association and Concept Formation," *Biol. Cybern.* 26(3):175–185 (1977).
17. Barto, A. G., R. S. Sutton, and C. W. Anderson. "Neuron-Like Adaptive Elements that Can Solve Difficult Learning Control Problems," *IEEE Trans. Syst., Man Cybern.* SMC-13(5):834–846 (1983).
18. Grossberg, S. and E. Mingolla. "Neural Dynamics of Perceptual Grouping: Textures, Boundaries, and Emergent Segmentations," *Percept. Psychophys.* 38(2):141–171 (1985).

19. Grossberg, S. "How Does a Brain Build a Cognitive Code?" *Psychol. Rev.* 87(1):1–51 (1980).

20. Grossberg, S. Ed. *Neural Networks and Natural Intelligence* (Cambridge, MA: MIT Press, 1988).

21. Hubel, D. H. and T. N. Wiesel. "Receptive Fields, Binocular Interaction, and Functional Architecture in the Cat's Visual Cortex," *J. Physiol.* 160(1):106–154 (1962).

22. von der Malsburg, C. "Self-Organization of Orientation Sensitive Cells in the Striate Cortex," *Kybernetik* 14(1):85–100 (1973).

23. Hopfield, J. J. "Neural Networks and Physical Systems with Emergent Collective Computational Abilities," *Proc. Natl. Acad. Sci.* 79(8):2554–2558 (1982).

24. Kohonen, T. "Self-Organized Formation of Topologically Correct Feature Maps," *Biol. Cybern.* 43(1):59–69 (1983).

25. Grossberg, S. and D. Levine. "Some Developmental Biases in the Contrast Enhancement and Short Term Memory of Recurrent Neural Networks," *J. Theor. Bio.* 53(2):341–380 (1975).

26. Grossberg, S. and N. A. Schmajuk. "Neural Dynamics of Pavlovian Conditioning: Conditioned Reinforcement, Habituation, and Opponent Processing," *Psychobiology* 15(3):195–240 (1987).

27. Cohen, M. A. and S. Grossberg. "Absolute Stability of Global Pattern Formation and Parallel Memory Storage by Competitive Neural Networks," *Trans. IEEE Syst., Man Cybern.* SMC-13(5):815–826 (1983).

28. Carpenter, G. A. and S. Grossberg. "The ART of Adaptive Pattern Recognition by a Self-Organizing Neural Network," *Computer* 21(3):77–88 (1988).

29. Levine D. S. and P. S. Prueitt. "Modeling Some Effects of Frontal Lobe Damage: Novelty and Perseveration," *Neural Networks* 2(2):103–116 (1989).

30. Bullock, D. and S. Grossberg. "Neural Dynamics of Planned Arm Movements: Emergent Invariants and Speed-Accuracy Properties During Trajectory Formation," *Psychol. Rev.* 95(1):49–90 (1988).

31. Levine D. S. and P. S. Prueitt. "Simulations of Conditioned Perseveration and Novelty Preference From Frontal Lobe Damage," in *Neural Network Models of Conditioning and Action*, M. Commons and S. Grossberg, Eds. (Hillsdale, NJ: Erlbaum Press, 1991).

32. Levine, D. S. "Neural Population Modeling and Psychology: A Review," *Math. Biosci.* 66(1):1–86 (1983).

33. Atlan, H. and I. R. Cohen. *Theories of Immune Networks* (New York: Springer-Verlag 1989).

34. Eisenfeld, J. "Switching Network Models," in *Immunology via Formal Interpretation of Diagrams. Biomedical Modeling and Simulation*, J. Eisenfeld and D. S. Levine, Eds. (Basel: J. C. Baltzer AG, 1989) pp. 189–195.

35. Hall, F. M. *An Introduction To Abstract Algebra* (Cambridge: Cambridge University Press, 1969).

36. Pribram, K. H., M. Nuwer, and R. J. Baron. "The Holographic Hypothesis of Memory Structure in Brain Function and Perception," in *Contemporary Develops in Mathematical Psychology*, Vol. 2, *Measurement, Psychophysics, and Neural Information Processing*, D. H. Krantz, R. C. Atkinson, R. D. Luce, and P. Suppes, Eds. (San Francisco: W. H. Freeman, 1974) pp. 416–457.

37. Schneider, W. "Connectionism: Is it a Paradigm Shift For Psychology?," *Behavioral Research Methods, Instruments, and Computers* 19(2):73–83 (1987).
38. Hameroff, S. R. *Ultimate Computing, Biomolecular Consciousness and Nanotechnology* (Amsterdam: North Holland, 1987).
39. Pribram, K. *Brain and Perception; Holonomy and Structure in Figural Processing* (Hillsdale, NJ: Erlbaum, 1991) chap 1.
40. Minsky, M. and S. Papert. *Perceptrons* (Cambridge: MIT Press, 1969) pp. 1–20.

CHAPTER 8

Ethology and Noninvasive Techniques

Peter H. Klopfer

8.0 History of Animal Behavior Studies

The study of animal behavior is hardly a modern development. The Greek philosophers, foremost among them Aristotle, articulated and formalized what was then the state of the art. Aristotle's span was prodigious. At least one noted psychologist and historian of science has claimed that there exists no single theme in modern psychology which had not previously been addressed by Aristotle. Not that Aristotle always had his facts right! Nonetheless, much of what he says does indeed have a modern ring, not least what he had to say about animals. For about 2000 years, from Aristotle to Darwin, almost nothing important was added to our understanding of animals, and indeed, a great deal of foolishness propounded: in 18th century England a pig that escaped into a neighbor's garden could be tried and hung for a deliberate act of trespass!

With the flowering of science in the next century, however, natural history and particularly behavior studies came into their own. Ethology, a term that had previously been applied to the portrayal of human characters on a stage, was redefined as "the study of animals, not as corpses reeking with formaldehyde—but as living things in their natural habitat".[1]

0-87371-504-7/93/$0.00+$.50
© 1993 by Lewis Publishers

Interestingly, this redefined sense of ethology did not immediately catch on. When its use did become more widespread, it was largely identified with the writings of ardent Lamarckians, those who believed in the inheritance of acquired traits. Biologists such as Alfred Giard* (in the mid-19th century) popularized both the term and Lamarck's views on how individual adaptations to the environment influenced the appearance (and hence evolution) of one's offspring. As Lamarck's views lost ground, so did the use of ethology. It was not until the 1940s that the term regained any measure of popularity, as noted below.

The term ethology aside, the field itself also underwent changes. Before Darwin, the study of behavior had largely practical goals: improved husbandry, or better sport. Indeed, breeders of racing pigeons contributed in no small way to the development of Darwin's views on the power of selective breeding in shaping a species. However, with the acceptance (at least by many biologists) of Darwin's evolutionary models the focus of ethologists shifted to more theoretical issues. Specifically, it was the evolution of mental capacities and the "laws" of mental evolution which became the topics of interest.

Foremost among the new, evolutionary-oriented breed of ethologists was surely the Englishman, Lloyd Morgan. He disdained as sterile the controversies as to whether a given behavior pattern was "innate" or "acquired", conscious or unconscious. He developed experimental methods that precluded consideration of factors not under the experimenter's control. "Never use a complex explanation if a simpler one will do" is a crude statement of Morgan's canon. A similar attitude pervaded the work of Jacques Loeb, who pioneered physiological (or mechanistic) approaches to the study of behavior. Neither man had patience for vague, nondemonstrable concepts such as "consciousness".

A host of other workers were also active in the last half of the 19th century, though to discuss them all might be tedious. Let us, however, at least mention the prodigious Herbert Spencer, who contributed a volume on the evolution of behavior, along with reams on every other conceivable topic. And let us not forget Charles Darwin himself, who wrote several books that dealt explicitly with the evolution of behavior, and his successor in this domain, George John Romanes. Finally, there was the sagacious William James, generally regarded as the founder of comparative psychology, and of whom it was said he was as good a novelist as his brother Henry was a psychologist. Yet, William James left us a far richer heritage than pleasantly written tracts. Indeed, he is the most "modern" of the 19th century's ethologists.

As the 19th century ended, behavioral studies on the two continents, the Old World and the New, diverged. How much of this was chance? How much a reflection of fundamental differences in the way of life and world view? This is an issue well suited to historical analysis, but we can avoid answering it here. The fact that the behavior studies in the U.S. were largely characterized by their experimental nature: homogeneous populations were selected as subjects (most

---

* For references to these and others mentioned, see Klopfer.[2]

often inbred mice and pigeons), environments were "simplified" and conditions systematically varied. Of course, this is a parody. Not only did the Skinner box (an automated device by which rats or pigeons were trained to peck or press bars in response to particular signals) not appear full blown on the scene in 1900, but a great many Americans continued studying behavior in the naturalistic tradition. Some were truly amateurs, as the author-explorer Earnest Thomas Seton, whose descriptions of wildlife behavior beguile all who read him, or the ornithologist Margaret M. Nice. Others, like Charles Whitman and William Wheeler, set standards of clarity, originality, and precision that continue to serve us today, though their work is more readily classified as "naturalistic" than "experimental". Some experimentalists, as for instance J. B. Watson, the "behavioristic psychologist", began scientific careers doing naturalistic studies. In Watson's case, his work on bird behavior with K. S. Lashley, later the founder of modern neurobiology, was as important a contribution in its time as were his later theories on how behavior can be controlled by the environment.

Still, in all, the U.S. became the home of the vigorous laboratory-minded study of behavior, usually under the aegis of "comparative" psychologists. Their goal, it must be noted, was less to understand the behavior of their subjects than to trace the course of mental evolution or to understand the mechanism underlying behavior.

By contrast, in Europe the naturalistic tradition continued to dominate the scientific scene, though here, too, the alternative camp was not without representation. Indeed, the mechanistic approach of the laboratory scientists had its start in the physiology labs of Germany, not in the U.S. The dominant figures in the 20th century Old World, however, were indisputably the naturalists, from Julian Huxley through David Lack in England, and Oscar Heinroth to Konrad Lorenz and Niko Tinbergen on the continent (though they performed experiments, too). Wolfgang Köhler and his studies of reasoning in apes, or Karl von Frisch with the dancing bees, combined the two traditions, naturalistic and experimental, so completely as to defy classification. Yet the two worlds did differ. Perhaps the major aspect of the difference was less in method than in goal: for the psychologists of the U.S., it was to understand the "structure" and "rules" of behavior; for the Old World counterparts it was issues of adaptive purpose and ecological significance that mattered most. How does the frequency of rewards alter behavior, as opposed to the question why is one substance more effective as a reward than another?[2]

8.1 Goals of Behavior Studies

Where the emphasis is on understanding mechanisms, it is perhaps inevitable that the animal comes to be viewed as a device which can be systematically altered so as to provide clues as to its construction. In contrast, when the questions relate to adaptive function ("what good is it?"), or evolution, the intact and normal animal itself becomes the focus. Classical ethology, in particular, though not eschewing issues of mechanism, was particularly committed to the latter. This, however, entailed seeing the world through the eyes of the subject. This notion is captured by the term *Umwelt*, introduced by J. von Üxkuell in his effort to describe the perceptual world of animals. Bees, with their sensitivity to ultraviolet light, obviously may see several white flowers, which appear to us as identical, as if they were of different hues. Cave fish, blind but sensitive to electromagnetic fields, "see" the world differently from their sighted brethren. In developing the capacity to appreciate such differences, the experimenter apparently comes to place the subject at the center of his/her interests, rather than just the physiological or behavioral mechanisms the organism embodies.

Should a specific date for the founding of ethology ("the objectivistic study of animal behavior") be required, it would most likely have to be the date of publication of Niko Tinbergen's article with that title in 1942.[3] The founding is, in any case, contemporaneous with the appearance of the works of Niko Tinbergen and Konrad Lorenz, whose Nobel awards (shared with Karl von Frisch) acknowledge the seminal importance of their work. But why do we study animals and their behavior? To what extent is intervention, from occasional disturbance of free-living individuals to vivisection, a necessary component of that study? What alternative to intrusive methodologies have ethologists to offer, both within their own domain and for scientists in other areas?

8.2 Ethological Techniques

A consequence of the ethological emphasis on understanding the functions and evolutionary history of behavior is that eschewal of techniques injurious to the subject becomes essential. At the same time, ethologists were not long satisfied with the crude, qualitative data to which naturalistic observation often limits one. Hence, ethologists have pioneered the development of a variety of unintrusive observational recording techniques.

Three major categories of ethological study can be recognized, though the distinctions are not absolute and grade into each other. At one extreme are direct observations of animals by a hidden observer, who interferes not at all. Next, come manipulations of the environment with observations of the subjects' responses to the changes. A further step entails more drastic alterations in the animals' perception of the environment, and includes some direct interference with what the animal might do or perceive. Some examples follow.

8.2.1 Direct Observations

Simple as these might seem, they are unlikely to be of value unless based on techniques which circumvent our human tendency to see what we expect to find. Thus, most western observers invariably record more "aggressive" encounters when the subjects they observe are identified to them as "male", and fewer when they are told the subjects are "female", irrespective of the actual sex. Protagonists of observational methods have spent considerable effort devising methodologies which avoid the various kinds of observer bias. Consider this study of "allo-parenting", the caretaking of an infant by an individual other than its parent, by Deanne Lee (Duke University Primate Center).

Lee's interest lay in discovering whether some individuals were more likely to alloparent than others, and if so, the attributes that were associated with this heightened likelihood of care. She had first to define the phenomenon so that anyone could recognize its occurrence; then she had to identify the attribute(s) which she would test for association with the alloparenting. Next came the task of developing a census method which would not be biased through her paying more attention to one individual in her sample than another. Finally, appropriate statistical procedures had to be selected for evaluation of her data. Following is her description of the procedure.

I. Materials and Methods

A. Subject and study site

The present study was conducted with a group of semi-free ranging ring-tailed lemurs (*Lemur catta*) that are living in an 8.2 acre, outdoor natural habitat area at the Duke University Primate Center (DUPC) in Durham, North Carolina with ten *Lemur fulvus rufus* and five *Varecia variegata variegate*. At the time of the present study, the ring-tailed lemur group consisted of twenty-three individuals. All animals were easily identifiable by individual neck collars and tags while their age and genealogical histories were obtained from the Primate Center records.

B. Data collection

Prior to the beginning of the birth season, all adult ring-tailed lemurs were placed in a dominance hierarchy on the basis of the outcome of agonistic interactions as defined by Pereira (in preparation). Each animal in the group was a focal animal for ten 10-minute sessions. A dominance index was calculated for each individual involved in either female-female or male-male agonistic interactions. Dominance indices were not calculated for female-male agonistic interactions, as *Lemur catta* possess separate male and female dominance hierarchies.

Upon birth of the infants, I recorded all interactions directed towards each mother-infant pair by all group members. Each pair was observed alternately for 15-minute focal samples from within 5 meters. Weather permitting, at least one focal session was conducted daily on each mother-infant pair for the infant's first four weeks of life.

All predefined interactions between the focal mother-infant pair and any group member were recorded on a checksheet along with the alloparent's identity, duration of the caretaking bout, and the mother and infant's reaction to the alloparent and/or behavior. Acceptance of the alloparent and its behavior by either mother or infant was recorded as "O". Reactions towards the alloparent and its behavior by the local mother was recorded as either aggressive or submissive (see above). Rejection of the alloparent and its behavior by the focal infant was recorded as one or a combination of the following types of behavior:

- Clinging (CL):   infant holds tightly onto its mother when the alloparent attempts to remove it from the mother's body.
- Moving away (MO):   while on its mother, the infant changes its position to increase the distance between it and the alloparent.
- Vocalization (VO):   infant vocalizes when the alloparent grooms too vigorously or attempts to remove it from the mother's body.

Changes in the behavior of the mother and/or infant towards the alloparent during the alloparental bout were also recorded. An infant's return to its mother after an infant-initiated transfer (IT) or a removal with locomotion (RM) was noted to facilitate future reconstruction of the sequence of alloparental bouts. Duration of periods of non-contact between the infant and either mother or alloparent was also recorded to document the infant's increasing independence from its mother. The nearest neighbor of each focal pair and the current maternal behavior exhibited towards the infant (i.e., grooming, nursing) were noted at 3-minute intervals. The duration and frequency of grooming bouts performed by the mother on her infant were recorded, where the end of one bout and the beginning of another bout were separated by at least five seconds without grooming.

C. Data analysis

All data were entered into the dBASE III Plus management system. To test the null hypothesis that no general relationship existed between the frequency of alloparenting and dominance in *Lemur catta*, I used the Spearman Rank Correlation test. Ranks were first assigned to each animal in which a rank of "1" signified the dominant individual and animals of the same dominance received an average rank. Ranks were assigned to the frequency of alloparent bouts performed by each individual where a value of "1" designated the lowest number of bouts.

To assess relationships between rank and the frequency of alloparental behavioral patterns of alloparenting that could not be examined thoroughly with the Spearman rank test, I applied the G-test to compare with expected and observed frequencies of the defined behavior patterns stated in the following null hypotheses:

1. All infants have equal chances of receiving all patterns of alloparental behavior.
2. The frequency of received alloparenting is independent of the rank of the mother-infant pair.
3. The frequency of performed alloparenting is equivalent for conspecifics of all ranks.
4. The frequency of performed alloparenting is the same for males and for females.

5. The frequency of performed alloparenting is equivalent for infants, juveniles, and adults.

The results of the application of this test are presented in the form of a histogram.

I used the non-parametric Mann-Whitney U-test to examine equivalence in the mean durations of alloparenting performed by males and females. I applied the non-parametric Kruskal-Wallis One-way Analysis of Variance by Ranks to test the following null hypotheses:

1. The duration of received alloparenting bouts is independent of the rank of the mother-infant pair.
2. The durations of performed alloparental bouts are equivalent for con specifics of all ranks.
3. The durations of performed alloparental bouts by infants, juveniles, and adults are equal.

The results of Ms. Lee's study indicated *inter alia* that higher ranking mother-infant pairs received more alloparenting.

8.2.2 Environmental Manipulations

When the events of interest occur infrequently, the impatient observer may need to induce their occurrence. If this is appropriately done, it may enhance one's ability to gain information about the subject's behavior. Consider this study by Pamela Yount (Duke University Primate Center), who wished to know if lemurs distinguished and recognized the calls of hawks, potential (but rare) predators on young lemurs. Given that only one of the above variables, call structure or rarity, is involved in discrimination between predatory and nonpredatory bird calls by *Lemur catta*, the following predictions were made:

Prediction 1: If call structure is the cue used to discriminate harmful from harmless avian stimuli, then playbacks of only the normal hawk call should elicit a response.

Prediction 2: If call rarity is the cue used to discriminate harmful from harmless avian stimuli, then the normal hawk call, the hawk call played backwards, and the backwards thrush call should elicit a response.

There were two other possible outcomes. First, if characteristics of hawk call other than call structure (such as call duration or frequency range) can be used to discriminate harmful from harmless avian stimuli even though the organization of the call structure has been rearranged by playing it backwards, then the reverse hawk call in addition to the forward hawk call should elicit a response. In this case, we would not be able to discern whether rarity of the variables of the call structure, or the variables themselves elicited a response. The elements making up the hawk call would still be rare, while those of the thrush would not be. A further study would be necessary to evaluate the role of rarity in the variable of the hawk call structure in eliciting a response. The second outcome was that the reverse thrush call, but not the reverse hawk call, might elicit a response; however, no logical reason for this outcome was obvious.

II. Methodology

A group of 21 ringtailed lemurs inhabiting a natural habitat enclosure (NHE) at the DUPC center were used in the study. This group inhabits a 3.5 ha. NHE(NHE-2) and consists of 6 female and 5 male adults (>3 years), 5 juveniles (1–2 years), and 5 infants (<1 year). All but the oldest male and female in this group were born in enclosure or have lived there since weaning. This group was originally released into the enclosure in 1981. Most members are related and a well-defined social system exists here.

The two bird species calls used in the playbacks were 1) a North Carolina hawk, the Redtailed hawk—*Buteo jamaicensis*—and the Wood Thrush—*Hylocichia mustelia*—also native to North Carolina. Both calls are in the range of 2 to 4 kHz. The volume of the playbacks was normalized to eliminate possible proximity effects. Playbacks were performed at 70 to 72 decibels, which is intermediate between natural volumes for the thrush call and the hawk call. The number of call repetition and the duration in which this set of calls takes place were also normalized for playbacks, to eliminate possible effects of these two variables on the extent of response. Five call repetitions within 30 seconds were made during each playback. Call playbacks were performed by a Sony TC-D5M cassette recorder through a Mineroff Electronic Field Speaker. Recordings of calls were played from TDK-ADX tape. Responses were recorded with a Curtis Mathis Video Camera onto TDK-HS videotape.

Playbacks were performed to animals in the trees, rather than to those on the ground. This decision was based on two reasons: 1) Animals in the trees (in contrast to those on the ground) should be less aware of the experimenters setting up speakers and performing videotaping on the ground, and thus may not show habituation effects to the experimental procedure that would otherwise occur; and 2) Most reactions seen previously in response to playbacks with animals on the ground involved standing bipedally or jumping into the trees—reactions that do not necessarily demonstrate an awareness of an aerial predator. Reactions of subjects in the trees to the playbacks might be more easily identified as antihawk behavior. An animal in the trees is most vulnerable to a hawk if it is high in the tree or on a peripheral branch. An animal is also in danger if it comes out of the tree onto the open ground. Reactions to playbacks where individuals moved in or down in the trees (but not out to the trees) could thus be considered as antihawk behavior. Unfortunately, it was not possible to record the identity of individuals because of the height animals were at during the playbacks. Thus, we could not discriminate between the reactions of juveniles and adults. This created the possibility of "diluting" adult reactions with reactions of inexperienced juveniles and exaggerating adult responses by including juvenile "overreactions".

Eleven trials, consisting of one playback type per trial, were conducted between April 2, 1989 and April 20, 1989. Playbacks were attempted each day, during this period where weather and scheduling conditions allowed. The minimum intertrial interval was 24 hours, although most intervals were longer. The four types of call playbacks were played in a random order which was assigned in advance. On dates where no playbacks occurred (and when weather conditions permitted), the researchers responsible for collecting data visited the group and carried out the experimental protocol in the absence of actual playbacks. Trials were usually conducted between 6:00 p.m. and 8:00 p.m. to minimize interference with other observations of the lemurs and to insure that a maximum number of animals would be in the trees during the playback.

The procedure for the playbacks involved first locating the *Lemur catta* group and following them until several members of the group went into the trees to feed. This activity usually occurred at a height of at least 10 meters. Performing the playbacks while the animals were feeding insured that they would be relatively stable, that is not moving up or down or from tree to tree. A group of 4 to 8 individuals in the trees was then selected. After this group had stabilized, the field speaker was concealed on the ground under brush and leaves at a minimum distance of ten meters from the trees occupied by the group. Operation of the speaker was performed at least five meters away from the speaker by means of an extended speaker wire connected to the tape recorder. One researcher focused on this group with the video camera. The group was filmed for 16 seconds before the playback, during the playback, and for 16 seconds after the playback.

Through videotape analysis, the proportion of individuals on the tape doing each of the following activities after each call repetition were determined: 1) moving down in the trees or from the periphery to the center of the tree before the playback, 2) moving down in the trees or from the periphery to the center of the tree after the playback, and 3) moving out of the trees. Data analysis involved the use of the G-Test in evaluating the proportion of individuals observed responding to a "call."

Ms. Yount did find evidence of a discriminative response to the hawk call.

8.2.3 Interference

Finally, we progress to studies in which some interference with the animals perceptions or actions takes place. For example, Schmidt-Koenig and Schlichte[4] fitted homing pigeons with contact lenses that interfered with their ability to form an image. In this way, they could rule out visual land marks in homing (the birds with frosted lenses still homed and their lenses were then removed). Interference need not involve physical alterations. To study the role of the solar clock in orientation, Schmidt-Koenig[5] merely advanced the onset of daybreak and sunset by 6 h (once using artificial light, another time by jetting the pigeons across country at high speed). The birds were unharmed, but the nature of the errors they made in compass orientation provided clues on how they managed navigational feats.

Other ethologists have occasionally employed more direct invasive techniques. Some early studies exploited electrophysiological methods, eliciting stereotyped (supposedly "innate" behavior) by stimulation of particular regions of the brain through chronically implanted electrodes. More commonly, however, ethologists exploited natural accidents, analyzing responses, e.g., of congenitally blind subjects in order to determine the role of visual inputs.[6] The rationale underlying the avoidance of surgical (and other) interventions assumes a deliberately damaged system is less likely to yield nonartifactual results than analyses of intact systems, or those deviations from the norm that result from natural processes. In all likelihood, an esthetic element is also involved: for those to whom understanding the subject animal is an end in itself, damaging the subject to gain knowledge is akin to cheating at solitaire. Indeed, this is a predominant trait of many "curious naturalists",[7] even those who believe that some questions are of an importance to justify invasive procedures. Ethologists, as a group, are, if anything, too inclined to identify with the subjects of their study! That, of course, is why ethological methodologies may be of general utility to those using animals.

8.3 Summary

Animal behavior studies have a history that can be traced to Aristotelian times, though experimental approaches date largely from Darwin's time. Naturalistic (observational) and laboratory studies (entailing direct interference, by behavioral, surgical, or other invasive means) developed relatively independently of each other, though a few investigators (viz, Lashley) availed themselves of both approaches.

Modern ethology, which became a distinct field of inquiry in the late 1940s and early 1950s, brought the experimental and observational approaches together, focusing on questions of function, evolution, mechanism, and development. An emphasis on sound experimental design still plays a major role in ethology, but increasingly these designs avoid treatments that traumatize the subjects. Many ethologists have been as much motivated by their love of animals as by their scientific zeal. This, and the realization that undamaged animals may be more informative, is leading to a decreasing dependence on invasive techniques.

REFERENCES

1. Jaynes, J. "The Historical Origins of 'Ethology' and 'Comparative Psychology'," *Anim. Behav.* 17(4):601–606 (1969).
2. Klopfer, P. H. *An Introduction to Animal Behavior: Ethology's First Century* (New Jersey: Prentice-Hall 1974).
3. Tinbergen, N. "An Objective Study of the Innate Behavior of Animals," *Biblioth. Biotheor.* 1(1):39–98 (1942).
4. Schmidt-Koenig, K. and H. T. Schlichte. "Homing in Pigeons with Improved Vision," *Proc. Nat. Acad. Sci. U.S.A.* 69(9):2446–2447 (1972).
5. Schmidt-Koenig, K. *Migration and Homing in Animals* (Berlin: Springer-Verlag, 1975).
6. Eibl-Eibesfeldt, I. *Ethology: the Biology of Behavior* (New York: Holt, Rinehard, and Winston, 1970).
7. Tinbergen, N. *Curious Naturalists* (London: Country Life, 1958).

ADDITIONAL READING

Alberts, A. "Ultraviolet Visual Sensitivity in Desert Iguanas: Implications for Pheromone Detection" *Anim. Behav.* 38(1):129–137 (1989).

Birke, L. "How Do Gender Differences in Behavior Develop? A Reanalysis of the Role of Early Experience," in *Perspectives in Ethology*, P. P. G. Bateson and P. Klopfer, Eds. (New York: Plenum, 1989) pp. 215–242.

Gendron, R. "Searching for Cryptic Prey: Evidence for Optimal Search Rates and the Information of Search Images in Quail," *Anim. Behav.* 34(3):898–912 (1986).

Gorden, D. "The Development of Flexibility in the Colony Organization of Harvester Ants," *Evolution of Social Behavior and Integrative Levels*, G. Greenberg and E. Toback, Eds. (New Jersey: Erlbaum, 1988) pp. 197–204.

Goss-Custard, J. D. and S. E. A. Durell. "Age-related Effects in Oyster-Catchers," *J. Anim. Ecol.* 56(2):549–558 (1987).

Hepper, P. G. "The Discrimination of Different Degrees of Relatedness in the Rat: Evidence for a Genetic Identifier?," *Anim. Behav.* 35(2):549–554 (1987).

Raleigh, M. J. and M. T. McGuire. "Female Influences on Male Dominance Acquisition in Captive Vervet Monkeys," *Anim. Behav.* 38(1):59–67 (1989).

Rowell, T. E. "What Do Male Monkeys Do Besides Competing?," in *Evolution of Social Behavior and Integrative Levels*, G. Greenbergand and E. Toback, Eds. (New Jersey: Erlbaum, 1988) pp. 205–212.

Theimer, T. C. "The Effect of Seed Dispersion on the Foraging Success of Dominant and Subordinant Dark-Eyed Juncos," *Anim. Behav.* 35(6):1883–1890 (1987).

Werner, D. I., E. M. Baker, E. C. Gonzalez, and I. R. Sousa. "Kinship Recognition and Grouping in Hatchling Green Iguanas," *Behav. Ecol. Sociobiol.* 21(1):83–89 (1987).

CHAPTER 9

Computation Modeling of Biological/ Medical Systems

Matthew Witten

9.0 Introduction

An apologetica is not an author's desire. However, the field of biological computing is so vast that, out of necessity, some editorial lines had to be drawn. Many of the subject areas in biological computing are subject areas unto themselves; artificial intelligence, image processing, computational chemistry/pharmacokinetics, and database/information systems, for example. As a consequence of this fact, I have chosen to focus upon a less-discussed facet of biocomputing, high-performance computing, and its role in biological modeling and simulation, interweaving other subject areas as necessary and relevant to the main discussion.

Why be involved in high-performance computing in the life sciences? We examine this question as part of the dual purpose of this chapter. First, it is important to understand the growing role of high-performance computing as it relates to computational modeling and simulation of complex biological systems. We will address this issue by examining the field of high-performance modeling and give examples or illustrations of what is being done in these areas of research. We will see how ultralarge-scale computing impacts the cost of medicine and why it is an extremely important discipline as the cost, the rigor, and the level of complexity of research increase. Second, having seen the various applications of high performance modeling of biological systems, we will examine the question of whether or not high performance computer modeling can help reduce and/or replace the use of animals in the research environment. Let us begin with a brief historical overview.

9.1 Modeling/Simulation of Living Systems

Circa the late 1800s the discipline of mathematics began to turn to biology/ecology as a source of intriguing mathematical problems. The very complexity that made life (pardon the pun) difficult for the experimental biologists, intrigued the mathematicians. The study of these varied complex biological systems lead to both simple and complex *mathematical biology* sprouted into being. The leading edge of computer technology moved forward and, as computers became more cost effective, simulation modeling became a more widely used mechanism for incorporating the necessary biological complexity into the original, often simplified, mathematical models. As an outgrowth of this phase of its development, mathematical biology added a strong component of computer modeling/simulation to its research toolbox.

Many factors discouraged belief in mathematical modeling as a viable tool. The experimentalists objected! The theoretical analyses were deficient in a variety of areas. The mathematical/computer models were still too simple to be useful in clinical and/or practical biological application. They lacked crucial biological/medical realism. In some instances, the necessary realism was barely understood by the practicing experimental physiologists. *How can we make models of things we don't understand? And, when we understand them, why will we need the models?* Mathematical modelers bawked at the demands for increased levels of biological complexity. The addition of the required biological reality often lead to significant alterations in the mathematical models; thereby making them intractable to formal mathematical analysis. Or else, the increase level of realism required extremely complex equations. And, such complexity required increased computational memory and ultrahigh computation speeds. In addition, the experimentalists often wanted a level of realism that demanded an understanding of the biological system well beyond known experimental results. In particular, the experimentalists were demanding a level of reality whose mathematical representation required building a model with numerous parameters; parameters whose values were not even known by the experimentalists.

With the advent of the new computer technologists, implementation capability for a more rich and complete biological reality is finally within the grasp of the mathematical/computer modeler. Mathematical complexity is no longer a serious issue as computation speeds are now practical enough to enable large large-modeling computations to be performed. Speeds are now measured in millions of instructions per second (MIPS) or in mega/giga flops (floating point operations per second), and mathematical/computational models with hundreds/thousands of equations are now routinely analyzed. Large memory is now routinely available. It is not unreasonable, for example, to consider memory sizes in the gigabyte range and to reasonably dream of terabytes of memory. In anticipation of these developments, highspeed, efficient, optimized numerical algorithms are routinely being developed.

Before we discuss the concept of high-performance computing and biological modeling/simulation, it is important to talk about the basic concept of *modeling*. In an excellent paper, Spanier[1] discusses some thoughts on the essentials of mathematical modeling. In this paper, he points out that a mathematical model is *a mathematical image of the physical process of interest which incorporates realistic assumptions and constraints*. Thus, a mathematical model is, in essence, one step removed from the reality that it is attempting to represent. Having stated the problem—*we wish to model a particular physical/biophysical system*—the first step of the modeling process involves translating the physical reality into a set of assumptions and constraints which are then, second step, represented by mathematical/simulation equations. This is a complex procedure which is, in many ways, as much an art as a science. (See References 2 through 57 for many useful examples and insights into the processes involved in mathematical/computer modeling.)

Oftentimes, the newly obtained model is exceedingly difficult to analyze; numerically, analytically, and/or biologically. This can arise for any number of reasons. At this point one has a variety of paths to follow: (1) brute force analysis,[25,28,39,42,47] (2) simulation,[2,16,54] (3) simplification and subsequent analysis,[54,55] or (4) recasting the model in a different, perhaps more tractable form. Brute force analysis may or may not lead to *useful* results. We italicize useful to emphasize the fact that what is useful to one party (say the mathematicians and/or computer scientists) may or not be useful to another party (say the biologists). A wonderful example of this dichotomy arises in the area of computational molecular biology and genetics.[58] The question of how efficient a particular database-search algorithm is gives rise to certain proofs that certain classes of search algorithm are NP complete. While this is of interest to the theoretical computer scientist, it is of little practical relevance to the biologist who still needs to perform the search/alignment match. The only useful information derivable from known NP completeness is that the search will be difficult to perform. We shall save simulation for a later point in the discussion. Simplification and subsequent analysis is often a saving approach. One returns to the original assumptions and attempts to make further, more simplifying and hopefully biologically meaningful/relevant assumptions concerning the real system. The hope is that the resulting model will be more tractable to the various tools of analysis. Additionally, one can recast the model in a different form/representation.

Having moved past the simplification stage, we attempt to analyze the model. This may involve analytical methods and/or simulation approaches. Once a solution is available, it is extremely important to *interpret* the solution. This requires comparison with the known biological dynamics. That is, we must compare our model results with the real world or experimental results. If there is a difference, the reasons for this difference must be ascertained and the model must be subsequently assessed and/or revised.

It cannot be overemphasized that the modeling/simulation process is an iterative process. It is iterative within itself and without itself. Within, there is the constant revision and analysis. Without, there is the constant comparison with the real-world dynamics: the experimental data, if you will. As a consequence, it is important to emphasize that models and simulations cannot live in a world disjoint from those systems they seek to represent. Each model must be compared against the available data (experimental) and constantly revised until it can be claimed to accurately mimic the reality it seeks to imitate.

Witten[2] discusses his thoughts about the essentials of simulation modeling and the various necessary approaches to formulating this class of representation/model. It is important to realize that a simulation model is, in a sense, two steps removed from the real world. This can be seen in the following way. There is the real world which we seek to represent. There is the understanding which we have of that reality. Then, there is our representation of that reality via mathematical equations. However, when these mathematical equations are translated into the computer, the computer must represent them so that it can understand them. The computer makes errors of representation in order to store such equations. Finally, when the equations are actually solved/simulated, there are errors of computation. Hence, simulation of biological process—processes which are not well understood—has numerous pitfalls and traps associated with it. It is crucial that all available biological data be integrated into these models so as to minimize as much error as is possible. This is illustrated in Figure 1. For further discussion on mathematical modeling philosophy see Avula.[3,4]

From the biological perspective, many new types of measurement systems have become available, with more methods being routinely developed. Model parameters once thought impossible to measure are now a routine measurement in the laboratory. There is an increasing improvement in the experimental data, both from the point of accuracy as well as repeatability. Hence, the new computer technology and the advances in the life sciences make biological modeling/simulation both practical and useful. With this brief history in mind, let us explore some of the diversity of biocomputing.

9.2 What Is High-Performance Computing?

The words high-performance computing imply a vision of some type of extremely fast computer quite able to leap tall buildings at a single bound. The typical vision is that of a very large mainframe machine with massive amounts of memory and an extremely rapid execution, cycle thereby allowing extensive amounts of calculations to be performed in a short period of time.

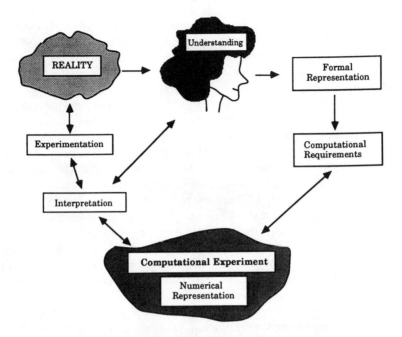

Figure 1.   The interplay of understanding, representation, and numerical simulation is illustrated by the multiple stages of this figure. In order to model reality, we must first have some level of understanding of that reality. This is gleaned by performing experiments and subsequently interpreting them. This forms our understanding of the reality. From here, a formal representation is developed. This can be in the form of a mathematical model or a computer simulation or any other alternative formal representation is developed, it is transformed into a computational model and computational experiments are performed. It is important to realize that, within such a model, there are many parameters. These parameters must be known accurately if the model is to give reliable results. A significant portion of the time, these parameter values can only be estimated by performing animal experiments of some sort. Once the parameters are known, the simulation results are then reinterpreted, perhaps suggesting new experiments and/or new understanding which can lead to further model refinements. It is important to emphasize that any mathematical/computer model of a biological system, particularly one that might have clinical relevance, must be well validated.

More recently, the *supercomputer* (vector/parallel) and the advanced architecture *workstation* have appeared on the scene. Suddenly, the researcher's ability to perform computations at rates of millions of floating point operations per second is within grasp. This new generation of machine is routinely 10 to 100 times as fast as the architectures of the 1960 and -70s. The new generation architectures approach speeds of 1000 times or more rapid as this same period.

What once occupied a rather large room now occupies a space less than a desktop. Hence, it behooves us to interpret high-performance computing in its most liberal manner; from large mainframes to tightly coupled networks of high-powered workstations, and down to single extremely fast single advanced architecture workstations. Thus, we constrain our definition of high-performance computing with respect to speed and memory, not by architecture and/or design. Within this context, we now consider the role of high-performance computing in the study of living systems.

The study of living systems implies the study of complexity and the necessary admission of incomplete knowledge as well as subjective observation and interpretation. Inherent in such a discipline as computational biology is the obvious and clear need to capture as much of the biological reality as is possible/known. Otherwise, the modeling effort becomes an exercise in mathematics and not in understanding the biology. As a consequence of these facts, computational models often contain vast amounts of complex equations which describe the various biological dynamics under study. There are, as we shall see, numerous examples of computational models having 10^1 to 10^6 or more equations.[59-63]

It follows that large, complex models generate large amounts of data. Data must be analyzed/visualized in order to ascertain the correctness of the modeling effort. Complex and/or massive data sets often require complex visualization/rendering techniques be applied in order to obtain useable scientific visualization.

Thus, we see that high-performance computing plays two important roles in the study of living systems: (1) modeling to obtain study data, and (2) subsequent analysis of that same data. We begin with the issues of data visualization/analysis.

9.3 Visualization

Visualization is a method of computing. It transforms the symbolic/numeric into the geometric, thereby enabling researchers to observe their simulations and computations. The life sciences are, by their very nature, visual/tactile sciences. They are visual in two ways: (1) directly, in that they handle data from images (X-ray, molecular modeling, and computational chemistry), and (2) indirectly, in that they handle complex data and transform it to a visual representation (mathematical and computer models, enzymic reaction simulations, physiological process models, image reconstruction, and medical diagnostics). When one looks at the various classes of medical data visualization problem, it is clear that they fall into the following three categories:

1. *Synthesis*—integration of information; preferably interactively and in real time
2. *Analysis*—interpretation and evaluation of the data by selectively displaying experimental and/or computational results within a comprehensible framework
3. *Communication*—bridging the gap between science and the people, between the sciences, and between the scientists themselves

In a sense, computer becomes the laboratory. And, as a consequence of this new development, *what was once done in the tube is now being done on the tube.*

9.3.1 Imaging

Perhaps the most obvious use of computers, in the visualization arena, is the handling of patient image data and/or the construction/reconstruction of medical image data for the purposes of clinical diagnosis and analysis. In the area of imaging, we recognize the following three major problem classes:

1. Simple rebuilding of two-dimensional (2-D) image (graphics) data into a useful/ useable 2-D image on a screen
2. Reconstruction of three-dimensional (3-D) images from 2-D scans, as well as direct 3-D full reconstruction/visualization
3. Visualization of an image in a realtime, interactive mode; given a 3-D image (say of the pelvis) can we manipulate it, in realtime, for the purposes of clinical examination?

As an outgrowth of attempts to address these three areas, from the computer science perspective, clinical medicine/clinical diagnosis has become more powerful. Nowhere has this been better demonstrated than in the areas of noninvasive medicine and image reconstruction; CAT, PET, and NMR scanners now inhabit most hospital complexes of any reasonable size. A further extension of this area of investigation may be found in the surgical planning systems (ANALYZE)[64] at the Mayo Clinic and at the Mallinkrodt Institute (Washington University at St. Louis). With these systems, physicians are now able to simulate a surgical procedure before it is performed on the patient, thereby minimizing potential hazard to the patient, and increasing surgical accuracy. Experimental science benefits as well. These same methods, when applied to experimental biology, allow us to begin to understand the biological and physiological functions of various organs and organ systems. For example, brain mapping studies have allowed us to investigate the cognitive function, as well as the physiological behavior of the brain.[65-67]

As an outgrowth of such analyses, we find that interesting questions arise in the area of visualization of multiple datasets of different types. For example, how can one effectively visualize the combined CAT, PET, NMR, and simulation data for a particular patient so that it is possible to visualize the bone, muscle, and metabolic data at the same time?

9.3.2 Realtime Visualization

Increasingly, the issue of real time visualization rears its head in other areas of research. Diverse biological disciplines turn to computer graphics and advanced imaging techniques as a means of studying (visualizing) subcellular, cellular, and supercellular biological phenomena. Molecular biologists study the dynamics of molecules and the issue of structure/function. Virologists use computer aided design techniques to study viral capsid structures and the dynamics of viral infection. Neurophysiologists/neurologists map the 3-D behavior of the brain, in an effort to understand questions of disease, behavior, and physiology. Bio-mechanicists study the behavior of muscles and bones as they attempt to investigate the healing process and the potential for using the computer to aid in bone replacement surgery.[68,69]

9.4 Computational Genetics

The analysis of genetic structure contains numerous interesting questions ripe for investigation. One of the more important of these questions is the issue of the evolution of the structure/complexity of the human genome. As experimental molecular biology sequences more and more of the genes in various species, we have a greater database of information which can be used to study evolutionary biology (see later section on the matrix of biological knowledge). Evolutionary biology questions are intensely scalar process, involving complex tree-search problems. Computational tree-search algorithms, implemented on parallel computers and on networks of smaller workstations (functioning in a parallel-like environment), can assist scientists in evaluating genetic evolutionary trees. And, in doing so, help them to understand the evolution of these genomic structures. In addition, these same algorithms can be used to study the related problem of the origin of the species. Linkage analysis, a complex mathematical analysis involving tree-search algorithms, is used to locate and to map gene structures, for the purposes of understanding inherited disorders.

At the gene sequencing level, mathematical and computational algorithms are utilized to align gene sequences, match gene sequences, to determine similarity between sequences to reconstruct gene sequences from sequence fragments, and to construct theoretical 3-D structures based upon those sequences. These hypothesized structures are subsequently compared to the experimental data and binding and/or transcription predictions can be made and/or analyzed for new insights into the biological dynamics of the gene. Harris et al.* (Abbot-Northwestern Hospital) have developed an hypothesis for a simple code for site specific recognition at the genetic level. Their work, based upon information derived from genetic sequence comparisons, X-ray crystallography data, and point mutation studies is intensely computer oriented at a number of levels. However, of great interest is that their predictions were substantiated by supercomputer simulations of the DNA-protein binding predicted by their model.

Beyond the issue of algorithms for searching, folding, alignment, and graphics, the gene sequencing problem gives rise to important questions in database design and analysis; particularly as related to the concept of integrated datasets. The incessant daily increase in biological information requires information systems that can handle massive amounts of data at rapid speeds. The integration of structural, sequence, biochemical, biological, genetic, and physicochemical datasets is not only increasingly important, but mandatory for effective pursuit of the new

---

* Personal communication.

generation of biological/medical research questions. In time, we will see artificial intelligence and neural net overlays to complex, high performance, database systems. These systems, learning from their users, will eventually be able to hypothesize biological questions and to search the database for possible examples/counter-examples. As their usage continues, it is possible to postulate that the systems will garner enough knowledge to formulate and/or deduce rules; thereby entering the *metaquery* stage of evolution.[70,71]

9.5 Computational Cell Biology

The dynamics of cell populations is of great interest to both biologists and clinicians. Understanding the cell cycle would have an impact upon our understanding of how to better control the development of various forms of cancer. From a therapeutic perspective, a mathematical model or enhanced simulation of cellular processes could be used to test treatment protocols and regimens before they were actually implemented upon the patient. Early work in this area was performed by Morrison, Aroesty, and Lincoln[119-123] at the RAND Corporation. These investigators developed a sophisticated mathematical model/computer simulation of cancer growth and treatment using ara-c. More recently, mathematical models of cell growth have been studied by Webb[124-125] (Vanderbilt University), Tucker and Zimmerman[96] (M.D. Anderson Cancer Center), Witten[73-77] (Univ. of Texas System–CHPC), Tyson (Virginia State), and others. These models have attempted to examine cell growth from a variety of perspectives.[72-133]

The early work, in the area of cell population dynamics, was based upon demographic construction (see Section 9.14 on computational population biology). The cells were treated as a fluid with an age/time structure. These models were unsatisfactory as they did not incorporate a number of relevant biological factors. Rubinow,[98] in a seminal treatise, proposed the introduction of a maturity variable μ as a means of overcoming this difficulty. And, while the *maturity/time* representation of cell models has had a reasonable amount of success, it still lacks sufficient detail to handle certain cell dynamics questions. More recently, Witten[77] and subsequently Zimmerman[97] have proposed that these models should be augmented with an additional variable called a *particle or property* variable. This *particle* may or may not be linked to flow through the cell cycle. These models lead to a class of generalized nonlinear stochastic hyperbolic partial differential equations in three variables. Of interest is the fact that the numerical issues arising in the study of these equations present highly complex as well as computer intensive problems.

Numerous investigators are examining cellular dynamics of neurons and other single cell types such as cardiac cells and intestinal cells. The flow of various intracellular and extracellular ions (calcium for example) is crucial to the correct behavior of these cells.

9.6 Computational Physiology

Human physiology attempts to explain the physical and the chemical factors that are responsible for the origin, the development, and the progression of human life. Human beings are complex machines built from equally complex systems (immune system, digestive system, nervous system, etc.). These systems contain multiple parts of organs (each a complex hierarchy of systems and subsystems). Realistic models of these systems can lead to a deeper understanding of the basic biology of these interacting bodily systems. And, as the models become more sophisticated, they can lead to a deeper understanding of the important synergism between the systems.[69]

9.7 Reproductive Biology

The ovaries are the repository of the female reproductive component, the follicles. Of the approximately 500,000 follicles present in the two ovaries at birth, only about 375 of these follicles will eventually develop into ova (eggs). World-wide, it has been demonstrated that there are increasing levels of infertility in both sexes. This is particularly true in the U.S. and in Poland. It is not at all clear what is causing such an increase to occur. As a consequence of this fact, it is of no small importance that the dynamics of the reproductive cycle be studied in detail. Such models might give insight into how the environment and/or other factors might play into the level of infertility displayed in a particular country or population. In addition, such models can be used to study the dynamics of aging in the mammalian reproductive system.

Mathematical models of the development of an egg have been made by a number of groups; Lacker (Courant Institute for Mathematical Sciences), Gosden et al. (England), and Witten (Univ. of Texas System–CHPC). These models represent various increasing levels of complexity in the mathematical modeling process. The basic premise of all of these models is that the follicle undergoes a series of stages or steps in its growth. These stages, and the transitions between them, are modeled by differential equations. This class of compartmental or Markov model can generate systems of equations that can be extremely large. The systems of equations range from fairly simple to fairly complex in their structure. The model system of Witten, for example, involves the solution of anywhere from 50,000 to over 200,000 nonlinear differential equations describing a probability distribution for a given number of eggs, in each stage (compartment) of development. The model is clearly computationally intensive in that it involves the solution of a large number of nonlinear differential equations.

On the male side, mathematical models of swimming tails (sperm without heads) have been studied by Fauci (Tulane University). This model is numerically intensive as it involves the solution of a swimming object in a viscous fluid; computational fluid dynamics.

9.8 The Heart of Supercomputing—Cardiac Dynamics

The cardiovascular system is fundamental to the life support of the human. Central to this system is the four chambered muscle called the heart. Arthur Winfree (University of Arizona) is involved in the mathematical modeling and computer simulation of nonlinear waves in excitable media. One particular example of an excitable medium is the heart muscle. Winfree has been studying circulating, vortex-like excitation (re-entrant tachycardia) in the heart as it is related to the onset of fibrillation—when the heart suddenly loses the rhythmic movement that allows it to pump blood. Within the context of his theory and simulations, Winfree has been able to show that two- and three-dimensional vortices arise in excitable media such as heart muscle and that they do so in ways that are predicted by his theory.[56,57,59]

At the University of Calgary, Wayne Giles[136,137] heads a research team that is investigating the electrical energy of the heart and its affect upon the organ's natural rhythm. He is particularly interested in how such a model could be utilized to study the interaction of cardiac function and cardiac drugs. Dr. Peter Backx, Dr. H. ter Keurs (University of Calgary) and Dr. S. Goldman (University of Guelph) have been involved in studying the property of propagated after-contractions in cardiac preparations.[135,136] Their mathematical model, involving up to 40,000 coupled ordinary differential equations, is numerically integrated to study the dynamics of calcium-mediated contractile waves in cardiac preparations.

Charles Peskin[139-144] (Courant Institute for Mathematical Sciences) is actively involved in cardiac modeling from a different perspective. He has been performing two- and now three-dimensional modeling of the heart, including valves, ventricles, and is now involved in adding atria and other vessels. This working model beats and moves the blood through the chambers of the heart. The model is a complex one involving a coupled system of equations modeling the wall, the blood, and the valve motion. The purpose of the Peskin research project is to develop a model that will allow for the design of artificial valves and their subsequent testing. In addition, he wishes to be able to study the affect of heart function on the valve design.

Peskin points out that such a model can be used for a number of other investigatory questions. For example, looking at the timing between the atrial and ventricular contraction—a clinically important facet of cardiac function, as sophisticated pacemakers can now separately pace the chambers. Finally, Peskin points out that such a model can be used to study heart disease and its affect on cardiac dynamics. He was able to use his model to show weakened capillary muscles, in the valve, lead to valve prolapse.[143,144]

Others have examined the issue of blood flow modeling. Dey* (Eastern Illinois University) has looked at viscous blood flow through an elastic tube, using conventional computational fluid dynamic models and techniques. Salathe (Rutgers

---

* Personal communication.

University) has been involved in issues of modeling and simulation as applied to the dynamics of the foot, both vascular and skeletal.

9.9 The Nervous System

The nervous system (along with the endocrine system) provides the control functions for the human body. The nervous system is responsible for the rapid activities of the body; muscular contraction, rapidly changing visceral events, and even the rates of secretion of some of the endocrine glands. It is a unique system in that it can control and perform a vast complex of actions. The human brain is estimated to contain approximately 10^{12} neurons. Many of these neurons are connected to 10,000 other neurons. Thus, in many ways, the brain is itself a sophisticated supercomputer.

At the single neuron level, Steve Young and Mark Ellisman (Laboratory for Neurocytology at the University of California, San Diego)[69] are using the supercomputer to reconstruct single neurons. The neurons are frozen, sliced into sections 0.25 to 5.0 μm thick, and photographed through a high voltage electron microscope. The computer is then used to reconstruct the slices and to subsequently view them on a graphics workstation. Ultimately such techniques can be integrated with advanced simulation modeling to allow the scientist to investigate and to simulate tissue activities and structure/function relationships. As these techniques are refined, researchers can envision methods for viewing, at the single cell level, Alzheimer's disease, which haunts the aged in our population. Perhaps, with these more sophisticated techniques, we will begin to understand how the disease progresses and how it might be treated.[69]

Chay (University of Pittsburgh)[145-148] has been studying the dynamics of excitable cells. In particular, she and her group have been trying to understand the behavior of channel gating in patch clamp data. Lagerlund (Mayo Clinic) has been examining the effects of axial diffusion on oxygen delivery in the peripheral nerve via mathematical modeling and computer simulation. It is known that victims of diabetes often suffer changes in their system of blood vessels. These changes reduce the supply of oxygen and nutrients to the tissue and subsequently damage the kidneys, retinas, and nerves. The work of Lagerlund has been to examine the mechanism of tissue damage in diabetes and how nutrients reach the cells. His work has been primarily concerned with diffusion of various nutrients and other substances through nerve tissue. A deeper understanding of these mechanisms could lead to a deeper understanding of and a subsequent treatment for a variety of nerve diseases caused by diabetes and other related conditions.

At a higher level of neural organization, Lagerlund, in addition to his kidney work, has developed computer models for modeling various features of the electroencephalogram (EEG) as recorded by scalp electrodes. Their model has been an attempt to understand the mechanisms that are responsible for the generation of the rhythmic fluctuations in potential.[151-152]

9.10 Computing the Kidney

The body fluids are extremely important to the basic physiology of the human being. The renal system, of which the kidneys are a part, is intimately tied to the dynamics of the body fluids. The kidneys perform two major functions: (1) they excrete most of the end-products of bodily metabolism; and (2) they control the concentrations of most of the constituents of the bodily fluids. Loss of kidney function can lead to death. Don Marsh (University of Southern California School of Medicine) is leading a group of investigators in large scale mathematical modeling and simulation of the kidney. He and his group have looked at two problems: (1) the concentrating mechanisms of the inner medulla of the kidney; and (2) the oscillation in tubular pressure initiated by the kidney's nonlinear control mechanism. The concentrating mechanism was modeled using a 3-D model of the kidney structure. It included longitudinal symmetry, tubules, and blood vessels. The group was able to demonstrate that the longitudinal symmetry played no part in the concentrating mechanism of the kidney. In their study of the oscillation in tubular pressure, Marsh's group is using a sophisticated system of partial differential equation models to describe the physiological control of the kidney tubular pressure. They have been able to show the existence of what appears to be a chaotic attractor in the system and that there is a period doubling bifurcation in the development of hypertension.[153,154]

9.11 Modeling the Dynamics of the Body

Mathematical/computer models of the limb motion are of importance in a number of areas, from robotics to biomechanics. Karl Newell (University of Illinois Urbana-Champaign) simulates limb movements using springmass models. Such models are currently used as a metaphor for the neuromuscular organization of limb motion. Other investigators, at the Illinois Institutes of Technology, are looking at modeling the biomechanics of the skeleton. Such models can then be used to study how collision forces are distributed through the skeletal structure. Hopefully, such understanding will lead to better ways to design sports equipment and other protective outer-wear. In addition, such models can better aid in the design of prosthetics and bioimplants.

At the cellular level, Frank and Rangayyan (University of Calgary) are examining ligament injuries and methods of treatment. Collagen fibrils, the basic building block of normal healthy ligament, are in nearly parallel arrangement when the ligament is healthy. In injured tissue, the arrangement is highly random. These investigators have been able to demonstrate that the randomness of the distribution depends upon the nature of the injury sustained and the stage of healing. As the tissues heal, the collagen fibrils realign in a process called collagen remodeling. Using the supercomputer for sophisticated and intense image processing, the investigators are attempting to interpret the realignment stages and to use such knowledge to more accurately treat trauma to the limbs.[155]

9.12 Patient-Based Physiological Simulation

Patient-based physiological modeling has come of age. More and more computer systems are being targeted at taking patient image data and reconstructing it so that a physician can view/review, in 3-D, a patient's X-ray, CAT, PET, NMR, as well as other clinical image data. Computerized surgery systems are currently in place at the Washington University of St. Louis, Mallincrodt Institute, and at the Mayo Clinic. Facial reconstruction and surgical simulation are no longer a pipe dream. They are a practiced reality. The day of the computer-enhanced mathematical scalpel has arrived.[59-62, 64-68]

Such workstation-based and mainframe-based systems allow one to dream of a new class of ultralarge-scale patient-based physiology simulations that could be performed with a high performance computing engine. At the VA Medical Center Minneapolis, Johnson and Vessella are developing a patient-based simulation of radioactive decay in the organs of the body. Such a problem is computer intensive in that it requires the mapping of the 3-D spatial distribution of radiolabeled compounds. In addition, the difficulty of the problem is enhanced by the fact that the radiation may travel a distance before it interacts with matter, and the irregular shapes of the organs do not lend themselves to simple dose–distance relationships.[156-158]

Project DaVinci (University of Illinois) is attempting to build a 3-D simulation of the human body. At the University of Texas System Center for High Performance Computing, we are looking at the problem of ultralarge-scale simulation of cellular system and the interaction between aging cellular system and cancerous ones. The increased graying of the U.S. population and the increased evidence of age-related cancer points to the fact that there will be increased healthcare costs to be borne by the healthcare system. Understanding of the dynamics of such a complex biological system will allow us to better understand how to treat cancer in an individual of advanced year.

9.13 Project Human

Beyond the complexity of such ultralarge-scale simulations and models is the no longer unreasonable goal of an ultralarge-scale simulation of a human being. Such a simulation would rely upon the patient's image data, noninvasive measurements of his physiological functions, and assorted clinical tests. One can begin to hypothesize scenarios in which chemotherapy can be simulated, in a given patient, before the therapy is performed. Radical and new-drug treatments can be simulated and the results can be examined and evaluated, not based upon an idealized mathematical model but rather, as based upon an integrated model and patient system. Eventually, one can envision the possibility of actually testing newly designed drugs (now designed in computers) in computer-based large-scale simulations. While it will be a long time before such a complex simulation/modeling system can be put into place, it is no longer a pipedream to imagine its existence. Project Human is slowly becoming a practical reality.

9.14 Computational Population Biology

The study of populations, particularly human populations, is called demography. Models in this area are general hyperbolic partial differential equations or their approximations. The canonical system is the McKendrick/Von Foerster[82-84] system given by

$$\frac{\partial n(t,a)}{\partial t} + \frac{\partial n(t,a)}{\partial a} = -\mu(t,a...)n(t,a)$$

$$n(t,0) = \int_0^\infty \gamma(t,a...)n(t,a)da$$

$$n(0,a) = n_0(a)$$

where $n(t,a)$ = the number (or density) of individuals of age a at time t
$\mu(t,a...)$ = the per capita mortality rate
$\gamma(t,a...)$ = the per capita birth rate
$n_0(a)$ = the initial population distribution and is a given

Should we choose to discretize "a" into a discrete age-class structure, we obtain a system of differential equations which approximate the original partial differential equation system.

The study of such models is of great interest for a number of reasons. In particular, given the increasing cost of healthcare and the associated increase of the aged component of the population, it is of great importance to understand the dynamics of the human population in an effort to hold down the cost of healthcare. In addition, models of this type arise in the study of toxicological effects of the environment upon a population (ecotoxicology). For example, how does PCB exposure (at the molecular-level computational physiology)? And, how is this result seen at the population level (the demographic-level computational population biology)?[71-135]

Mathematical modeling of diseases, particularly of such diseases as AIDS and Lyme disease, requires the use of computational methods. The models are routinely complex, often stochastic in nature, and quite frequently intractable to analytic solution methods. Models of this class have been studied by Hyman et al. (Los Alamos National Laboratories) and Levin et al. (Cornell University).

Epidemiology and biostatistics study population dynamics and characteristics from a probabilistic perspective. Clinical trials often generate large datasets. Statistical analysis of these datasets is often intense, due to the sample size and the complexity of the interactions. In addition, there are often issues of multicenter trials and the more recent problems arising in metastatistical analysis; the integration of originally disjoint datasets for the purposes of statistical analysis. In general, this class of problem is both computer dependent and computer intensive;

not only from the point of view of numerical computation, but also from the point of graphic visualization of the resultant computations.

9.15 Computational Chemistry

In his Philosophie Positif, A. Comte stated

> Every attempt to employ mathematical methods, in the study of chemical questions, must be considered profoundly irrational and contrary to the spirit of chemistry. If mathematical analysis should ever hold a prominent place in chemistry—an aberration which is happily almost impossible—it would occasion a rapid and widespread degeneration of that science.

Needless to say, the field of computational chemistry is a burgeoning field which is readily divided into the following major topic areas: (1) *biophysical properties* such as crystallographic reconstruction and molecular visualization, (2) *molecular biochemistry* which encompasses such areas as structure/function studies, enzyme/substrate studies (reaction studies, pathway analysis), and protein dynamics and their properties, (3) pharmacokinetics/pharmacodynamics, and (4) *nuclear chemistry/medicine*, which encompasses such areas as interactive molecular modeling, drug design/drug interactions (cancer chemotherapy, orphan drugs), binding studies (binding site properties), structure/function relationships as applied to drug effectiveness, and cell receptor structures. All of these areas involve intensive numeric computation and subsequent real-time graphics for the visualization of the final molecular/chemical structures. The computations are so intensive that a number of specialty high-speed super-workstations dedicated to real-time rapid visualization of chemistry/pharmacology oriented problems are currently being marketed. Of interest is the fact that, within the discipline of computational chemistry, the field of neutral nets is taking hold. Neutral nets (Wilcox at Minnesota Supercomputing Center, Liebman at Amoco Technology Corporation) are being used to learn to identify similar protein structures based upon recognition of pattern representations for the 3-D structure of proteins. This work is so intensive, particularly in the early learning stages, that it is performed on a vector supercomputer.[45]

While super-workstations and supercomputers are used for molecular visualization and dynamics, another computational issue is that of large-scale pharmacologic simulation; both at the molecular and the physiological levels. Here, we wish to assess the impact of a particular drug upon the given biological and/or physiological system or systems. Such problems involve large-scale numeric and symbolic databases, numerous systems of nonlinear differential/partial differential equations (with possible stochastic factors), and sophisticated numerical techniques for handling the numerical computations related to their solution; not to mention the associated visualization problems.

Computational fluid dynamics intertwines with computational chemistry in an effort to understand the structure of blood and to aid in the design of artificial blood.

9.16 Agricultural/Veterinary Applications

It is clear that the same issues that arise in human populations, in such areas as disease spread, environmental impact analysis, and epidemiology also arise in animal/insect populations. In addition to the obvious areas of investigation, one can investigate, via simulation modeling, such issues as crop yield, milk yield, nutritional demands, and more complex problems such as the interaction between genotype and environment as it relates to dairy-herd location. Other investigators have looked at breeding scheme problems in an effort to study the effects of genetic changes and genetic drift, with the goal of maximizing milk yield in a dairy herd or meat yield in a swine population. Finally, other investigators have been examining the question of how competing plants interact in an environment containing limited resources. These models/simulations have been extended to include pest management methods. Similar models exist for fisheries and for forestry management.

9.17 Computational Dentistry

What can be done with visualizing the bones and muscles in the torso can also be done with the jaw and the facial muscles. Many dental schools are collaborating with mechanical and biomedical engineers for the purpose of finite element modeling of the jaw (Day at the University of Louisville, Hart at Tulane University). The resultant models are then applied to examining the problems of orthodonture and of computer automated patient-based, dental prosthetics design.

One of the greatest dental healthcare costs is TMJ (temporal mandibular joint) syndrome. ETA Systems, in collaboration with the School of Dentistry at the University of Texas Health Science Center, San Antonio, is developing a neuro-muscular joint model, in an effort to study TMJ syndrome. The model involves, not only the use of sophisticated mathematical equations to describe the dynamics of the bones and muscles of the jaw, but also patient-based data as the input for describing these same structures. Thus, the models will be based upon real-patient data rather than hypothesized and/or idealized dental structures. Such models require the supercomputer to be used, not only as a computation engine for model simulation, but also as an image processing system to facilitate the handling of patient-based image data (CAT, NMR, PET, etc.).

Second only to the problem of TMJ syndrome is the problem of periodontal disease. This complex interplay between the bacterial ecology of the patient's mouth and the basic physiology of the patient is not very well understood. In a newly instigated and embarked upon project between the University of Texas

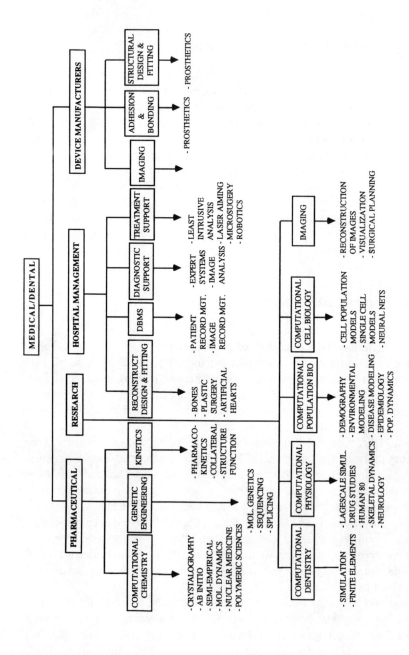

Figure 2.   In this figure we illustrate, in flow chart form, various aspects of medical/dental research and development using high performance computing tools. This is not exhaustive, but rather serves as a fairly condensed overview of the field.

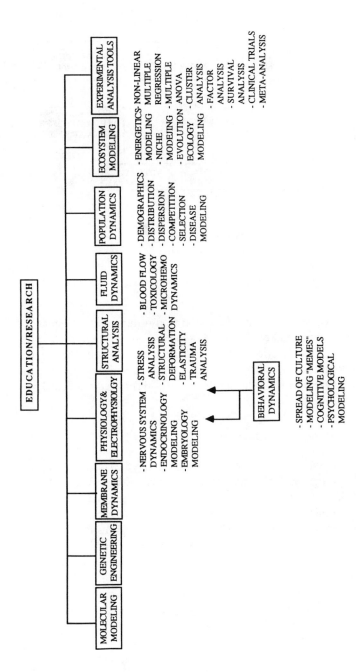

Figure 3. In this figure we illustrate, in flow chart form, various aspects of research and development, in the life sciences, performed in the educational (university/college) environments. Again, this is not an exhaustive list.

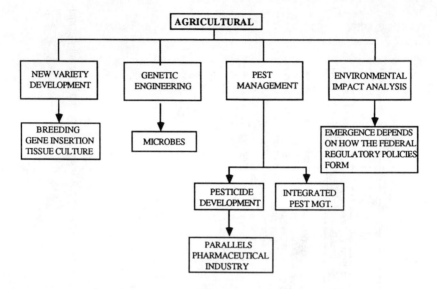

Figure 4.   This final figure illustrates agricultural applications of high performance computing.

Health Science Center, the University-Industrial Consortium, and University of Texas System Center for High Performance Computing, an ultralarge-scale simulation of the mouth and its bacterial environment is being developed. The purpose of this project is to develop a method for better understanding how periodontal disease occurs, what factors may influence the progression of the disease, and how it can be better treated.[159]

9.18 Matrix of Biological Knowledge

We close our discussion of biocomputing by addressing the issue of the matrix of biological knowledge and by returning to our original discussions; briefly addressing both databases and artificial intelligence. Current understanding of biology involves complex relationships rooted in enormous amounts of data; data obtained from numerous experiments and observations, and gleaned from diverse disciplines. As a consequence of these harsh realities, few scientists are capable of staying abreast of the ever increasing knowledge base, let alone searching that database for new and/or unsuspected biological phenomena. Yet, hidden within the *complete database of published biological experiments—the matrix of biological knowledge*, lies the potential for developing a new and powerful tool for the investigation of biological principles. Many databases of biological information already exist. Perhaps the best known of these is GenBank, the database of all known gene sequences. This project is, in some sense, an outgrowth of the Human Genome Project, a worldwide effort to sequence the entire human genome. The Human Genome Project will require massive computer support in such areas as numerical computation, searching algorithms, and database design. As these databases increase in size and complexity, it becomes increasingly important that effective and efficient user interfaces be developed. One can envision user interfaces incorporating knowledge engineering, advanced graphics and mathematical capabilities, and simulation engines.[160]

9.19 Conclusions

Biocomputing has, very rapidly, gone from its conception to its infancy. The technological advances of recent years carry with them the necessary fuel to allow this field to grow into adulthood. Once thought of as unnecessary, the computer has gained a strong foothold in the biosciences. As technology emerges from its annual metamorphosis, the need for biocomputing becomes stronger, the problems being tackled become more complex, and the technology more ready and able to handle both the needs and the demands of the biosciences.

Biological computing and high performance modeling have taught us numerous lessons as scientists. We have seen that a good model/simulation can aid us in testing hypotheses that might be extremely expensive to test in the laboratory and/or might be impossible to test. We have seen that we ask the all important *what if question*; thereby allowing us to investigate what might happen under various experimental conditions. We have also learned to face the limitations of this approach.

Good models and good simulations must depend upon *good data*! We must return to the living system and check our findings. Certain measurements must be made, experimentally, in order for the mathematical/computer model to have validity. We have seen that many forms of model can give rise to similar quantitative results. Hence, careful hypotheses must be involved in the formative modeling stages, lest ambiguity be introduced. As we increase the size and complexity of the models, we often introduce more parameters. These parameters must be known in order for the model to be an effective tool. Statisticians are fond of the warning: "Give me enough parameters and I can model the world." However, even with enough parameters, one must know their values if one is to study the dynamics of the world. And, while measurement techniques are getting better, there will always be parameters that cannot be known and/or easily measured. Thus, like any tool, one must take the good with the bad; refining the tool so that it can be more effective. Still, models depend upon computational speed, size, and mathematical complexity. This can and does hinder our ability to include all known biological factors.

Thus, computational simulations and mathematical models are not replacements for animals. Rather, as J. Mailen Kootsey put it, "they are partners with animal research." Complementing each other, neither can exist independently of the other. The future of biocomputing is one of great excitement. Experimentation and computational modeling can work hand-in-hand to improve the quality of life for all living species.

REFERENCES

1. Spanier, J. "Thoughts about the Essentials of Mathematical Modeling," *Math. Modeling* 1(1):99–108 (1980).
2. Witten, M. "Thought about the Essentials of Simulation Modeling," *Math. Modeling* 2(4):393–397 (1980).
3. Avula, X. J. R. "Mathematical Modeling," in *Encyclopedia of Physical Science and Technology* (New York: Academic Press, 1987).
4. Avula, X. J. R. "Mathematical Modeling in Biomedical Systems," preprint (1988).
5. Andres, J. G. and R. R. McLone. *Mathematical Modelling* (London: Butterworths, 1976).
6. Cross, M. and A. O. Moscardini. *Learning The Art of Mathematical Modeling* (New York: John Wiley & Sons, 1985).
7. Dym, C. L. and E. S. Ivey. *Principles of Mathematical Modeling* (New York: Academic Press, 1980).
8. Saaty, T. L. and J. M. Alexander. "Thinking with Models: Mathematical Models," in *The Physical, Biological, and Social Sciences* (New York: Pergamon Press, 1981).
9. Aris, R. *Mathematical Modeling Techniques* (London: Pitman and Company, 1978).
10. Lotka, A. J. *Elements of Mathematical Biology* (New York: Dover Publications, 1956).
11. Riggs, D. S. *The Mathematical Approach to Physiological Problems* (New York: Dover Publications, 1963).
12. Grodins, F. S. *Control Theory and Biological Systems* (New York: Columbia University Press, 1963).
13. Milsum, J. J. *Biological Control Systems Analysis* (New York: McGraw Hill, 1966).
14. Carson, E. R., C. Cobelli, and L. Finkelstein. *The Mathematical Modeling of Metabolic and Endocrine Systems* (New York: John Wiley & Sons, 1983).
15. Aris, R. and M. Penn. "The Mere Notion of a Model," *Math. Modeling* 1(1):1–12 (1980).
16. Yates, F. E. "Good Manners in Good Modeling: Mathematical Models and Computer Simulations of Physiological Systems," *Am. J. Physiol.* 3:R159–R160 (1978).
17. Noble, R. D. "Mathematical Modeling in the Context of Problem Solving," *Math. Modeling* 3(2):215–219 (1982).
18. Klir, G. J. "Complexity: Some General Observations," *Systems Res.* 2(2):131–140 (1985).
19. Rosen, R. "Second W. Ross Ashby Memorial Lecture 1984 the Physics of Complexity," *Systems Res.* 2(2):171–175 (1985).
20. Kinston, W. "Measurement and Structure of Scientific Analysis," *Systems Res.* 2(2):95–104 (1985).
21. Eisenfeld, J. and M. Witten, Eds. *Modeling of Biomedical Systems* (Amsterdam: North-Holland, 1986).
22. Rosen, R. Ed. *Foundation of Mathematical Biology* (New York: Academic Press, 1972).
23. Rosen, R. Ed. *Theoretical Biology and Complexity* (New York: Academic Press, 1985).

24. Rosen, R. *Anticipatory Systems* (New York: Pergamon Press, 1985).

25. Berger, J., W. Buhler, R. Repges, and P. Tautu. Eds. *Mathematical Models in Medicine* (New York: Springer-Verlag, 1976).

26. Heinmets, F. Ed. *Concepts and Models of Biomathematics* (New York: Marcel Dekker, 1969).

27. Meyer, W. J. *Concepts of Mathematical Modeling* (New York: McGraw Hill, 1969).

28. Goel, N. S. and N. Richter-Dyn. *Stochastic Models in Biology* (New York: Academic Press, 1974).

29. Rosen, R. *Dynamatical System Theory in Biology* (New York: J. Wiley & Sons, 1970).

30. Roach, G. F. Ed. *Mathematics in Medicine and Biomechanics* (Boston: Birkhauser 1984).

31. Finkelstein, L. and E. R. Carson. *Mathematical Modeling of Dynamic Biological Systems* (New York: J. Wiley & Sons, 1986).

32. Giordano, F. R. and M. D. Weir. *A First Course in Mathematical Modeling* (Pacific Grove, CA: Brooks/Cole, 1985).

33. Cherruault, Y. *Mathematical Modeling in Biomedicine* (Boston: D. Reidel, 1960).

34. Ingram, D. and R. F. Bloch. *Mathematical Methods in Medicine*, Vol. 1 (New York: J. Wiley & Sons, 1984).

35. Ingram, D. and R. F. Bloch. *Mathematical Methods in Medicine*, Vol. 2 (New York: J. Wiley & Sons, 1984).

36. Jones, D. S. and B. D. Sleeman. *Differential Equations and Mathematical Biology* (Boston: G. Allen & Unwin, 1983).

37. Cullen, M. R. *Mathematics for the Biosciences* (Boston: PWS Publishers, 1983).

38. Marmarelis, V. Z., Ed. "Advanced Methods of Physiological System Modeling," Biomedical Simulation Resource, University of Southern California, Los Angeles, CA (1987).

39. Jacques, J. A. Compartmental Analysis in Biology and Medicine (Ann Arbor, MI: University of Michigan Press, 1985).

40. Godfrey, K. *Compartmental Models and Their Application* (New York: Academic Press, 1983).

41. Savageau, M. A. *Biochemical Systems Analysis* (MA: Addison-Wesley, 1976).

42. Cronin-Scanlon, J. *Mathematical Aspects of Hodgkin-Huxley Neutral Theory* (England: Cambridge University Press, 1987).

43. Koch, C. and I. Segev, Eds. *Methods in Neuronal Modeling* (MA: MIT Press, 1989).

44. Wasserman, P. D. *Neural Computing: Theory and Practice* (New York: Van Nostrand Reinhold, 1989).

45. McCammon, J. A. and S. C. Harvey. *Dynamics of Proteins and Nucleic Acids* (England: Cambridge University Press, 1987).

46. Segel, L. A., Ed. *Mathematical Models in Molecular and Cellular Biology* (England: Cambridge University Press, 1980).

47. Swan, G. W. *Optimization of Human Cancer Radiotherapy* (New York: Springer-Verlag, 1979).

48. Eisen, M. *Mathematical Models: In Cell Biology and Cancer Chemotherapy* (New York: Springer-Verlag, 1979).

49. Thompson, J. R. and B. W. Brown. Eds. *Cancer Modeling* (New York: Marcel Dekker, 1987).

50. Perelson, A. S. Ed. *Theoretical Immunology* (New York: Addison-Wesley, 1988).

51. Hoppensteadt, F. C. *Mathematical Methods of Population Biology* (England: Cambridge University Press, 1982).

52. Frauenthal, J. C. *Mathematical Modeling in Epidemiology* (New York: Springer-Verlag, 1980).

53. Guyton, A. C. *Textbook of Medical Physiology* (Philadelphia: W. B. Saunders Company, 1971).

54. Witten, M. Ed. *Advances in Mathematics and Computers in Medicine*. 1 (New York: Pergamaon Press, 1987).

55. Witten, M. Ed. *Advances in Mathematics and Computers in Medicine*. 2 (New York: Pergamon Press, 1989).

56. Winfree, A. T. *The Geometry Of Biological Time* (New York: Springer-Verlag, 1980).

57. Winfree, A. T. *When Time Breaks Down* (New Jersey: Princeton University Press, 1987).

58. Witten, M., S. Barron, R. Harkness, and J. Driver. "Computational Molecular Biology and Genetics," Advances In Mathematical and Computers in Medicine, in press (1990).

59. Winfree, A. T. "Electrical Instability in Cardiac Muscle: Phase Singularities and Rotors," *J. Theor. Biol.* 138(3):353–405 (1989).

60. Witten, M. "Modeling the Aging-Cancer Interface: Some Thoughts on a Complex Biological Dynamics," *J. Gerontology* 44(6):72–80 (1989).

61. Murphey, C. R., J. W. Clark, and W. R. Giles. "A Model of Slow Conduction in Bullfrog Atrial Strands," preprint (1989).

62. Lagerlund, T. D. and F. W. Sharbrough. "Computer Simulation of the Generation of the Electroencephalogram," *Electroencephalog. Clin. Neurophysiol.* 72:31–40 (1989).

63. Johnson, T. K. and R. L. Vessella. "On the Possibility of Real-Time Monte Carlo Calculations for the Estimation of Absorbed Dose in Radioimmunotherapy," *Comput. Methods Programs BioMed.* 29(3):205–10 (1989).

64. Robb, R. "At Mayo, Healers Digitally Peer into the Human Machine," *Comput. Graphics Today* December 8, 1988.

65. Centofani, M. "Pinpoint the Problem: Tailor the Answer," *Hopkins Med. News* 11(3):16–23 (1988).

66. Fuchs, H., M. Levoy, and S. M. Pizer. "Interactive Visualization of 3D Medical Data," *IEEE Comput.* 22(8):46–51 (1989).

67. Spitzer, V. M. and D. G. Whitlock. "A 3-D Database of Human Anatomy," *Adv. Imaging* 4(3):48–49 (March, 1989).

68. Witten, M. "Peering into the Body: Physiology in the Supercomputer," *Supercomput. Revi.* in press (1990).

69. Maisel, M. "Reconstructing Neurons in the Computer," *San Diego Supercomput. Cent. Newsl.* 17 (1988).

70. Bell, G. and T. Marr. Eds. *The Interface Between Computational Science and Nucleic Acid Sequence* (Reading, MA: Addison-Wesley, in press, 1989).

71. Witten, M. "Modeling Cellular Systems and Aging Processes: I. Mathematics of Cell System Models-A Review," *Mech. Aging Dev.* 17(1):53–94 (1981).

72. Luria, S. E. and M. Delbruck. "Mutations of Bacteria from Virus Sensitivity to Virus Resistance," *Genetics* 28(6):491–511 (1943).

73. Witten, M. "*In vitro* Clonal Mutagenesis: A Brief Mathematical Model," in *Advances In Computer Methods for Partial Differential Equations*, R. Vichnevetsky and R. S. Stepelman. Eds. (New Brunswick, NJ: IMACS, Rutgers University, 1984).

74. Witten, M. *On Stochasticity in the McKendrick/VonFoerster Hyperbolic Partial Differential Equation System, Advanced Hyperbolic Partial Differential Equations*. 1 (New York: Pergamon Press, 1983).

75. Witten, M. and R. Kalaba. "Quasilinearization of a Von Foerster Distributed System: Simulation and Parameter Estimation. I. Issues of Principle," *Proc. 1981 Summer Simulation Symp.* 49–53 (1981).

76. Witten, M. "Modeling Cellular Aging and Tumorigenic Transformation," *Math. Comput. Simulation*, 24:572–584 (1982).

77. Witten, M. "Modeling Cellular Systems and Aging Processes. II. Towards Describing an Asynchronously Dividing Cellular System," in *Proc. Third International Conference Nonlinear Mathematics*, V. Laksmikantham. Ed. (New York: Academic Press, 1980).

78. Tucker, S. L. and S. O. Zimmerman. "A Nonlinear Model of Population Dynamics Containing an Arbitrary Number of Continuous Structure Variables," *SIAM J. Appl. Math.* 48(3):549–591 (1988).

79. Lopez, L. and D. Trigiante. "A Hybrid Scheme for Solving a Model of Population Dynamics," preprint (1983).

80. Kostova, T. V. "Numerical Solutions of a Hyperbolic Differential-Integral Equation," *Comput. Math. Appl.* 15(6–8):427–36 (1988).

81. Barr, T. "Approximation for Age-Structured Population Models Using Projection Methods," preprint (1989).

82. McKendrick, A. G. and M. K. Pai. "The Rate of Multiplication of Micro-organisms: a Mathematical Study," *Proc. Roy. Soc. Edinburgh* 31:649–655 (1910).

83. McKendrick, A. G. "Applications of Mathematics to Medical Problems," *Proc. Math. Soc.* 44:98–130 (1926).

84. Von Foerster, H. *Some Remarks on Changing Populations: The Kinetics of Cellular Proliferation* (New York: Grune, Stratton, 1959).

85. Scherbaum, O. and G. Rasch. "Cell Size Distribution and Single Cell Growth in *Tetrahymena pyriformis G.L.*," *Acta Pathol. Microbiol. Scand.* 41(1):161–182 (1957).

86. Nooney, G. C. "Age Distributions in Dividing Populations," *Biophys. J.* 7(1):69–76 (1967).

87. Trucco, E. "Mathematical Models for Cellular Systems: The Von Foerster Equation—Part 1," *Bull. Math. Biophys.* 27(3):285–304 (1965).

88. Trucco, E. "Mathematical Models for Cellular Systems: The Von Foerster Equation—Part 2," *Bull. Math. Biophys.* 27(4):449–471 (1965).

89. Trucco, E. "On the Use of the Von Foerster Equation for the Solution and Generalization of a Problem in Cellular Studies," *Bull. Math. Biophys.* 27:S39–48 (1965).

90. Trucco, E. "Mathematical Approaches to the Study of Cellular Populations," in *Biomathematics and Computer Science in the Life Sciences* (Springfield, IL: Charles C Thomas, 1965).

91. Trucco, E. "On the Average Cellular Volume in Synchronized Cell Populations," *Bull. Math. Biophys.* 32(4):459–473 (1970).

92. Schweitzer, D. G. and D. J. Dienes. "A Kinetic Model of Population Dynamics," *Demography* 8(3):389–400 (1971).

93. Hirsch, H. R. and J. Engelberg. "Decay of Cell Synchronization: Solutions of the Cell Growth Equation," *Bull. Math. Biophys.* 28:391–401 (1966).

94. Gurtin, M. E. and R. C. MacCamy. "Nonlinear Age-Dependent Population Dynamics," *Arch. Rat. Mech. Anal.* 54(1):281–300 (1974).

95. Gyllenberg, M. "Stability of a Nonlinear Age-Dependent Population Model a Control Variable," *SIAM J. Appl. Math.* 43(6):1418–1438 (1983).

96. Tucker, S. L. "Cell Population Models with Continuous Structure Variables," in *Cancer Modeling,* J. R. Thompson and B. W. Brown, Eds. (New York: Marcel Dekker, 1987).

97. Zimmerman, S. and R. A. White. "Generalizations of a Fluid Dynamic Model for Analyzing Multiparameter Flowcytometric Data," in *Biomathematics and Cell Kinetics*, M. Rotenberg, Ed. (Amsterdam: Elsevier/North-Holland, 1981).

98. Rubinow, S. "A Maturity-Time Representation for Cell Populations," *Biophys. J.* 8(10):1055–1073 (1968).

99. Lebowitz, J. L. and S. I. Rubinow. "A Theory for the Age-Time Distribution of a Microbial Population," *J. Math. Biol.* 1(1):17–36 (1974).

100. Rubinow, S. I. "Age-Structured Equations in the Theory of Cell Populations," in *A Study In Mathematical Biology,* S. Levin, Ed. (Washington, D.C.: Mathematical Association of America, 1978).

101. Rubinow, S. I. "Cell Kinetics," in *Mathematical Biology*, L. A. Segel, Ed. (Cambridge: Cambridge University Press, 1980).

102. Diekmann, O., H. Heijmans, and H. Thieme. "On the Stability of the Size Distribution," *J. Math. Biol.* 19(2):227–248 (1984).

103. Diekmann, O., H. Lauwerier, T. Aldenberg, and H. Metz. "Growth, Fission, and the Stable Size Distribution," *J. Math. Biol.* 18(2):135–148 (1983).

104. Kimmel, M., Z Darzynkiewicz, O. Arino, and F. Traganos. "Analysis of a Model of Cell Cycle Based on Unequal Division of Mitotic Constituents to Daughter Cells During Cytokinesis," preprint (1984).

105. Lasota, A. and M. Mackey. "Globally Asymptotic Properties of Proliferating Cell Populations," *J. Math. Biol.* 19(1):43–62 (1984).

106. Prescott, D. M. "Variations in the Individual Generation Times of *Tetrahymena gelii HS*," *Exp. Cell Res.* 16(2):279–291 (1959).

107. Bell, G. I. and E. C. Anderson. "Cell Growth and Division. I. A Mathematical Model with Applications to Cell Volume Distributions in Mammalian Suspension Culture," *Biophys. J.* 7(4):329–351 (1967).

108. Anderson, E. C. and D. F. Peterson. "Cell Growth and Division. II. Experimental Studies of Cell Volume Distributions in Mammalian Suspension Cultures. *Biophys. J.* 7(4):353–364 1967.

109. Bell, G. I. "Cell Growth and Division. III. Conditions for Balanced Exponential Growth in a Mathematical Model," *Biophys. J.* 8(4):431–444 (1968).

110. Anderson, E. C., G. I. Bell, D. F. Peterson, and R. A. Tobey. "Cell Growth and Division. IV. Determination of Volume Growth Rate and Division Probability," *Biophys. J.* 9(2):246–263 (1969).

111. Oldfield, D. G. "A Continuity Equation for Cell Populations," *Bull. Math. Biophys.* 28(4):545–554 (1966).

112. Bernardi, M. L., A. C. Capelo, and P. Periti. "A Mathematical Model for the Evolution of Cell Populations under the Action of Mutagenic Agents," *Math. Biosci.* 71(1):19–39 (1984).

113. Bertuzzi, A., A. Gandolfi, and M. A. Giovenco. "Mathematical Models of the Cell Cycle with a View to Tumor Studies," *Math. Biosci.* 53(3/4):159–188 (1981).

114. Periti, P., C. Baiocchi, A. C. Capelo and V. Comincioli. "Mathematical Models of Neoplastic Growth Control," *Med. Biol. Environ.* 7:183–214 (1979).

115. White, R. A. "A Review of Some Mathematical Models in Cell Kinetics," in *Biomathematics and Cell Kinetics*, M. Rotenberg, Ed. (Amsterdam: Elsevier/North-Holland, 1981).

116. Bronk, B., G. J. Dienes, and A. Paskin. "The Stochastic Theory of Cell Proliferation," *Biophys. J.* 8(11):1353–1398 (1968).

117. Langhaar, H. L. "General Population Theory in the Age-Time Continuum," *J. Franklin Inst.* 293(3):199–213 (1972).

118. Fredrickson, A. G., D. Ramkrishna, and H. M. Tsuchiya. "Statistics and Dynamic of Procaryotic Cell Populations," *Math. Biosci.* 1(3):327–374 (1967).

119. Aroesty, J., T. Lincoln, P. Morrison, and G. Carter. "Cell Kinetic Models of Transient States: A Preliminary Investigation of Lymphocyte Stimulation," in *Growth Kinetics and Biochemical Regulation of Normal and Malignant Cells,* B. Drewinko and R. M. Humphrey, Eds. (Baltimore: Williams & Wilkins, 1976).

120. Creekmore, S. P., S. M. Johnson, J. Aroesty, T. L. Lincoln, K. L. Willis, and P. F. Morrison. "New Mathematical Models of Cell Kinetics Including Heredity Differentiation, Regulatory Control," *Proc. Summer Comput. Simulation Conf.* Chicago, IL, 1977.

121. Aroesty, J., T. Lincoln, N. Shapiro, and G. Boccia. "Tumor Growth and Chemotherapy: Mathematical Methods, Computer Simulations, and Experimental Foundations," *Math. Biosci.* 17(1):243–300 (1973).

122. Creekmore, S. P., J. Aroesty, K. L. Willis, P. F. Morrison, and T. L. Lincoln. "A cell Kinetics Model which Includes Heredity, Differentiation and Regulatory Control," in *Biomathematics and Cell Kinetics,* A. J. Valleron and P. D. M. MacDonald, Eds. (Amsterdam: Elsevier/North-Holland, 1978).

123. Lincoln, T. L., P. Morrison, J. Aroesty, and G. Carter. "Computer Simulation of Leukemia Therapy: Combined Pharmacokinetics, Intracellular Enzyme Kinetics, and Cell Kinetics of the Treatment of L1210 Leukemia by Cytosine Arabinoside," *Cancer Treat. Rep.* 60(12):1723–1739 (1976).

124. Webb, G. F. *Theory of Non-Linear Age-Dependent Population Dynamics* (New York: Marcel Dekker, 1985).

125. Webb, G. F. "A Model of Proliferating Cell Populations with Inherited Cycle Length," *J. Math. Biol.* 23(2):269–282 (1986).

126. Yamaguti, M. and M. Hata. "Chaos Arising from the Discretization of an Old and an Age-Dependent Population Model," in *Nonlinear Partial Differential Equations in Applied Science U.S.-Jpn. Sem.* (Amsterdam: North Holland, 1982).

127. Horwood, J. W., R. C. A. Bannister, and G. J. Howlett. "Comparative Fecundity of North Sea Plaice," *Proc. R. Soc. Lond* B 228(1253):401–431 (1986).

128. Saleem, M. and R. K. Pandey. "Egg-Eating Age-Structured Predator and Prey Interactions: Some Simple Cases," *Math. Biosci.* 89(2):209–224 (1988).

129. Smith, J. R. and R. G. Whitney. "Intraclonal Variation in Proliferative Potential of Human Diploid Fibroblasts: Stochastic Mechanisms for Cellular Aging," *Science* 207(4426):82–84 (1980).

130. Rotenberg, M. "Theory of Distributed Quiescent State in the Cell Cycle," *J. Theor. Biol.* 96(3):495–509 (1982).

131. Rotenberg, M. "Transport theory for growing cell population," preprint (1982).

132. Frenzen, C. L. and J. D. Murray. "A Cell Kinetics Justification for Gompertz' Equation," *SIAM J. Appl. Math.* 46(4):614–629 (1986).

133. Witten, M. "A Mathematical Model for the Effects of a Lymphokine-like Ring Shaped Particle on the Dynamics of a Conjoint Tumor-Normal Cell Culture: Some Implications for the Aging-Cancer Question," in *Mathematics and Computers in Biomedical Applications,* J. Eisenfeld and C. DeLisi, Eds. (Amsterdam: Elsevier/ North-Holland, 1985).

134. Witten, M. "Modeling the Dynamics of a Conjoint Tumor-Normal Cell Culture Systems. II. Further Thoughts on the Aging-Cancer Question," in *Modeling of Biomedical Systems,* J. Eisenfeld and M. Witten, Eds. (Amsterdam: Elsevier/North-Holland, 1986).

135. Witten, M., Ed. *Advances in Hyperbolic Partial Differential Equations* (New York: Pergamon Press, 1983).

136. Murphey, C. R., J. W. Clark, W. R. Giles, R. L. Rasmusson, J. Halter, K. Hicks, and B. Hoyt. "Conduction in Bullfrog Atrial Strands: Simulations of the Role of Disk and Extracellular Resistance," preprint (1989).

137. Backx, P. H., P. O. De Tombe, J. H. K. van Deen, B. J. M. Mulder, and H. E. D. J. Ter Keurs. "A Model of Propagating Calcium-Induced Calcium Release by Calcium Diffusion," *J. Gen Physiol.* 93(5):963–977 (1989).

138. Schouten, V. J. A., J. H. K. van Deen, P. P. De Tombe, and A. A. Verveen. "Force-Interval Relationship in Heart Muscle of Mammals," *Biophys. J.* 51(1):13–26 (1987).

139. Peskin, C. S. "The Fluid Dynamics of Heart Valves: Experimental, Theoretical, and Computational Methods," *Annu. Rev. Fluid. Mech.* 14(1):235–259 (1982).

140. Peskin, C. S., D. M. McQueen, and S. Greenberg. "Three Dimensional Fluid Dynamics in a Two Dimensional Amount of Central Memory," in *Wave Motion: Theory, Modeling, and Computation* (New York: Springer-Verlag, 1987).

141. McQueen, D. M and C. S. Peskin. "A Three Dimensional Computational Method for Blood Flow in the Heart: Contractile Fibers," *J. Comput. Phys.* 82(2):289–97 (1989).

142. Peskin, C. S. and D. M. McQueen. "A Three Dimensional Computational Method for Blood Flow in the Heart: Immersed Elastic Fibers in a Viscous Incompressible Fluid," *J. Comput. Phys.* 81(2):372–405 (1989).

143. McQueen, D. M. and C. S. Peskin. "Computer-Assisted Design of Butterfly Bileaflet Valves for the Mitral Position," *Scand. J. Thor. Cardiovasc. Surg.* 19(2):139–148 (1985).

144. Meisner, J. S., D. M. McQueen, Y. Ishida, H. O. Vetter, U. Burtolotti, J. A. Strom, R. W. M. Frater, C. S. Peskin, and E. L. Yellin. "Effects of Timing of Atrial Systole on LV Filling and Mitral Valve Closure: Computer and Dog Studies," *Am. J. Physiol.* 249(3):H604–H619 (1985).

145. Lambert, M. H. and T. R. Chay. "Cardiac Arrhythmias Modeled by Ca_i-Inactivated Ca^{2+} Channels," *Biol. Cybern.* 61(1):21–28 (1989).

146. Chay, T. R. "Kinetic Modeling for the Channel Gating Process from Single Patch-Clamp Data," *J. Theor. Biol.* 132(4):477–493 (1988).

147. Chay, T. R. "Analyzing Stochastic Events in Multi-Channel Patch-Clamp Data," *Biol. Cybern.* 58(1):19 (1988).

148. Chay, T. R. "Complex Periodic Oscillations in Four-Variable Model of an Excitable Cell," *Physica D* preprint (1988).

149. Lagerlund, T. D. and P. A. Low. "A Mathematical Simulation of Oxygen Delivery in Rat Peripheral Nerve," *Microvascular Res.* 34(2):211–22 (1987).

150. Lagerlund, T. D. and P. A. Low. "Mathematical Simulation of the Effects of Axial Diffusion and Non-Zero-Order Kinetics on Oxygen Delivery in Rat Peripheral Nerve," preprint (1989).

151. Lagerlund, T. D. and F. W. Sharbrough. "Computer Simulation of Neuronal Circuit Models of Rhythmic Behavior in the Electroencephalogram," *Comput. Bio. Med.* 18(4):267–304 (1988).

152. Lagerlund, T. D. and F. W. Sharbrough. "Computer Simulation of the Generation of the Electroencephalogram," *Electroencephalog. Clin. Neurophysiol.* 72(1):31–40 (1989).

153. Layton, H. E. "Distribution of Henle's Loops may Enhance Urine Concentrating Capability," *Biophys. J.* 49(5):1033–1040 (1986).

154. Pitman, E. B. and H. E. Layton. "Tubuloglomerular Feedback in a Dynamic Nephron," *Comm. Pure and Appl. Math.* 42:49–97 (1989).

155. Chaudhuri, S., H. Nguyen, R. M. Rangayyan, S. Walshi, and C. B. Frank. "A Fourier Domain Directional Filtering Method for Analysis of Collagen Alignment in Ligaments. *IEEE Trans. Biomed. Eng.* BME-34 (7):509–518 (1987).

156. Johnson, T. K. and R. L. Vessella. "On the Application of Parallel Processing to the Computation of Dose Arising from the Internal Deposition of Radionuclides," *Comput. Physics* 3(3):69–72 (1989).

157. Johnson, T. K. "MABDOS; A Generalized Program for Internal Radionuclide Dosimetry," *Comput. Meth. Progr. BioMed.* 27(2):159–167 (1988).

158. Moyers, M. F., J. L. Horton, and A. L. Boyer. "A Scatter Model for Fast Neutron Beams Using Convolution of Diffusion Kernals," *Radiat. Prot. Dosimetry* 23 (1–4):475–478 (1988).

159. Weiss, R. "High-Tech Tooth Repair," *Sci. News* 134(24):376–379 (1988).

160. Morowitz, H. R. and T. Smith. "Report of the Matrix of Biological Knowledge Workshop," Santa Fe Institute, New Mexico (1987).

161. Koshland, D. E. "Frontiers in Neuroscience (editorial)," *Science* 242(4879):641 (1988).

162. Sejnowski, T. J., C. Koch, and P. S. Churchland. "Computational Neuroscience," *Science* 241(4871):1299–1306 (1988).

163. Garwood, M., K. Ugurbil, A. R. Rath, M. R. Bendall, B. D. Ross, S. L. Mitchell, and H. Merkle. "Magnetic Resonance Imaging with Adiabatic Pulses Using a Single Surface Coil for RF Transmission and Signal Detection," University of Minnesota Supercomputing Institute, 88/72 (1988).

164. Greene, A. S., P. J. Tonellato, J. Lui, J. H. Lombard, and A. W. Crowley, Jr. "Microvascular Rarefaction and Tissue Vascular Resistance in Hypertension," *Am. J. Physiol.* 256(1 Pt. 2):H126–H131 (1989).

CHAPTER 10

The Human Genome Project: An Overview of Computational Issues in Molecular Biology and Genetics

Sarah Barron, Matthew Witten, Robert Harkness,
Fang Wang, and Jesse Driver

10.0 The Promise of the Human Genome Project

It is projected that the effort to sequence the human genome will lead to major understandings and contributions in the areas of growth and development, and that it will open new avenues for the therapy of a variety of genetic diseases. The fact that the entire AIDS virus sequence was known shortly after the virus was discovered has enabled this disease to be one of those addressed by the more than 100 biotechnology-derived therapeutics currently in the developmental or approval process.[1] Approved genetically engineered therapeutics can already be used to treat some diseases, including diabetes, growth hormone deficiency, anemia of kidney dialysis, myocardial infarction, pulmonary embolism, leukemia, kidney transplant rejection, and hepatitis B. Full translation of the built-in genetic message would allow medical researchers to identify, to study, and to potentially cure thousands of still largely mysterious inherited disorders, both physical and behavioral—diseases like cystic fibrosis, heart disease, and cancer.

10.1 The Human Genome Effort—Not Just Computers, Not Only Animals

In animal testing, *Homo sapiens* are often overlooked. Nonetheless, sufferers of genetic disease especially may well become "guinea pigs" even though both the therapy and the drugs to treat these disorders exist. For example, even though animal insulin is no longer required since human insulin is now available via recombinant DNA (deoxyribonucleic acid) techniques, any diabetic individual can relate how a number of *trials* were necessary before insulin dosage or other drug therapy particularly suited to his or her genetic makeup was determined. Those with hypertensive disease are another instance of individuals who often go through numbers of different drug regimes before one with acceptable *side effects* that works is found for that individual. Would it not be better if one could simply carry a CD-ROM of his/her own genotype into a pharmacy and receive medicines *customized* by genotypes?

It is one of the goals of the Human Genome Project that this very scenario of individualized drug therapy will come to pass. If successful, the Human Genome Project will enable the final animal testing lineup to be tested in drug trials which are free of both pain and the suffering of *trial-and-error* therapies. Yet, many computational issues must be solved before *in vivo* drug testing can become accurate and reliable in the computer testing; before what is done *in the tube* becomes what is done *on the tube*. It is the purpose of this chapter to provide a general overview of these computational challenges. For additional discussion on the role of computational modeling see Chapter 9.

10.2 The Data

The human genome project comprises a worldwide, multibillion dollar effort to determine (map) the human genome. The human genome is the entire set of instructions for making a human being, and it is encoded in the nucleus of cells in the form of the DNA molecule. The ongoing research effort in molecular and cellular genetics has led to the creation of a variety of computer databases of nucleic acid and amino acid sequences. These databases now dominate the major biotechnology databases (Table 1). Further, advances in rapid automated sequencing have allowed experimental/laboratory investigators to accelerate their respective sequencing efforts and therefore, to increase the knowledge held in these molecular genetic databases. The most commonly used database is GenBank. Currently, over 2×10^7 nucleotides are entered into the GenBase database per year.[2] In addition, the sequencing effort is proceeding at more than 7×10^6 nucleotides per year. Satellite data repositories are being set up in order to facilitate rapid access to the data by experimentalists.

In a typical laboratory experiment, an investigator obtains a DNA or amino acid sequence. They then wish to compare this newly obtained sequence to the various sequences already known. In order for the biologist to search effectively

Table 1.   Major Databases in Biotechnology

Database	Type of Data
GenBank	Genetic sequences from virtually all phylogenetic groups and synthetic sequences
EMBL	European Molecular Biology Laboratory nucleotide sequences which largely overlap GenBank
PIR	Protein sequence data bank operated by the National Biomedical Research Foundation in Washington, D.C.
PDB	Brookhaven structural Protein Data Bank on proteins, nucleic acids, viruses, and polysaccharides, including sets of atomic coordinates
Cambridge structural database	Data on X-ray and neutron studies of organocarbon compounds including carbohydrates, steroids, amino acids, peptides, and antibiotics
CARBBANK	Carbohydrate Data Bank of primary structural information about complex carbohydrates, operated as part of the Complex Carbohydrate Research Center at the University of Georgia

for a comparison of their DNA or amino acid sequence to all known sequences, a comprehensive, highspeed, integrated database (or database format) needs to be built (designed). While there are nationally organized databases (Table 1), other organizations are also creating their own databases. This increasing abundance of databases raises a number of important questions. For example, how will the future spread of data between and across databases be better handled when there is currently no real standardization of data entry formats; formats which are usually different for various databases. In addition, there should be an increasing emphasis placed upon open architecture systems and data portability. Development of information retrieval systems, using more powerful and general techniques than provided through the current relational models is needed, as well as new techniques for storage and organization of the data in those databases. Having data is great. However, if one cannot easily access the data, it is not scientifically useful to have a collection of data. One such solution is a logical data language (LDL) that provides a rule-based query system for recursive, content, and other types of previously atypical data extractions from rational databases.[3] Another issue is data quality or integrity. It is important to know how accurate the database data actually is. Problems of data integrity could be checked electronically with the development of expert systems and sophisticated parsers.[4] The role of artificial intelligence in molecular biology and genetics needs to be seriously and continually researched. Development of special-purpose hardware/chips for the human genome databank will probably be required (and is being currently investigated), through optimization of current codes for existing supercomputers (vector, scalar, parallel) would considerably speed up current computations, as has been witnessed for the FASTA algorithm.[5]

    Visualization, certainly at the three dimensional (3-D) level, extensively used by protein and nucleic-acid chemists, needs to be interfaced to databases and database-retrieval systems. Such systems are being developed at such drug companies as Eli Lilly and Smith, Kline, and French. As with any research effort that gathers various forms of data, the data must be presented in a way that allows for the communication of meaning.

10.3 Biology

Inside each cell of any given individual is a nucleus. This nucleus contains 46 chromosomes, 24 of which are termed the genome. Each genome, in males, consists of 22 autosomes and 2 sex chromosomes, one X and one Y (the Y chromosome is not present in females). Each chromosome can be roughly termed a molecule of DNA and is twisted into a double helix shape. The critical components of DNA are four bases: adenine (A), thymine (T), cytosine (C), and guanine (G). The sequence of these bases determines the order in which building block amino acids are linked to form the all-important proteins. A segment of the DNA that contains the instructions for a complete protein is called a gene. DNA is the pattern from which the proteins that comprise the body are built, and it could be considered the template from which to *build* a particular individual.

The human genome is estimated to contain 3.5 billion base pairs or approximately 100,000 genes; however, only about 1500 are represented as mapped genes and markers, cloned DNA segments, fragile sites, cloned genes, and neoplasia-associated break points.[6] James Watson who, with Francis Crick, determined the structure of DNA, predicted the effort to map and sequence the entire human genome would be completed by September 30, 2005. If this effort (which began October 1, 1990) is to be accomplished, new technologies will need to be developed. These technologies will involve crucial and exciting interdisciplinary cooperation among biologists, mathematicians, computer scientists, physicists, chemists, and engineers. The day of the computational molecular biologist and/or the mathematical molecular geneticist has arrived. If we are to be truly effective in this effort, we must see beyond the narrow old niches of pigeonhole traditional science and allow ourselves to explore the boundaries between many sciences.

The first step in the human genome effort will be to construct complete maps— that is, ordered linear arrays of genes, markers, or nucleotides—on representative chromosomes. Maps vary according to the level of genome organization, resolution, and the experimental techniques used to obtain the data. It is the physical map of the genome that must first be addressed (Figure 1). A gross physical map assigns genes to chromosomes or parts of chromosomes and has a resolution of 10^7 to 10^8 bases.[7] Once the physical map is determined, individual bases or nucleotides that compose DNA can be identified and ordered (sequenced).

Obtaining the DNA nucleotide sequence is only the beginning of the investigative process. Once one has a sequence, there are many further questions to be asked. For example, how similar is this sequence to other known sequences? Can we assign our newly obtained sequence to a particular class of already determined sequences and, in doing so, begin to understand some of its biological characteristics?

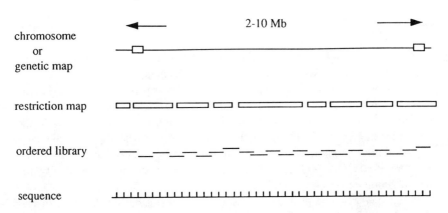

Figure 1. Types of maps. (From Cantor, C. R. and C. L. Smith, in *Molecular Genetic Approaches to Neuropsychiatric Diseases*, J. Brosius and R. T. Freeman, Eds. [New York: Academic Press 1991]; and Bell, G. I., in *Computers and DNA: Proceedings of the Interface Between Computation Science and Nucleic Acid Sequencing Workshop*, Vol. 7, G. I. Bell and T. G. Marr, Eds. [Reading, MA: Addison-Wesley 1990].)

Similarity searches align sequences so that corresponding residues are alike or nearly so; from similarities found in sequences, homology inferences about common ancestry can be deduced. But, similarity searches for comparison and alignment of a new sequence require extremely efficient handling of the data stored in our electronic databases; databases whose structures are not necessarily comparable/compatible in format. Although there are a number of nucleic acid and protein databases in existence, no public databases of physical maps currently exists. Current search and comparison algorithms, as well as computational methods, are not expected to be able to deal with the growth projections in database size in the near future. Additionally, not all of the DNA molecule codes for a protein. Part of the problem in analyzing DNA sequences is to distinguish between coding regions and noncoding or *junk* DNA regions. Assuming that a nucleotide sequence is identified, the scientific investigator often wishes to visualize the 3-D structure of the coded molecule. That is, they would like to translate the given sequence into a 3-D structure of the molecule coded by that given sequence. Computational methods to predict protein structures (secondary/tertiary) and structure/function relations from these coding regions are obviously a sorely needed component of genetic research involving a close collaboration/cooperation between the theoretical and the experimental investigator communities. At this point in time, little is understood about how even the simple linear arrangement of amino acids of a protein fold into their complicated 3-D structure.[8] The abilities of computers to fold more complex structures, for example, tRNAs (transfer ribonucleic acids), are only in their infancy. And even the simplest folding algorithms require enormous amounts of computer time for the shortest of sequences.

10.4 Sequence and Search Algorithms

Molecular biology applications rank among the most challenging applications of computers today.[9] Not even current supercomputers, using current software, can efficiently deal with the expected growth in data as part of the human genome effort. Nor will the addition of more manpower, more current machines, and other resources solve the problem. In particular, there must be advancements in the current technology for handling all classes of DNA and protein sequence analyses—similarity (homology) searches, signal searches, statistical analyses, and structural predictions[10]—if any sense is to be made of the data generated by the human genome project.

When the sequence of a given molecule is known, but the function of that molecule is not, a comparison of that sequence to all known sequences may identify commonality among molecules and, therefore, help to classify the molecule. Entire sequences may be compared or specific determinants of structure and function may be emphasized. **Sequence alignment** places the residues of the sequences into the best one-to-one correspondence. Current search and alignment algorithms[11-13] generally have one of two faults; they either are not sensitive enough to find all the possible alignments or they require excessive computational power.

Global alignments, where an attempt is made to align an entire sequence, are typically done by the *Needleman-Wunsch-Sellers (NWS)*,[14,15] but increasing sequence length makes the combinatorics of this approach unmanageable. When multiple alignments are desired, the computation using the NWS algorithm becomes the fifth power of the mean sequence length[13] and may not even give consistency for pairwise comparisons![16] Additionally, global alignments may fail to find common subsequences. Clearly, global alignments are not always efficient and/or effective. Hence, another approach is to use **local alignments** in which the attempt is to align short but highly similar subsequences. Several different methods for local alignment have been adopted. The most widely used is by Smith and Waterman.[17] The *Smith and Waterman* algorithm modified the NWS algorithm in several ways by including negative scores for mismatches and by setting the minimum score in the score matrix as zero. A similar strategy was developed by Goad and Kanehisa.[18]

Although the best alignments are found by **dynamic programming techniques**,[19] their computationally intensive nature along with other problems, including storage requirements, led to the development of **hash coding algorithms** for performing local alignments.[20-23] A hashing table is constructed from the locations of subsequences which are called *words* or *tuples*. Segments of the database are then sequentially compared against the hashing table. This method has been embodied into the fast-search program FASTA;[23,24] however, to make the hash coding algorithms more sensitive involves picking a smaller word length (nucleic acid string) or *tuple* value. A tuple value of one will solve the sensitive issue, but cause the computational time to increase substantially, even on parallel machine architectures where decrease in CPU (central processing unit) time may result in a relative increase in input/output (I/O) time.[5,25] If one desires to know the significance of an alignment, additional computations may range from simple counts of bases to the use of highly compute intensive Markov chain theory.[26,27] Evolutionary analyses[28] by maximum likelihood methods, especially with the addition of molecular clocks as typlified by the program PHYLIP,[29] may tax the computational power of even the most powerful of Cray computers. Even currently published algorithms that have yet to be implemented, such as the d^2 metric for sequence searches and dissimilarity measurements[30] will not be adequate for the expected 10^{12} nucleotide database.[31]

With the exponentially increasing size of sequence databases, it is additionally necessary to develop search methods which balance the search sensitivity and search specificity. Karlin and Altschul[32] derived a rigorous theory for the significance of upgapped sequence alignments. Based on the results, a rapid similarity search algorithm, BLAST was developed to directly approximate alignments that optimize a measure of local similarity.[33,34] Additionally, fast Fourier transforms (FFTs) show some promise over dynamic programming in dealing with insertions and deletions vs. substitutions when databases are large.[35]

Given an anonymous DNA sequence, locating the exons or portions of DNA which code for a protein and predicting the amino acid sequence from that original DNA is no small task. Fields and Soderlund[36] attempt to address this with their *gm* (gene modeler) interactive tool kit. Once the DNA is appropriately translated into amino acids, the range of functions mediated by proteins from the diversity and versatility of only 20 amino acids results in the need for new measures of similarity—those especially for amino acids. Karlin and Ghandour[37] grouped amino acids into four different alphabets according to their structural, functional, charge, and chemical properties. They further aligned immunoglobulin k-chain constant domains and scored matches and mismatches in the chosen alphabet. Taylor,[38] on the other hand, based on the known crystallographic coordinates, selected physicochemical properties of amino acids that are important in tertiary structure determination. By incorporating a Venn diagram, he divided amino acids into two major sets, polar and hydrophobic. The amino acids found in the overlap are considered to be ambivalent. Amino acids were also grouped into sets in light of their size, charge, etc. Measuring amino acids similarity also provides practical procedures of aligning protein sequences. But, most alignment programs use similarity matrices with graded scales/weighting. Commonly used weighted methods include: Unitary (UM), Genetic Code (GC), Structure-Genetic (SG), and Dayhoff's log-Odds percent accepted mutation (PAM).

10.5 Visualization

In light of the lack of data regarding the 3-D conformation of genetic sequences, other **visualization techniques** are used. These methods help the researcher visually detect similarities or dissimilarities in sequences. An example of one such technique is **dot matrix analysis**. Dot matrix analysis is a simple yet powerful technique for sequence analysis. A comparison of two sequences should start with a dot matrix analysis.[39] Yet, no present implementation of dot matrix analysis takes full advantage of modern computer hardware and graphic user interface (GUI) technology. Thus, dot matrix analysis would benefit from integration with other types of analysis such as image display tools. For instance, *XSauci* is a correlation image generating program used for comparing two nucleotide sequences.[40] A more comprehensive integration is done in NCSA (National Center for Supercomputing Applications). The matrix of values like local alignment scores are imported as text files into NCSA Datascope and associated images representing traditional dot matrix plots as well as numerical values are generated. Data can also be opened in NCSA Image which provides a set of scientific visualization tools, including color raster, 3-D, contour, shape, and dither plots. Another approach is to use different colors to represent various amino acids and nucleotides. Thus, one uses a color mapping technique to display results of sequence comparisons (personal communication with Vinod Nair).

Unlike sequence visualization, visualization of molecular data has become common place in recent years. Molecules stored in the Protein Data Bank (PDB) format can be exchanged among researchers, or stored in databases for later retrieval. Rendering of the molecule may be different depending on the level of hardware assistance to visualization available. Wire frame renditions of molecules can be rotated in real time on mid-range Sun systems, while the rendering of the isosurfaces of a molecular probability density volume can be rotated in real time on the higher end graphics stations such as Stardent and Silicon Graphics Iris. PDB serves as an adequate data format for much of the information resulting from computations on molecules; however, standards are beginning to evolve at the application level for the data structures to be shared between packages. As an example, Stardent has promoted the use of their Chemistry Development Kit (CDK) data structure for chemistry. This structure has all of the information of the PDB format and more optional fields which can contain additional information which may be useful to keep along during the course of a computation. Better standards will need to be implemented for the storage of molecular data, due partly to the fact that so many diverse packages exist for this purpose today.

PDB formatted data customarily contains all of the x,y,z coordinates for all of the atoms in a molecule. Thus, there is no guess work as to the locations of atoms in the molecule prior to rendering. This 3-D geometric information about the molecule can be obtained in two major ways. X-ray crystallography and Nuclear Magnetic Resonance (NMR) are methods for obtaining empirical data concerning the conformation of a molecule. Minimizations and dynamic simulations of the computer are another way of predicting the 3-D locations of atoms within a molecule. Unfortunately, the size of the sequences encountered in genetics research causes the determination of tertiary structure by use of minimization and dynamics to be intractable. Therefore, researchers are forced to rely on data which has been gathered empirically. Since empirical data may not be available for most sequences with which a researcher may be interested, all of the powerful insights that could be obtained from molecular visualization cannot be realized.

10.6 Communication

Since genetic research and the human genome project has become an international effort, there is, a need for greater integration of worldwide scientific intercommunications and data exchange over computer networks. Clearly, the need for higher-speed network communications and network systems is of growing concern. It is still open to question whether the efforts of Open Standards Initiative (OSI) to spread X.400 worldwide will finally succeed.[41]

10.7 Hardware

The computational tasks associated with the human genome project place it among the grand challenges in computing for the 1990s. It is widely stated that computers with Teraflop (TF) performance (one trillion floating point operations per second, 10^9) will be required if true breakthroughs in modeling and visualization of real biological systems is to occur. In order to obtain a feeling for this level of performance, consider that today's machines run in the gigaflop (GF, 10^6 floating point operations per second) range. Further consider the following exercise: write down two 13-digit numbers at random. Enter them into the computer. Multiply them together. Store the results. Enter another random 13-digit number. Add the new random number to the stored result of the previous multiplication. Store that final result. A GF machine can perform this sequence of operation 10^6 times per second. A TF machine could do it 10^9 times a second. Performing this 100 times on a pocket calculator could average 20 s to do it once! It is highly unlikely that TF performance can be achieved, using conventional computer architectures, since clock cycle times of less than 1 psec would be required to attain the aforementioned goals. It is therefore apparent that the future of high performance computing lies in the domain of massively parallel architectures, coupled with symbolic/numeric machines and machines that have yet to be imagined.

Parallelism, in one form or another, has been steadily introduced into computing since the mid 1960s, but often in ways which were transparent to the user. IBM introduced instruction pipelining and several Control Data Corp. (CDC) machines appeared with multiple functional units which could operate concurrently. The first commercially successful vector pipeline computer, the Cray-1, was introduced in 1976. The Cray-1 has been the model for several vector supercomputers of the 1980s, and variations of this basic architecture with relatively small number of CPUs (in the range 8 to 64) will probably dominate the supercomputer market in the short term. Vector architectures can still be enhanced by adding multiple floating point pipelines or other new independent functional units but they are also approaching fundamental limitations. In particular, as Dr. Carl Ledbetter,* formerly of ETA Systems, points out, "the speed of light is the same on both sides of the Pacific Ocean." Increasing logic density may reduce the number of machine cycles needed to perform a basic function (such as a floating point multiplication); but, at most, a vector machine can deliver one result per pipeline per clock period and we are rapidly approaching the limit of the clocking technology. It is important to note, however, that even a machine like a Cray Y-MP with apparently only eight processors actually has a degree of parallelism comparable to 2560 one-bit processing elements.[42] Most of this parallelism is hidden from the user. The Cray can be effective on codes which may not have been designed with explicit parallelism but nonetheless vectorizeable. Unfortunately, a great many existing codes do not contain opportunities for vectorization, let alone parallel/vector execution.

It has taken 15 years to develop efficient vectorizing compilers. Essentially the same ideas are used by vendors with moderately parallel products. Some vendors are now offering compilers which can both vectorize and automatically parallelize codes for execution on multiple vector CPUs (e.g., Cray Autotasking). The Thinking Machines Corporation CM-2 and Active Memory Technologies DAP massively parallel architectures both rely on extensions to Fortran (or C), many of which are embodied in the proposed Fortran 8X standard.

There has also been many attempts to provide parallel programming tools and languages for managing parallel tasks. Examples include Strand, Linda, Schedule, etc. These products were conceived in an effort to address the portability problem and to provide parallel process management at a high level. None of these systems is widely available, and it may be that greater utilization of parallel systems will depend upon a further generation of advanced parallel compilers.

The success of parallel computing will lie, in part, in the nature of the problem to be solved. The supercomputers of the 1960s and early 1970s allowed researchers to attack mainly one-dimensional problems, and parallelism was hardly an issue. The Cray-1 and its successors, with memories up to 512 megawords have allowed today's researchers to perform detailed two-dimensional problems (fluid flow in two dimensions, for example) and some 3-D problems (flow over an airfoil, bloodflow in a heart, 3-D nerve conduction models; see Witten,[43-45] for biological examples). When more than one dimension is involved, the inherent parallelism in a problem usually becomes much more obvious. One-dimensional parallelism may be exploited by vector architecture, although it is quite often the case that a vector computer is not efficiently utilized until two or more dimensions are involved. With multiple-CPU vector machines like the Cray Y-MP, a further dimension of parallelism is apparent at the hardware level. In principle, manufacturers could continue this line, adding more very high performance CPUs but the ever increasing sophistication of very low cost microprocessors and custom very large scale integration (VLSI) chips has made it possible to contemplate parallel machines with millions of processors at a reasonable cost.

---

* Personal communication

10.8 Summary

The discovery of new molecular structures of new drugs has never been easy. Yet within the last century profound changes in pharmaceutical development have enabled the common person to have access to a wealth of medicines for the treatment of many serious diseases. Many of these drugs were designed without real understanding of the molecular biology and genetics underlying the disease. Now, with the advances in mathematical and computational algorithms, and with the increasing capability of the new hardware technologies, we will begin to see more rapidly developed and more effectively designed pharmaceuticals. Meeting the computational issues of sequencing the human genome necessitates new techniques in data storage and retrieval, sequence and search algorithms visualization, and network communications, as well as the construction of advanced computer hardware. But, if the computational challenges of the Human Genome Project can be met, what occurred over a century before can happen in as little as one or two decades. And this article only hints at how therapeutics will be directly affected by the solutions of these problems. What genetically engineered tools for drug discovery resulting from the work on the human genome can do remains for other authors. Indeed, in the incredibly farsighted words of Julian Huxley, "...biotechnology will in the long run be more important than mechanical and chemical engineering."[46]

REFERENCES

1. Venuti, M. C. "Molecular Genetics in Drug Discovery," in *Molecular Genetic Medicine*, T. Friedmann. Ed. (San Diego: Academic Press, 1991).
2. Cinkosky, M. J., J. W. Fickett, P. Gilna, and C. Burks. "Electronic Data Publishing and GenBank," *Science* 254(5036):1273–1277 (1991).
3. Naqvi, S. and S. Tsur. A Logical Language for Data and Knowledge Bases (New York: W. H. Freeman, 1989).
4. Read, R. L., D. Davidson, J. E. Chappelear, and J. S. Garavelli. "GBPARSE: A Parser for the GenBank Flat-File Format with the New Feature Table Format," *CABIOS*, 8(4):407–408 (1992).
5. Miller, P. L., P. M. Nadkarni, and N. M. Carriero. "Parallel Computation and FASTA: Confronting the Problem of Parallel Database Search for a Fast Sequence Comparison Algorithm," *CABIOS* 7(1):36 (1991).
6. Barnhart, B. J. "The Human Genome Project," in *Biotechnology and the Human Genome*, A. D. Woodhead and B. J. Barnhart, Eds. (New York: Plenum Press, 1988), pp. 161–166.
7. Bell, G. I. "The Human Genome: An Introduction," in *Computers and DNA: Proceedings of the Interface Between Computation Science and Nucleic Acid Sequencing Workshop*, Vol. 7, G. I. Bell and T. G. Marr., Eds. (Reading, MA: Addison-Wesley, 1990).
8. Fasman, G. D. Ed. *Prediction of Protein Structure and the Principles of Protein Conformation* (New York: Plenum Press, 1989).

9. Lesk, A. M. Ed. *Computational Molecular Biology: Sources and Methods for Sequence Analysis* (New York: Oxford University Press, 1988).

10. von Heijne, G. "Getting Sense Out of Sequence Data," *Nature* 333(16):605–607 (1988).

11. Waterman, M. S. "General Methods of Sequence Comparisons," *Bull. Math. Biol.* 46(4):473–500 (1984).

12. Goad, W. B. "Computational Analysis of Genetic Sequences," *Annu. Rev. Biophys. Chem.* 15(1):79–95 (1986).

13. von Heijne, G. *Sequence Analysis in Molecular Biology* (New York: Academic Press, 1987).

14. Needleman, S. B. and C. D. Wunsch. "A General Method Applicable to the Search for Similarities in the Amino Acid Sequence of 2 Proteins," *J. Mol. Biol.* 48(3):443–453 (1970).

15. Sellers, P. "An Algorithm for the Distance Between Two Finite Sequences," *J. Combinatorial Theor. (A)* 16(2):253–258 (1974).

16. Murata, M., J. S. Richardson, and J. L. Sussman. "Simultaneous Comparison of Three Protein Sequences," *Proc. Natl. Acad. Sci. U.S.A.* 82(10):3073–3077 (1985).

17. Smith, T. F. and M. S. Waterman. "Identification of Common Molecular Subsequences," *J. Mol. Biol.* 147(1):195–197 (1981).

18. Goad, W. B. and M. I. Kanehisa. "Pattern Recognition in Nucleic Acid Sequences. I. A General Method for Finding Local Homologies and Symmetries," *Nucleic Acid Res.* 10(1):247–263 (1982).

19. Gotoh, O. "Pattern Matching of Biological Sequences with Limited Storage," *CABIOS* 3(1):17–20 (1987).

20. Dumas, J. P. and J. Ninio. "Efficient Algorithm for Folding and Comparing Nucleic Acid Sequences," *Nucleic Acids Res.* 10(1):197–206 (1982).

21. Lipman, D. J. and W. R. Pearson. "Rapid and Sensitive Protein Similarity Searches," *Science* 227(4693):1435–1441 (1985).

22. Wilbur, W. J. and D. J. Lipman. "Rapid Similarity Searches of Nucleic Acid and Protein Data Banks," *Proc. Natl. Acad. Sci. U.S.A.* 80(3):726–730 (1983).

23. Pearson, W. R. and D. J. Lipman. "Improved Tools for Biological Sequence Comparison," *Proc. Natl. Acad. Sci. U.S.A.* 85(8):2444–2448 (1988).

24. Pearson, W. R. "Rapid and Sensitive Sequence Comparison with FASTP and FASTA," in *Methods of Enzymology 183*, R. F. Doolittle, Ed. (New York: Academic Press, 1990), pp. 63–98.

25. Deshpande, A. S., D. S. Richards, and W. R. Pearson. "A Platform for Biological Sequence Comparison on Parallel Computers," *CABIOS* 7(2):237–247 (1991).

26. Nussinov, R. "Theoretical Molecular Biology: Prospectives and Perspectives," *J. Theor. Biol.* 125(2):219–235 (1987).

27. Weir, B. S. "Statistical Analysis of DNA Sequences," *J. Natl. Cancer Inst.* 80(6):395–406 (1988).

28. Felsenstein, J. "Phylogenies From Molecular Sequences: Inference and Reliability," *Annu. Rev. Genet.* 22(1):521–565 (1988).

29. Felsenstein, J. "Evolutionary Tree from DNA Sequences: A Maximum Likelihood Approach," *J. Mol. Evol.* 17(6):368–376 (1981).

30. Torney, D. C., C. Burks, D. Davidson, and K. M. Sirotkin. "Computation of d^2—A Measure of Sequence Dissimilarity," in *The Interface Between Computational Science and Nucleic Acid Sequencing, SFI Studies in the Sciences of Complexity*, G. Bell and T. Marr, Eds. (Reading, MA: Addison-Wesley, 1990).

31. Proceedings of the Workshop on Advanced Computer Technologies and Biological Sequencing. ANL-88-45, November 3–5, 1988.

32. Karlin, S. and S. F. Altschul. "Methods for Assessing the Statistical Significance of Molecular Sequence Features by Using General Scoring Scemes," *Proc. Natl. Acad. Sci. U.S.A.* 87(6):2264–2268 (1990).

33. Altschul, S. F., W. Gish, W. Miller, E. W. Myers, and D. J. Limon. "A Basic Local Alignment Search Tool," *J. Mol. Biol.* 215(3):403–410 (1990).

34. Myers, G. "Practical and Theoretical Advances in Similarity Searching," Genome Sequencing Conference II, (Abstract Only) September 30 – October 3, 1990.

35. Benson, D. C. "Fourier Methods for Biosequence Analysis," *Nucleic Acids Res.* 18(21):6305–6310 (1990).

36. Fields, C. A. and C. A. Soderlund. "GM: A Practical Tool for Automating DNA Sequence Analysis," *CABIOS* 6(3):263–270 (1990).

37. Karlin, S. and G. Ghandour. "Multiple Alphabet Amino Acid Sequence Comparisons of the Immunoglobulin κ-Chain Constant Domain," *Proc. Natl. Acad. Sci. U.S.A.* 82(24):8597–601 (1985).

38. Taylor, W. R. "The Classification of Amino Acid Conservation," *J. Theor. Biol.* 119(2):205–218 (1986).

39. Davison, D. "Sequence Similarity ('Homology') Searching for Molecular Biologists," *Bull. Math. Biol.* 47(4):437–474 (1985).

40. Ward, M. O. and D. S. Adams. "Nucleotide Sequence Analysis Using Correlation Images," in *First Conference on Visualization in Biomedical Computing* (Atlanta: IEEE Computer Society Press, May 22–25, 1990), TH0311.

41. Faden, M. "The Rise of OSI," *Unix Today* pp. 17,23,25,26, May 13, 1991.

42. Lazou, C. *Supercomputers and Their Use* (Cambridge: Oxford University Press, 1988).

43. Witten, M. "Mathematical Modeling and Computers in Medicine: Editor's Remarks," *Advances in Mathematics and Computers in Medicine* 1: 653–659 (1986).

44. Witten, M. "Computational Biology: An Overview," Institute for Mathematics and Its Applications, University of Minnesota. Reprint #586 (1989).

45. Witten, M. "Biocomputing," in *Encyclopedia of Computer Science,* A. Ralston and E. D. Reilly, Eds. (New York: Van Nostrand Reinhold, 1992).

46. Huxley, J. in *Retreat From Reason*, L. T. Hogben. Ed. (New York: Random House, 1938).

ADDITIONAL READING

Barron, S., M. Witten, R. Harkness, and J. Driver. "A Bibliography on Computational Algorithms in Molecular Biology and Genetics," *CABIOS* 7(2):269 (1991).

Bishop, M. J. and C. J. Rawlings, Eds. *Nucleic Acid and Protein Sequence Analysis: A Practical Approach* (Oxford: IRL Press, 1987).

Burks, C. "GenBank: Current Status and Future Directions," in *Methods of Enzymology 183,* R. F. Doolittle, Ed. (New York: Academic Press, 1990).

Burks, C. "The Flow of Nucleotide Sequence Data into Data Banks: Role and Impact of Large-Scale Sequencing Projects," in *Computers and DNA*, G. Bell and T. Marr, Eds. (Reading, MA: Addison-Wesley, 1990).

Burks, C. "How Much Sequence Data the Databanks Will Be Processing in the Near Future," in *Biomolecular Data: A Resource in Transition*, R. R. Colwell, Ed. (Oxford: Oxford University Press, 1989).

Burks, C., J. W. Fickett, W. B. Goad, M. Kanehisa, F. I. Lewitter, W. P. Rindone, C. D. Swindell, C-S. Tung, and H. S. Bilofsky. "The GenBank Nucleic Acid Sequence Database," *CABIOS* 1(4):225–33 (1985).

Cameron, G. N. "The EMBL Data Library," *Nucleic Acids Res.* 16(5):1865–7 (1988).

Cantor, C. R. and C. L. Smith. "Mapping and Sequencing the Human Genome," in *Molecular Genetic Approaches to Neuropsychiatric Diseases*, J. Brosius and R. T. Freeman, Eds. (New York: Academic Press, 1991).

Church, G. M. and W. Gilbert. "Genomic Sequencing," *Proc. Natl. Acad. Sci. U.S.A.* 81(7):1991–95 (1984).

Churchill, G. A. "Stochastic Models for Heterogeneous DNA Sequences," *Bull. Math. Biol.* 51(1):79–94 (1989).

Clementi, E., S. Chin, G. Corongiu, J. H. Detrich, M. Dupuis, D. Folsom, G. Lie, G. C. Logan, and V. Sonnad. "Supercomputing and Supercomputers: For Science and Engineering in General and for Chemistry and Biosciences in Particular," in *Biological and Artificial Intelligence Systems*, E. Clementi and S. Chin, Eds. (Holland: ESCOM Science, 1988).

Collins, J. F. and S. F. Reddaway. "High-Efficiency Sequence Database Searching: Use of the Distributed Array Processor," in *Computers and DNA, SFI Studies in the Science of Complexity, VII*, G. Bell and T. Marr, Eds. (New York: Addison Wesley, 1990).

Colwell, R. R., Ed. *Biomolecular Data: A Resource in Transition* (Oxford: Oxford University Press, 1989).

Committee on Mapping and Sequencing the Human Genome. *Mapping and Sequencing the Human Genome* (Washington, D.C.: National Academy Press, 1988).

Coulson, A. F., J. F. Collins, and A. Lyall. " Protein and Nucleic Acid Sequence Database Searching: A Suitable Case for Parallel Processing," *Comput. J.* 30(5):420–4 (1987).

Cowin, J. E., C. H. Jellis, and D. Rickwood. "A New Method of Representing DNA Sequences which Combines Ease of Visual Analysis with Machine Readability," *Nucleic Acids Res.* 14(1):509–15 (1986).

Davison, D. B. "Sequence Searching on Supercomputers," in *Computers and DNA, SFI Studies in the Sciences of Complexity*, Vol. 7, G. Bell and T. Marr, Eds. (Reading, MA: Addison-Wesley, 1990).

DeLisi, C. "Computers in Molecular Biology: Current Applications and Emerging Trends," *Science* 240(4848):47–52 (1988).

Diamond, R. "Applications of Computer Graphics in Molecular Biology," *Comput. Graphics Forum* 3:3–11 (1984).

DOE Human Genome Steering Committee Report, January 16, 1989.

DOE/NIH Human Genome Contractors/Grantee Workshop, Santa Fe Institute, Santa Fe, NM, November 3–4, 1989 (abstracts only).

Department of Energy Office of Health and Environmental Research. Sequencing the Human Genome, Summary Report on the Santa Fe Workshop, March 3–4, 1986.

Feng, D. F. and R. F. Doolittle. "Progressive Sequence Alignment as a Prerequisite to Correct Phylogenetic Trees," *J. Mol. Evol.* 25(4):351–360 (1987).

Fickett, J. W. and C. Burks. "Development of a Database for Nucleotide Sequence," in *Mathematical Methods for DNA Sequences*, M. Waterman, Ed. (Boca Raton, FL: CRC Press, 1989).

Gotoh, O. and Y. Tagashira. "Sequence Search on a Supercomputer," *Nucleic Acids Res.* 14(1):57–64 (1986).

Gray, N. "A Program to Find Regions of Similarity Between Homologous Protein Sequences Using Dot-Matrix Analysis," *J. Mol. Graphics* 8(1):11–5 (1990).

Gribskov, M., J. Devereux, and R. R. Burgess. "The Codon Preference Plot: Graphic Analysis of Protein Coding Sequences and Prediction of Gene Expression," *Nucleic Acids Res.* 12(1):539–49 (1984).

Hamori, E. "Graphic Representation of Long DNA Sequences by the Methods of H Curves—Current Results and Future Aspects," *BioTechniques* 7(7):710–20 (1989).

Hamori, E., G. Varga, and J. J. LaGuardia. "HYLAS: Program For Generating H Curves (Abstract 3-D Representation of Long DNA Sequences)," *CABIOS* 5(4):263–69 (1989).

Hao, M-H. and W. K. Olson. "Molecular Modeling and Energy Refinement of Supercoiled DNA," *J. Biomol. Struct. Dynamics* 7(3):661–92 (1989).

Hao, M-H. and W. K. Olson. "Modeling DNA Supercoils and Knots With B-Spline Functions," *Biopolymers* 28(4):873–900 (1989).

Harr, R., P. Hagblom, and P. Gustafsson. "Two-Dimensional Graphic Analysis of DNA Sequence Homologies," *Nucleic Acids Res.* 10(1):365–74 (1982).

Havel, T. and K. Wuthrich. "A Distance Geometry Program for Determining the Structures of Small Proteins and Other Macromolecules for Nuclear Magnetic Resonance Measurements of Intramolecular ¹H–¹H Proximities in Solution," *Bull. Math. Biol.* 46(4):673–98 (1984).

Hockney, R. W. and C. R. Jesshope. *Parallel Computers 2* (New York: Adam Hilger, 1988).

Hodgman, T. C. "The Elucidation of Protein Function by Sequence Motif Analysis," *CABIOS* 5(1):1–13 (1989).

Holley, L. H. and M. Karplus. "Protein Secondary Structure Prediction for a Neural Network," *Proc. Natl. Acad. Sci. U.S.A.* 86(1):152–6 (1989).

Hozier, J., T. Nuttall, H. Newman, and W. Shoaff. "Supercomputer Assembly and Analysis of a Digitally Simulated Human Chromosome," preprint (1990).

Jaeger, J. A., D. H. Turner, and M. Zuker. "Improved Predictions of Secondary Structures for RNA," in *Methods in Enzymology—Neuroendocrine Peptide Methodology* (San Diego: Academic Press, 1989).

James, B. D., G. J. Olsen, and N. R. Pace. "Phylogenetic Comparative Analysis of RNA Secondary Structure," *Meth. Enzymol.* 180(1):227–39 (1989).

Jaroff, L. "The Gene Hunt," *TIME*, March 20, 1989, p. 62–7.

Jimenez-Montano, M. A. "On the Syntactic Structure of Protein Sequences and the Concept of Grammar Complexity," *Bull. Math. Biol.* 46(4):641–59 (1984).

Jones, R., W. Taylor, X. Zhang, J. P. Mesirov, and E. Lander. "Protein Sequence Comparison on the Connection Machine CM-2," in *Computers and DNA, SFI Studies in the Sciences of Complexity.* Vol. 7, G. Bell and T. Marr, Eds. (New York: Addison-Wesley, 1990).

Jungck, J. R. and R. M. Friedman. "Mathematical Tools for Molecular Genetics Data: An Annotated Bibliography," *Bull. Math. Biol.* 46(4):699–744 (1984).

Kanehisa, M. "Use of Statistical Criteria for Screening Potential Homologies in Nucleic Acid Sequences," *Nucleic Acids Res.* 12(1):203–13 (1984).

Karlin, S. "Comparative Analysis of Structural Relationships in DNA and Protein Sequences," in *Evolutionary Processes and Theory*, S. Karlin and E. Nevo, Eds. (New York: Academic Press, 1986).

Karlin, S. "Significant Potential Secondary Structures in the Epstein-Barr Virus Genome," *Proc. Natl. Acad. Sci. U.S.A.* 83(18):6915–9 (1986).

Karlin, S. and G. Ghandour. "The Use of Multiple Alphabets in Kappa-Gene Immunoglobulin DNA Sequence Comparisons," *EMBO J.* 4(5):1217–23 (1985).

Karlin, S., M. Morris, G. Ghandour, and M-Y. Leung. "Algorithms for Identifying Local Molecular Sequence Features," *CABIOS* 4(1):41–51 (1988).

Karlin, S., M. Morris, G. Ghandour, and M-Y. Leung. "Efficiency Algorithms for Molecular Sequence Analysis," *Proc. Natl. Acad. Sci. U.S.A.* 85(3):841–45 (1988).

Karlin, S., F. Ost, and B. E. Blaisdell. "Patterns in DNA and Amino Acid Sequences and Their Statistical Significance," in *Mathematical Methods for DNA Sequences,* M. Waterman, Ed. (Boca Raton, FL: CRC Press, 1989).

Karp, P. "A Process Oriented Model of Bacterial Gene Regulation," Stanford University Knowledge Systems Laboratory Report No. KSL-88-18 (1988).

Karp, P. "Hypothesis Formation as a Design," Stanford University Knowledge Systems Laboratory Report No. KSL-89-11 (1989).

Kingsbury, D. T. "Computational Biology for Biotechnology: Part I. The Role of the Computational Infrastructure," *Trends Biotech.* 7(4):82–7 (1989).

Kollman, P. "Molecular Modeling," *Annu. Rev. Phys. Chem.* 38(1):303–16 (1987).

Konopka, A. K. "Toward Mapping Functional Domains in Indiscriminately Sequenced Nucleic Acids: A Computational Approach," in *Human Genome Initiative and DNA Recombination*, R. Sarma, Ed. (New York: Adenine Press, 1990).

Konopka, A. K. and J. Owens. "Complexity Charts Can Be Used to Map Functional Domains in DNA," *Gene Anal. Tech.* 7(4):35–88 (1990).

Konopka, A. K., G. W. Smythers, J. Owens, and J. V. Maizel. "Distance Analysis Helps to Establish Characteristic Motifs in Intron Sequences," *Gene Anal. Tech.* 4(2):63–74 (1987).

Krawczak, M. "Algorithms for the Restriction-Site Mapping of DNA Molecules," *Proc. Natl. Acad. Sci. U.S.A.* 85(19):7298–7301 (1988).

Kriskal, J. B. "An Overview of Sequence Comparison," in *Time Warps, String Edits, and Macromolecules: The Theory and Practice of Sequence Comparison*, D. Sankoff and J. B. Kriskal, Eds. (Reading, MA: Addison-Wesley, 1983).

Lander, E. S. "Analysis with Restriction Enzymes," in *Mathematical Methods for DNA Sequences*, M. Waterman, Ed. (Boca Raton, FL: CRC Press, 1989).

Lapedes, A., C. Barnes, C. Burkes, R. Farber, and K. Sirotkin. "Application of Neural Networks and Other Machine Learning Algorithms to DNA Sequence Analysis," in *Computers and DNA*, G. Bell and T. Marr, Eds. (Reading, MA: Addison-Wesley, 1989).

Lathrop, R. H., T. A. Webster, T. F. Smith, and P. H. Winston. "ARIEL: A Massively Parallel Symbolic Learning Assistant for Protein Structure/Function," preprint (1989).

Lawton, J. R., F. A. Martinez, and C. Burks. "Overview of the LIMB Database," *Nucleic Acids Res.* 17(15):5885–99 (1989).

Le, S-Y., J-H. Hsiang, M. J. Braun, M. A. Gonda, and J. V. Maizel. "Stability of RNA Stem-Loop Structure and Distribution of Non-Random Structure in the Human Immunodeficiency Virus (HIV-1)," *Nucleic Acids Res.* 16(11):5153–68 (1988).

Le, S-Y., R. Nussinov, and J. V. Maizel. "Tree Graphs of RNA Secondary Structures and Their Comparisons," preprint.

Le, S-Y., J. Owens, R. Nussinov, J-H. Chen, B. Shapiro, and J. V. Maizel. "RNA Secondary Structures: Comparison and Determination of Frequently Recurring Substructures by Consensus," *CABIOS* 5(3):205–10 (1989).

Liebman, M. N. "Molecular Modeling of Protein Structure and Function: A Bioformatic Approach," *J. Comp. Aided Mol. Design* 1(4):323–41 (1988).

Linsley, J. "Mobility Models and Experimental Data for Lambda Phage Concatamers during Field Inversion Gel Electrophoresis," First International Conference on Electrophoresis, Supercomputing, and the Human Genome, preprint (1990).

Lipman, D. J., W. J. Wilbur, T. F. Smith, and M. S. Waterman. "On the Statistical Significance of Nucleic Acid Similarities," *Nucleic Acids Res.* 12(1):215–26 (1984).

Lipton, R. J. and D. Lopresti. "A Systolic Array for Rapid String Comparisons," in *Chapel Hill Conference on Very Large Scale Integration*, H. Fuchs, Ed. (Rockville, MD: Computer Science Press, 1985).

Luckow, V. A., R. K. Littlewood, and R. H. Round. "Interactive Computer Programs for the Graphic Analysis of Nucleotide Sequence Data," *Nucleic Acids Res.* 12(1):665–73 (1984).

Maizel, J. V. "Supercomputing in Biomedical Research," *Cray Channels* 10:3 (1988).

Mapping the Human Genome. Lawrence Berkeley Laboratory, University of California (1989).

McKusick, V. A. "The Human Genome Organisation: History, Purpose, and Membership," *Genomics* 5(2):385–87 (1989).

Milne, R. Computer Array Interprets the Human Genome," *New Scientist* 122(36):36 (1989).

Milosavljevic, A., D. Haussler, and J. Jurka. "Informed Parsimonious Inference of Prototypical Genetic Sequences," Proceedings Second Workshop on Computational Learning Theory, preprint (1989).

Miura, R. M., Ed. *Some Mathematical Questions in Biology: DNA Sequence Analysis, Lectures on Mathematics in the Life Sciences* (Providence, RI: American Mathematical Society, 1986).

Mizraji, E. and J. Ninio. "Graphical Coding of Nucleic Acid Sequences," *Biochimie* 67(5):445–8 (1985).

Moon, J. B. and W. J. Howe. "A Fast Algorithm for Generating Smooth Molecular Dot Surface Representation," *J. Mol. Graphics* 7(2):109–12 (1989).

Morowitz, H. J. and T. Smith. "Report of the Matrix of Biological Knowledge Workshop," Santa Fe Institute, Santa Fe, NM, July 13–Aug 14, 1987.

Morris, G. M. "The Matching of Protein Sequences Using Color Intrasequence Homology Displays," *J. Mol. Graphics* 6(3):135–40 (1988).

Mott, R. F., T. B. Kirkwood, and R. N. Curnow. "A Test for the Statistical Significance of DNA Sequence Similarities for Application in Databank Searches," *CABIOS* 5(2):123–31 (1989).

Norman, C. "Bush Budget Highlights R & D," *Science* 247(4942):517–19 (1990).

Nussinov, R. "Some Indicators for Inverse DNA Duplication," *J. Theor. Biol.* 95(4):783–91 (1982).

Nussinov, R. "Efficient Algorithms for Searching for Exact Repetition of Nucleotide Sequences, *J. Mol. Evol.* 19(3/4):283–5 (1983).

Pabo, C. O. "New Generation Databases for Molecular Biology," *Nature* 327(6122):467 (1987).

Palca, J. "Genome Projects Are Growing Like Weeds," *Science* 245(4914):131 (1989).

Papanicolaou, C., M. Gouy, and J. Ninio. "An Energy Model that Predicts the Correct Folding of Both the tRNA and the 5S RNA Molecules," *Nucleic Acids Res.* 12(1):31–44 (1984).

Patton, P. C. "Performance Limits for Parallel Processors," in *Parallel Supercomputing: Methods, Algorithms and Applications*, G. F. Carey, Ed. (New York: J. Wiley, 1989).

Pickover, C. A. "DNA Vectorgrams: Representation of Cancer Genes as Movements on a 2D Cellular Lattice," *IBM J. Res. Develop.* 31(1):111–9 (1987).

Pietrokovski, S., J. Hirshon, and E. N. Trifonov. "Linguistic measure of taxonomic and functional relatedness of nucleotide sequences," *J. Biomol. Struct. Dynamics*, 7:1251–1268 (1990).

Porter, B., L. Acker, J. Lester, K. Murray, and A. Souther. "The Construction of a Large-Scale Multifunctional Knowledge Base in Botany," preprint (1989).

Powell, P. A. "RESIM: Fast Algorithms for Finding the Similarity of Regular Expression Based Patterns and Sequences," University of Minnesota Computer Science Department Technical Report #90-16 (1990).

Pustell, J. and F. C. Kafatos. "A High Speed, High Capacity Homology Matrix: Zooming Through SV40 and Polyoma," *Nucleic Acids Res.* 10(15):4765–82 (1982).

Qian, N. and T. J. Sejnowski. "Predicting the Secondary Structure of Globular Proteins Using Neural Network Models," *J. Mol. Biol.* 202(4):865–884 (1988).

Rechid, R., M. Vingron, and P. Argos. "A New Interactive Protein Sequence Alignment Program and Comparison of Its Results with Widely Used Algorithms," *CABIOS* 5(2):107–13 (1989).

Reddaway, S. F. and R. M. Page. "High Speed Data Searching with a Processor Array," *Microproc. Microprogr.* 24(F-3):655–60 (1988).

Richards, F. M. and C. E. Kundrot. "Identification of Structural Motifs from Protein Coordinate Data: Secondary Structure and First-Level Supersecondary Structure," *Proteins: Structure, Function, Genetics* 3(2):71–84 (1988).

Roberts, L. "New Chip May Speed Genome Analysis," *Science* 244(4905):655–56 (1989).

Sankoff, D. and J. B. Kriskal, Eds. *Time Warps, String Edits, and Macromolecules: The Theory and Practice of Sequence Comparison* (Reading, MA: Addison-Wesley, 1983).

Sankoff, D. and M. Goldstein. "Probabilistic Models of Genome Shuffling, *Bull. Math. Biol.* 51(1):117–24 (1989).

Singh, A. K. and R. Overbeek. "Derivation of Efficient Parallel Programs: An Example from Genetic Sequence Analysis," ANL Mathematics and Computer Science Division, preprint MCS-P104-0989 (1989).

Soll, D. and R. J. Roberts. Eds. *The Applications of Computers to Research on Nucleic Acids II*, Parts 1 and 2. (Washington, D.C.: IRL Press, 1984).

Staden, R. "Computer Methods to Locate Signals in Nucleic Acid Sequences," *Nucleic Acids Res.* 12(1):505–19 (1984).

Staden, R. "Methods for Discovering Novel Motifs in Nucleic Acid Sequences," *CABIOS* 5(4):293–98 (1989).

Stormo, G. D. "Computer Methods for Analyzing Sequence Recognition of Nucleic Acids," *Annu. Rev. Biophy. Chem.* 17(1):241–63 (1988).

Subbiah, S. and S. C. Harrison. "A Method for Multiple Sequence Alignment with Gaps," *J. Mol. Biol.* 209(4):539–48 (1989).

Subcommittee on Human Genome of the HERAC for the U.S. Department of Energy, Office of Energy Research, Office of Health and Environmental Research, April 1987.

Tavare, S. and B. W. Giddings. "Some Statistical Aspects of the Primary Structure of Nucleotide Sequences," in *Mathematical Methods For DNA Sequences*, M. Waterman, Ed. (Boca Raton, FL: CRC Press, 1989).

Tavare, S. and B. Song. "Codon Preference and Primary Sequence Structure in Protein-Coding Regions, *Bull. Math. Biol.* 51(1):95–115 (1989).

Taylor, W. R. "Multiple Sequence Alignment by a Pairwise Algorithm," *CABIOS* 3(2):81–7 (1987).

Taylor, W. K. and C. A. Orengo. "Protein Structure Alignment," *J. Mol. Biol.* 208(1):1–22 (1989).

Tomboulian, S. "Introduction to a System for Implementing Neural Net Connections on SIMD Architectures," in *Neural Information Processing*, D. Z. Anderson, Ed. (New York: American Institute of Physics, 1988).

Trifonov, E. N. "Codes of Nucleotide Sequences," *Math. Biosci.* 90(1/2):507–17 (1988).

Trifonov, E. N. "Nucleotide Sequences as a Language: Morphological Classes of Words," in *Classification and Related Methods of Data Analysis*, H. H. Bock, Ed. (Amsterdam; Elsevier, 1988).

U.S. Congress, Office of Technology Assessment. *Mapping Our Genes—The Genome Projects, How Big, How Fast?,* OTA-BA-373 (Washington, D.C.: U.S. Gov. Print Office, 1988).

Vingron, M. and P. Argos. "A Fast and Sensitive Multiple Sequence Alignment Algorithm," *CABIOS* 5(2):115–21 (1989).

Waterman, M. S. "Mathematical Analysis of Molecular Sequences," *Bull. Math. Biol.* 51(1):1–4 (1989).

Waterman, M. S., Ed. "Consensus Methods for Folding Single-Stranded Nucleic Acids," in *Mathematical Methods for DNA Sequences* (Boca Raton, FL: CRC Press, 1989).

Waterman, M. S. and M. Eggert. "A New Algorithm for Best Subsequence Alignments with Application to tRNA–rRNA Comparisons," *J. Mol. Biol.* 197(4):723–28 (1987).

White, J. H. "Introduction to the Geometry and Topology of DNA Structure," in *Mathematical Methods for DNA Sequences*, M. Waterman, Ed. (Boca Raton, FL: CRC Press, 1989).

Wilcox, G. L. and M. O. Poliac. "Generalization of Protein Structure from Sequence Using a Large Scale Backpropagation Network," *Proc. IJCNN* II: 609 (1989).

Witten, M. "Some Mathematics of Recombination: Evolution of Complexity and Genotypic Modification in Somatic Cells: A Possible Model for Aging and Cancer Effects," *Mech. Aging Develop.* 13(2):185–97 (1980).

Witten, M. and A. Gross. "Modeling DNA: Some Applications of Error Correcting Codes and Information Theory," Notices of the AMS, August, 1980.

Woodhead, A. D. and B. J. Barnhard, Eds. *Biotechnology and the Human Genome* (New York: Plenum Press, 1988).

Wu, C. H., G. M. Whitson, and J. W. McLarty. "Artificial Neural System for Gene Classification Using a Domain Database," Proceedings 1990 ACM 18th Annual Computer Science Conference, (1990), pp. 288–292

Yamamoto, K., Y. Kitamura, and H. Yoshikura. "Computational of Statistical Secondary Structures of Nucleic Acids," *Nucleic Acids Res.* 12(1):335–46 (1984).

Zuker, M. "RNA Folding Prediction: The Continued Need for Interaction Between Biologists and Mathematicians," in *Lectures on Mathematics in the Life Sciences: Some Mathematical Questions in Biology—DNA Sequence Analysis*, R. Miura, Ed. (Providence, RI: American Mathematical Society, 1986).

Zuker, M. "The Use of Dynamic Programming Algorithms in RNA Secondary Structure Prediction," in *Mathematical Methods for DNA Sequences*, M. Waterman, Ed. (Boca Raton, FL: CRC Press, 1989).

Zuker, M. and R. L. Somorjai. "The Alignment of Protein Structures in 3 Dimensions," *Bull. Math. Biol.* 51(1):55–78 (1989).

CHAPTER 11

Epidemiology as an Alternative to Animal Research

Jennifer L. Kelsey and Susan Parker

11.0 Introduction

Epidemiology is the study of the distribution and determinants of health-related states or events in specified populations, and the application of this study to the control of health problems.[1] Epidemiologic studies are most frequently undertaken to learn about the causation, natural history, pathogenesis, clinical course, and control of disease in humans. The methods of epidemiology are also applicable to other fields studying associations between one characteristic and another in groups of individuals, including groups of animals. Epidemiologists bring expertise in study design to such collaborative efforts. This paper discusses the various types of studies commonly used in epidemiology, with emphasis on the general strengths and weaknesses of each type of design. How epidemiologists make causal inference is discussed. Finally, one specific aspect of epidemiologic study design, that is, determining the sample size needed for a given study, will be briefly covered, since if animal studies continue to be undertaken, it is imperative that as few animals as possible be used. More detailed discussion of these issues can be found in standard epidemiologic textbooks.[2-5]

Learning about causes and courses of diseases through epidemiologic studies is generally a gradual process that requires different types of study designs in various situations, depending upon the current state of knowledge and upon the nature of the disease and possible etiologic agents or other characteristics being considered. Study designs can be broadly divided into descriptive studies and analytic studies.

11.1 Descriptive Epidemiology

Descriptive epidemiology is the study of the distribution of diseases and other characteristics in population groups by such attributes as person, place, and time. In regard to "person", it might be of interest to determine the age distribution of people with a given disease or characteristic, or to learn whether risk for disease differs by gender, race, or socioeconomic status. For instance, descriptive studies undertaken several years ago showed that cervical cancer occurs most commonly in women of lower social class, and more often in married women than in women who have never married, observations that generated hypotheses linking cervical cancer to sexual behavior.

Regarding "place", disease occurrence within natural or political boundaries can be studied, or other distinctions such as urban vs. rural or variation by latitude can be made. Epidemiologists often use maps to represent graphically the geographic differences that are observed. For example, maps of cancer mortality rates in the U.S. according to county of residence were published in 1975.[6] These cancer atlases focused attention on certain geographic areas with unusually high cancer mortality rates, which led to further research into the reasons for high rates in areas such as New Jersey.

Studies of the distribution of disease by "time" can use units ranging from years to time of day. Changes in disease occurrence over long periods of time are called secular trends. Large increases in lung cancer rates in the past 50 years in males (and more recently in females), and marked decreases in stomach cancer rates over the same time period in both males and females, are examples of secular trends that have suggested environmental and lifestyle etiologic factors in these cancers. Knowledge of one or more of these epidemiologic characteristics of person, place, and time can also be of interest in clinical and health planning contexts.

11.2 Analytic Epidemiology

Analytic studies are designed to identify determinants of distributions of diseases and other conditions in populations. Whereas descriptive epidemiology describes *how* a disease is distributed in a population, analytic epidemiology goes one step further and tries to explain *why*.

Most analytic epidemiologic studies in humans are observational; that is, the investigator observes what is occurring in the study populations of interest. In

Table 1.   Distribution of Lung Cancer Cases and Controls According to Average
            Number of Cigarettes Smoked per Day During the Ten Years Preceding
            Onset of Present Illness (England, 1948–1950)

Cigarettes per day	Cases				Controls			
		No.		%		No.		%
0		7		0.5		61		4.5
1–4		55		4.1		129		9.5
5–14		489		36.0		570		42.0
15–24	1350	475	99.5	35.0	1296	431	95.5	31.8
25–49		293		21.6		154		11.3
≥50		38		2.8		12		0.9
Total		1357		100.0		1357		100.0

From Doll and Hill[15]

experimental studies, the investigator intervenes and assigns members of the study
population to one exposure or treatment category or another (as in a randomized
clinical trial). Experimental studies will not be covered here. Observational analytic studies are generally classified as case–control, cohort, or cross-sectional.

11.2.1 Case–Control Studies

   Case–control studies are those in which the investigator selects persons with a
given disease (cases) and persons without the given disease (controls) for study.
The cases are generally persons seeking medical care for the disease: newly
diagnosed cases are usually specified in order to be more certain that the risk
factor preceded the disease rather than being a consequence of it, and so that
rapidly fatal cases or cases of short duration are appropriately represented. The
controls may be selected from the general population, from people who live in the
same neighborhoods as the cases, from among patients seeking medical care for
other diseases or conditions at the same facility, or from other sources. The
proportions of cases and controls with certain characteristics or past exposure to
possible risk factors are then determined and compared. (For a numerical measurement such as blood pressure or weight, the mean level of the characteristic of
interest in the cases is compared to the mean level of the characteristic in the
controls.) The first epidemiologic studies to test the hypothesis that smoking
increases the risk for developing lung cancer, for instance, compared the proportion of smokers among lung cancer cases to the proportion of smokers in a control
group comprising patients of the same gender and similar age admitted to the same
hospitals with other diseases (Table 1).[7] The percentage of smokers among lung
cancer cases was found to be higher than the percentage of smokers among the
control subjects. Further, there was a strong tendency for the cases to have smoked
more cigarettes per day than the controls, and cases had on the average smoked
a greater number of years than the controls. All of these trends are consistent with
a causal link between smoking and lung cancer.

Table 2. **Diethylstilbestrol (DES) Use During Pregnancy in Mothers of Cases of Adenocarcinoma of the Vagina and Matched Controls**

Case no.	Case	Matched Controls			
		1	2	3	4
1	Y	N	N	N	N
2	Y	N	N	N	N
3	Y	N	N	N	N
4	Y	N	N	N	N
5	N	N	N	N	N
6	Y	N	N	N	N
7	Y	N	N	N	N
8	Y	N	N	N	N

Note: Use of DES designated by Y = yes and N = no. p <0.00001.

From Herbst et al.[8]

Identification of the association between exposure to diethylstilbestrol (DES) and vaginal cancer in young women provides an example of how a small number of case–control studies, with very few subjects, can sometimes provide enough evidence that an important public health measure can be implemented. In 1970 and 1971, seven cases of clear-cell carcinoma of the vagina and one case of the closely related endometrioid carcinoma were reported from Boston among women whose ages ranged from 15 to 22 years. Previously this condition had rarely been seen in young women. The mothers of seven of the eight cases reported having taken DES during the first trimester of pregnancy, while none of the mothers of 32 matched controls had used it (Table 2).[8] The association was soon confirmed in two other case–control studies, and in 1971 the U.S. Food and Drug Administration (FDA) banned the use of DES for maintenance of pregnancies.

Another recent example of a case–control study is one in which oral contraceptive use in women of ages 20 to 54 years with (a) breast cancer,[9] (b) endometrial cancer,[10] and (c) ovarian cancer[11] in eight geographic areas of the country was compared to oral contraceptive use among women of similar age from the general population in the same parts of the country. In this study, histories of oral contraceptive use were similar or slightly higher in breast cancer cases as compared to controls, suggesting at most a slight increase in risk. However, prior oral contraceptive use was greater in controls than in cases of endometrial cancer or ovarian cancer, suggesting that oral contraceptive use diminishes the risk of these two cancers.

Appropriate choice and sufficiently large numbers of cases and controls are obviously critical to the quality of case–control studies, unless the association is so strong, as in the instance of DES and vaginal cancer, that it can be seen even with small numbers. In the studies of oral contraceptives and female reproductive cancers, cases were all women of ages 20 to 54 years reported by hospitals to tumor registries covering eight relatively large geographic areas, and controls were selected by randomly dialing telephone numbers in the same geographic areas until a sufficient number of women were identified with an age distribution similar to that of the cases. Thus, it is unlikely that biases related to how cases and controls were selected could account for the results. Also, the participation rates among both the cases and the controls were relatively high (for example, 83 and 86%, respectively, for breast cancer cases and controls) and the proportion of households with telephones has been reported to be 94% in the U.S.[12] The early studies of cigarette smoking and lung cancer identified cases from selected hospitals in large cities. Since it would be impossible to specify the population from which the cases arose, a logical comparison group would be patients admitted to the same hospitals with other conditions, preferably conditions not thought to have any association (either positive or negative) with smoking. This, in fact, was what was done in several studies.

Choice of an inappropriate control group can call into question the results of a study. In a case–control study of risk factors for cancer of the pancreas reported some years ago,[13] cases were patients with a histologic diagnosis of cancer of the exocrine pancreas diagnosed in 11 large hospitals in the Boston metropolitan area and Rhode Island. Controls consisted of other patients under the care of the same physicians in the same hospitals as the patients with pancreatic cancer. The control group accordingly consisted mainly of persons with other cancers and gastro-enterologic conditions, since those were the diseases most commonly seen by these physicians. A strong association between coffee consumption and pancreatic cancer was found. However, some questioned whether an excess of coffee consumption among the cases really existed; an alternative explanation was that the controls, who included many people with gastrointestinal illnesses, could have reduced their coffee consumption below that of the general population.

In summary, in many instances case–control studies can provide useful information, but one must be aware of many possible pitfalls. Sackett[14] has given a lengthy list of potential biases in case–control studies; a few of the most important concerns are mentioned here. (1) Are the selected cases representative of all cases with the disease, and were the cases selected in such a way that the results will be tilted neither for nor against the hypothesis of interest? (2) Are the controls selected such that they are likely to give a fair estimate of the proportion of people with the characteristics of interest in the population from which the cases came? (3) Did the exposure or characteristic of interest precede or follow the disease under study? (4) Is information on the exposure or characteristic of interest equally likely to be detected in cases and controls? (5) Are there any other factors that could have independently caused both the exposure of interest and the disease under study, thus creating a connection between the exposure and the disease that is not causal? Such factors are called confounding variables by epidemiologists and will be discussed later.

11.2.2 Cohort Studies

In a prospective cohort study, individuals who are free of the disease at the time of entry into the study are classified according to whether they are exposed or not exposed to the factors of interest. The cohort is then followed for a period of time (which may be many years) and the incidence rates (number of new cases of disease per population at risk per unit time) or mortality rates (number of deaths per population at risk per unit time) in those exposed or not exposed are compared. Cohort studies thus have the major advantage over case–control studies that the exposure or characteristic of interest is measured before the disease has developed. However, prospective cohort studies generally require large sample size, long-term follow-up of study subjects, large monetary expense, and elaborate administrative and organizational arrangements. The outcome of interest must be relatively common, or prohibitively large numbers of subjects will be required in order to ensure adequate numbers experiencing that outcome. Therefore, prospective cohort studies are usually initiated under two circumstances: first, when sufficient (but not definitive) evidence has been obtained from less expensive studies to warrant a more expensive cohort study, and, second, when a new agent (e.g., oral contraceptives) that may alter the risk for several diseases is introduced into the environment.

An observational prospective cohort study of the association between cigarette smoking and lung cancer would involve assembling a cohort of individuals free of lung cancer, some of whom are smokers, some of whom are nonsmokers. These individuals would then be followed over time and the incidence rate of lung cancer in the smokers compared to that in the nonsmokers. In such studies the incidence rate in all smokers combined is about ten times greater than in nonsmokers.[15] The smokers can be subdivided according to the amount that they smoke, the length of time they have smoked, and into former and current smokers. It has been found (Table 3) that the greater the number of cigarettes smoked per day and the greater the number of years smoked, the higher the risk of lung cancer. Among former smokers, after a few years have elapsed the risk of lung cancer decreases as the number of years since quitting increases.

A more recent cohort study was concerned with the relationship between a high-fat diet and breast cancer.[16] Experimental studies in animals had strongly suggested that a high-fat diet promotes mammary tumors (reviewed by Prentice et al.[17]). Furthermore, descriptive epidemiologic studies found that countries with the greatest per capita fat purchases tend to have the highest breast cancer incidence rates. Many other differences between countries could, of course, explain the international variation in breast cancer incidence rates, so that the analytic epidemiologic studies were needed to test the hypothesis. Most case–control studies in humans found little or no association between a high-fat diet and breast cancer. This lack of an association was thought possibly to be attributable to the difficulty of accurately measuring fat intake in the past; a cohort study in women would provide more definitive evidence on this issue. Such a study was undertaken by Willett et al.[16] in a cohort of nurses. The results of the study actually showed a slight negative association between fat intake and breast cancer (Table 4), a reminder that what is found in animals is often of limited relevance to humans.

Table 3. Annual Mortality Rates Per 1000 from Lung Cancer in Relation to Amount Smoked by Physicians in the U.K., by Age

Age (yrs)	No. of deaths	Nonsmokers	1–14 g	15–24 g	>25 g
				Amount smoked	
35–54	10	0.00	0.09	0.17	0.28
55–64	24	0.00	0.32	0.52	3.10
65–74	31	0.00	1.35	3.34	4.81
≥75	19	0.70	2.78	2.07	4.16
All ages	84	0.07	0.47	0.86	1.66

From Doll and Hill[15]

Table 4. Age-Adjusted Relative Risk of Breast Cancer According to Quantile of Calorie-Adjusted Intake of Total Fat

Quantile of intake	Age-adjusted relative risk	95% Confidence limits
1(low)	1.0	
2	0.8	0.6–1.0
3	0.9	0.7–1.1
4	0.8	0.6–1.0
5 (high)	0.8	0.6–1.1

From Willett et al.[16]

A variation on the prospective cohort study is the retrospective cohort study (also called an historical cohort study or a nonconcurrent prospective study), in which investigators assemble a cohort by reviewing records to identify exposures in the past (often decades ago). Based on their recorded exposure histories, subjects are divided into exposed and unexposed groups. The investigator then reconstructs their subsequent disease experience up to some defined point in the more recent past or up to the present time. Typical of epidemiologic retrospective cohort studies are those in which individuals with occupational exposures (such as asbestos) many years ago are followed up to determine their subsequent mortality experience (such as from cancer of the lung[18] and cancer of the larynx[19]). A retrospective cohort study was also used to examine the connection between dietary fat intake and breast cancer. In a study linking data on fat consumption previously collected in the U.S. Health and Nutrition Examination Survey of 1971–75 with subsequent occurrence of breast cancer, Jones et al.,[20] obtained results similar to those of the prospective cohort study of Willett et al.,[16] that is, a slight negative association between dietary fat intake and breast cancer. The consistency of the findings in these two cohort studies, one prospective and one retrospective, in different populations, lends credence to the results.

Retrospective cohort studies have many of the advantages of prospective cohort studies, but can be completed in a much more timely fashion and are therefore much less expensive. However, only when the necessary information on past exposure and other characteristics of interest has been reliably recorded is a retrospective cohort study a viable option. Furthermore, the investigator must be able to trace a large proportion of the study subjects in order to determine whether they in fact developed the disease of interest.

Similarly to prospective cohort studies, it is usually feasible to carry out a retrospective cohort study only when the outcome of interest is relatively common. It is often important to obtain information on characteristics of the study subjects other than exposure and outcome (i.e., potential confounding variables, to be discussed later), so as to make sure that those with and those without the exposure of interest are comparable in other relevant respects; this may not be possible in many situations. Thus, retrospective cohort studies are economical and useful when the relevant information can be obtained and when the outcome of interest is relatively common; in many situations, however, the necessary information is simply not available.

11.2.3 Cross-Sectional Studies

In a cross-sectional or prevalence study, exposure to a hypothesized risk factor, or other characteristic of interest, and the occurrence of a disease are measured at one point in time (or over a relatively short period of time) in a population group. Prevalence rates of disease (number of cases of existing disease per population at risk at a given point in time or time period) among those with and without the exposure or characteristic of interest are then compared. For instance, a prevalence study might be used to determine whether obese individuals are more likely to have osteoarthritis than non-obese individuals. In prevalence studies, however, it is often difficult to differentiate between cause and effect. If obesity and osteoarthritis were associated, it would not be clear whether obesity predisposes to osteoarthritis or whether people with osteoarthritis tend to get less exercise and therefore become obese. Interpretation of cross-sectional studies is clear only for potential risk factors that will not change as a result of the disease, such as ABO blood groups or HLA antigens.

Prevalence means all cases, new and old. Therefore, a second limitation of cross-sectional studies is that the case group tends to be weighted towards individuals with disease of long duration, since the chances are greater for cases of long duration to be included than cases who recover or die quickly. Thus, any relationships found apply more to subjects with disease of long duration than to those with disease of short duration, since the latter group is not adequately represented in the study group. The only way to avoid this problem is to avoid cross-sectional studies, and to include only newly diagnosed cases, as is done in cohort studies or in many case–control studies.

11.3 Epidemiologic Methods in Studying Behavioral Variables

The general principles of epidemiologic study design described above can be readily applied to the study of psychological and sociological variables as risk factors for diseases and other conditions. Psychosocial risk factors for disease might be stress, depression, anxiety, demoralization, lack of social support, or some other variable. Considerable attention has been given to the construction of measures of these variables; perhaps best known are the inventories of stressful life events,[21] which are then related to disease occurrence. Examples of other specific associations that have been studied extensively (although for the most part not definitively) are Type A behavior and coronary heart disease,[22] depression and cancer,[23] and lack of social networks and mortality from all causes.[24] Measurement of the variables of interest can be challenging in these studies; increasing emphasis is being placed on specific narrowly defined concepts rather than general phenomena such as "stress".[25] Even within the concepts of Type A behavior, investigators are beginning to focus on its individual components such as hostility, time urgency, anger, need for control, self-esteem, and hardiness.[26]

In most studies of psychosocial variables and disease, it is important that cohort studies be undertaken. In case–control and cross-sectional studies, it is generally difficult to know which came first, the disease or the psychological variable. For instance, if stress, anxiety, or depression is measured in people who have had a heart attack, it will be impossible to know whether these psychological factors brought about the heart attack or whether the heart attack caused a person to feel stressed, anxious, or depressed. Many studies showing associations between stressful life events and disease inquire about the events after the occurrence of disease; the results of such studies are suspect because people with a disease may be much more likely to reconstruct the occurrence of past events to explain their disease than healthy people.[26] Given that a cohort study is to be done, the same issues of choice of study population, measurement and control of confounding variables, detection of effect modification, estimation of required sample size, and other considerations need to be taken into account just as in studies of physical variables.

11.4 Other Useful Epidemiologic Concepts

11.4.1 Confounding Variables

A statistical association between exposures or other characteristics and diseases does not necessarily mean they are *causally* connected. In ruling out variables other than causal explanations, "confounding" variables need to be considered. A confounding variable, if not adequately accounted for, can lead to finding an apparent causal association that does not really exist, or failing to find one that is, in fact, real. For instance, the literature prior to 1970 contains reports of an inverse association between length of lactation and risk for breast cancer.[27]

This apparent protective effect of lactation, however, at least in postmenopausal women, has since been found in several studies to have occurred because women who breast fed for long periods of time tended to have had their first child at a young age. Early full-term pregnancy, rather than lactation, is the true protective factor.[28] In other words, the apparent protective effect of lactation against breast cancer disappeared once age at first full-term pregnancy was taken into account.

A confounder is defined as a variable (e.g., age at first birth) that (1) is causally related to the disease (e.g., breast cancer) under study independently of the exposure or characteristic of primary interest (e.g., lactation), and (2) is associated with the exposure or characteristic of primary interest in the study population, but (3) is not a consequence of this exposure. Confounding can be controlled for either by matching cases to controls (in a case–control study, for instance) on the confounding variable or by controlling for the confounding variable in the statistical analysis.[3]

11.4.2 Effect Modification

Effect modification, sometimes referred to as statistical interaction, also needs to be considered when studies are designed, analyzed, and interpreted. It occurs when the magnitude of the association between one variable and another differs according to the level of a third variable. Many studies show that the association between obesity and breast cancer depends upon a woman's age (and presumably menopausal status). In women older than about 50 years of age, obesity is associated with an increased risk for breast cancer, while in younger women no association, or possibly an inverse association, is found.[29] Detecting effect modification is an important component of the analysis of epidemiologic data.

11.4.3 Relative Risk

In cohort studies, the strength of the association between a putative risk factor (or other characteristic) and a disease is often measured by what is commonly called a relative risk (or, more technically, a rate ratio or risk ratio; a discussion of the difference between a rate ratio and a risk ratio is beyond the scope of this paper). A relative risk is simply the risk (or rate) of disease in one group divided by the risk (or rate) of disease in another group. For instance, in the smoking–lung cancer association shown in Table 3, the following relative risk estimates can be made for the row "all ages"; smokers of 25 or more grams per day compared to nonsmokers, 1.66 per 1000 divided by 0.07 per 1000, or a relative risk of 23.7; smokers of 15 to 24 g/d compared to nonsmokers, 0.86/0.07 = 12.3; and smokers of 1 to 14 g/d, compared to nonsmokers, 0.47/0.07 = 6.7. These relative risks can be interpreted to mean that light smokers have about 7 times the risk of nonsmokers of developing lung cancer, moderate smokers, about 12 times the risk, and heavy smokers, about 24 times the risk. Relative risk estimates thus give a meaningful idea of the extent to which an exposure elevates risk for a disease and are important in assessing whether a causal relationship between an exposure and a disease exists. Relative risks can be estimated controlling for the effects of confounding variables.

11.4.4 Odds Ratio

In case–control studies, incidence rates are generally not available, so relative risks cannot be calculated. Instead the "odds ratio" (ratio of exposed to nonexposed among cases divided by the ratio of exposed to nonexposed among controls) is calculated. It can be shown[5] that for all but the most common diseases (>10% of the population affected, for instance), the odds ratio is a good approximation to the relative risk, and can be interpreted similarly. In the early case–control study of smoking and lung cancer shown in Table 1, the odds ratio for all smokers combined was computed as (1350/7)/(1296/61), or 9.1, while for smokers of 50 or more cigarettes per day, the odds ratio is (38/7)/(12/61) = 27.6, associations quite consistent with those described above. Odds ratios can also be computed controlling for the effects of other variables.

11.5 Criteria for Causation

Because most epidemiologic studies are observational rather than experimental, study subjects will differ on many variables besides the exposure and disease of primary interest to the investigator. Sometimes these variables can be recognized, measured, and accounted for (see *Confounding Variables,* above), but often they are unknown or only vaguely hypothesized. Also, the ideal methodology to be used in studying an exposure–disease relationship may not be clear cut. Therefore, seldom will a single observational epidemiologic study provide definitive evidence for or against a hypothesis. Even results from several studies may not be convincing. For example, despite strong associations between lung cancer and cigarette smoking observed in early case–control studies, critics postulated that the people who chose to smoke tended to be destined to develop lung cancer anyway, or that some other factor (such as heredity) caused people both to smoke and to develop lung cancer.

In lieu of the more definitive evidence for causality that experiments provide in the physical sciences, for instance, epidemiologists have developed causal criteria to evaluate studies in the context of current knowledge. Not all criteria need be fulfilled in all instances, nor are all equally important, but taken together they provide useful guidelines for determining whether an association between a given exposure and disease is causal. These criteria are described and illustrated by the example of smoking and lung cancer.

1. *Strength of association:* The measure of association (relative risk or odds ratio) should be elevated, indicating that the exposed are at increased risk of disease over the nonexposed, or that those with disease are more likely to have histories of exposure than those without the disease. The greater the magnitude of these measures, the more likely the association is to be causal. As a rough rule of thumb, a relative risk or odds ratio of 2 is moderate, of 3 or more, strong. If there is no association between exposure and disease, the issue of causality does not arise, so that establishing an association is an essential first step; the stronger the association, the more convincing is this aspect of the argument. Cigarette smokers are, overall, 10 times more likely to develop lung cancer than nonsmokers, and people with lung cancer much more frequently report histories of smoking than those without lung cancer.

2. *Statistical significance:* A finding of statistical significance means that the result is unlikely to be a consequence of chance. Statistical significance depends on both the strength of association and on the number of study subjects. If sample size is inadequate, even relatively strong associations may not be statistically significant. Conversely, a tiny, biologically meaningless elevated risk can become "significant" with a very large sample size. Large numbers of studies have found substantial, statistically significant associations between smoking and lung cancer.

3. *Ruling out alternative explanations:* Once a significant association has been established (i.e., the exposure and disease are related, and the relationship is unlikely to be due to chance), other explanations for the observed association, such as methodologic deficiencies and confounding, should be carefully considered and ruled out. For instance, perhaps people who smoke cigarettes tend to live in areas of high air pollution and it is really air pollution that is causing the lung cancer. Such explanations have, in fact, been considered and ruled out for the smoking–lung cancer association.

4. *Dose–response relationship:* If increasing dose or length of exposure correlates with increasing risk, a strong case is made for causality, because the likelihood is considerably reduced that such a pattern could arise by chance or be attributable to confounding. However, the absence of a dose–response relationship does not disprove causality since other patterns of association (e.g., threshold effects) also can occur. Smokers of two packs a day are about 20 times more likely to develop lung cancer than nonsmokers, a relative risk that declines steadily as the number of cigarettes per day decreases. The risk also increases with years smoked, given the same number of cigarettes smoked per day.

5. *Removal of exposure:* If the presence of an exposure increases risk of disease and removing the exposure reduces risk, a causal explanation is strengthened. The risk for lung cancer decreases in persons who stop smoking a few years after they quit, and continues to decrease with additional years of abstinence.

6. *Time order:* Although it may seem trivially obvious that a cause must precede an effect, determining time order unambiguously can present problems in some studies. In case–control studies of diseases of insidious onset or long induction periods (such as many cancers), the appropriate timing of exposure may be decades before ascertainment. This problem is particularly notable in cross-sectional studies, where prevalent disease and exposure are determined simultaneously, as illustrated by the association between osteoarthritis and obesity described above. Time order is unique among the causal criteria in that if disease can be shown to precede exposure, causality is definitively ruled out. Generally, the time lapse between beginning

smoking and occurrence of lung cancer is on the order of 20 years or more, making it unlikely that lung cancer causes a person to smoke.

7. *Predictive power:* Hypotheses deduced from a presumed causal association that can in turn be shown to predict future occurrences lend strong support to the causality of the original association. If smoking causes lung cancer, it might be expected that those groups of people with high per capita cigarette consumption would have high lung cancer rates. One early argument against the hypothesis that smoking causes lung cancer was that women who smoked seemed to be at a fraction of the risk of men. However, it was argued that women began smoking in large numbers much later than men, and it was predicted than an increase in lung cancer rates would be seen after an appropriate induction period. Sadly, this has turned out to be all too true; lung cancer is now the leading cause of cancer death among women, surpassing breast cancer in the mid-1980s.

8. *Consistency:* If associations of similar magnitude are found in different populations by different study methods, the likelihood of causality is increased substantially, since all studies are unlikely to have the same methodologic limitations or study population idiosyncrasies. Cigarette smoking has been associated with lung cancer among both males and females, all races, and many nationalities in a variety of cohort and case–control studies, all showing approximately a tenfold increase in risk overall.

9. *Coherence with experimental data:* When available, the results of a well designed experiment in which exposures are assigned at random are very convincing, because the only factor on which groups differ, except by chance, is the exposure of interest. However, many exposures, including smoking, cannot ethically be assigned at random. In addition, some well controlled experiments on a few carefully selected subjects (e.g., dietary experiments on metabolic wards) may have little relevance to free-living populations. Good observational studies usually have the advantage of being more generalizable to the larger population.

10. *Biologic plausibility:* When a new finding fits well with the currently known biology of a disease, it is more plausible than if a whole new theory must be developed to encompass the new finding. Certainly, it is logical that smoking, which delivers the products of burning tobacco directly into the lungs, might cause lung cancer. Conversely, when epidemiologic studies first showed smoking to be associated with an increased risk of cervical cancer, no direct mechanism could be postulated, and it was assumed that a confounding variable, perhaps sexual activity, which is associated with both smoking and cervical cancer, was the true cause. Since that time metabolites of cigarette smoke have been identified in cervical mucus,[30] adding credence to the possibility that smoking itself increases the risk of cervical cancer. Another possible means of enhancing biologic plausibility is through animal experiments. Animals can be randomly assigned to many exposures where humans usually cannot, so that if an association in humans is replicated in animals, the belief in causality may be enhanced. However, agents are often species- and even organ-specific, making extrapolation from animals to humans and from humans to animals tenuous at best. By the time lung tumors had been induced in beagles that had been taught to smoke,[31-33] the causal criteria had already been fulfilled beyond any reasonable doubt.[34] Had these dogs not developed bronchio-alveolar tumors, the conclusion that smoking causes lung cancer in humans, given the overwhelming evidence, would hardly have been affected.[34,35]

As implied by the sort of reasoning inherent in assessing the causal criteria, any decision on the likelihood of causality is necessarily judgmental. For this reason, Lilienfeld[36] divided the degree of evidence for causation into three levels. At the first level, the evidence is considered sufficient for further study. For instance, the descriptive epidemiologic and animal studies suggesting a relationship between a high-fat diet and breast cancer demonstrated the need for analytic epidemiologic studies specifically to test this hypothesis. At the second level, the evidence is considered sufficient to warrant public health action, even if the causal association has not been definitively established. The banning of DES for prevention of miscarriages on the basis of just a few case–control studies would fall into this category. At the third level, the evidence is so strong that the causal association is considered part of the body of scientific knowledge. Most people would consider the smoking–lung cancer association in this category, and by now most would also consider the DES–vaginal carcinoma association established.

11.6 AIDS: An Epidemiologic Paradigm

Even if it were desirable, animal models are not available for all diseases, and research must proceed without them. Tremendous effort and large sums of money have been expended on the attempt to develop an animal model for AIDS, so far with little success. Chimpanzees can be infected with the human immunodeficiency virus (HIV), but they do not develop symptomatic disease; transgenic mice that carry the HIV genome in every cell of their bodies have been bred, but whether they will provide a useful model is still unknown; Asian macaques are susceptible to simian immunodeficiency virus (SIV), a retrovirus closely related to HIV that causes an AIDS-like syndrome in these primates, but it is not the same agent.[37] Meanwhile, since the epidemic was recognized in 1981, great strides have been made in the identification and elucidation of the distribution, modes of transmission, causal agent, myriad manifestations, and possible interventions in AIDS. Epidemiologic studies have contributed substantially to this current knowledge.[38]

What was to become AIDS first came to medical attention when a cluster of cases of *pneumocystis carinii* pneumonia (PCP), a rare pneumonia previously found mainly in immunosuppressed cancer patients and transplant recipients, was reported in a group of otherwise healthy, young homosexual men in Los Angeles.[39] Then a rare cancer, Kaposi's sarcoma, also usually associated with immunosuppressive therapy, was reported in similar men in New York and California.[40] Other conditions associated with immunosuppression, such as chronic lymphadenopathy and non-Hodgkin's lymphoma, were appearing in the same population, and indeed, laboratory tests showed these men to have impaired immune function. This early descriptive epidemiology involving person (young, mostly white, homosexual men), place (San Francisco, New York, Los Angeles), and time (record reviews indicated that these cases began to appear in the late 1970s), was the first signal of the AIDS epidemic.

Following these leads, risk factors were sought in case–control studies of gay men with and without AIDS. Number and frequency of sexual partners and receptive anal intercourse were found to increase risk. Then cases began appearing among recipients of blood transfusions, hemophiliacs receiving blood products, and intravenous drug users, all of whom shared intravenous exposure to blood. Thus, a transmissible infectious agent present in blood, semen, and perhaps other body fluids became the likeliest cause of AIDS, shifting attention away from toxic causes. Soon thereafter HIV was isolated in French and American laboratories, and a test to identify HIV antibodies in blood made it possible to detect infection in asymptomatic people and to screen blood donors. Similar studies later identified heterosexual partners of intravenous drug users, hemophiliacs, and bisexual men, as well as infants born to infected women, as additional risk groups. These and other case–control studies, in addition to identifying exposures that increased risk, demonstrated that casual contact was not a risk factor for HIV infection.

The HIV antibody test also made it possible to assemble cohorts of gay men, hemophiliacs, and intravenous drug users known to be exposed and unexposed to the virus (HIV positive and negative), none of whom had symptoms of AIDS, and to follow them to determine incidence rates of new infections and of progression from infection to AIDS, as well as to identify other opportunistic infections associated with HIV. Especially valuable were retrospective cohort studies of gay men in New York and San Francisco who had originally been recruited for clinical trials of the hepatitis B vaccine in the late 1970s; for many of these men, stored sequential serum samples were available. These subjects contributed data on when the virus first appeared in the population, its rate of spread, its current prevalence, the clinical course of the infection, as well as risk factors and other characteristics. Because the stored serum samples could be used to identify men infected in the past, the follow-up period was shortened considerably.

Clinical trials (a type of experimental study not covered in this chapter) are currently underway to test promising AIDS drugs and vaccines and were crucial to demonstrating the efficacy of AZT, DDI, and DDC, the only FDA-approved drugs for treating AIDS and HIV infection at present. Clinical trials have also shown the efficacy of a number of drugs used to treat various opportunistic infections associated with AIDS, prolonging the lives and improving the quality of life of people infected with HIV. As can be seen from this example, epidemiology has much to contribute to medical research, and substantial progress can and does occur in the absence of animal experiments.

11.7 Sample Size Considerations

If animal studies are to be undertaken, they should be based on study designs that include the smallest possible number of animals that are needed to produce meaningful results. In many instances, the number of animals seems to be chosen without much rhyme or reason. Many statistical and epidemiologic textbooks give formulas for sample size estimation.[3-5,38] The sample size required depends upon a number of factors, all of which enter the equations below: (1) how sure one wants to be that one does not reject a null hypothesis (no difference) that is true— this is the α value, usually taken to be 0.05, or a willingness to reject incorrectly a null hypothesis once out of 20 times; the lower the value of α selected, the larger the sample size that will be required; (2) how sure one wants to be that one does not fail to reject a null hypothesis that should be rejected—this is the β value, usually taken to be 0.10 or 0.20, corresponding to power $(1-\beta)$ of 90 and 80%, respectively, to correctly reject a null hypothesis; the greater the power (and the smaller the β) that is desired, the larger the sample size that is required; (3) the magnitude of the difference that one wants to be able to detect—the smaller the difference, the larger the sample size that will be needed; (4) if a proportion is the outcome of interest rather than a continuously distributed variable, the smaller the proportion, the larger the sample size that will be needed; and (5) the variance of what is being measured in the population—the greater the variance, the larger the sample size that will be needed.

Two formulas for use in estimation of required sample size are given here when the objective is to detect differences between two groups. To detect differences between means, the appropriate formula is

$$n = \frac{(Z_{\alpha/2} + Z_\beta)^2 \sigma^2 (r+1)}{(d^*)^2 \ r}$$

To detect differences between proportions, the appropriate formula is

$$n = \frac{(Z_{\alpha/2} + Z_\beta)^2 \bar{p}(1-\bar{p})(r+1)}{(d^*)^2 \ r}$$

where values for $Z_{\alpha/2}$ and Z_β can be looked up in tables for given values of α and β.

d^* = the value of the difference in means or proportions that one wishes to be able to detect

n = the number of exposed individuals in a cohort or cross-sectional study or the number of cases in a case–control study

r = the ratio of the number of unexposed individuals to the number of exposed individuals in a cohort or cross-sectional study, and the ratio of the number of controls to the number of cases in a case–control study

σ = the standard deviation in the population for a continuously distributed variable

p_1 = the proportion of exposed individuals who develop (or have) the disease in a cohort study (or a cross-sectional study), and the proportion of cases who are exposed in a case–control study

p_2 = the proportion of unexposed individuals who develop (or have) the disease in a cohort (or cross-sectional) study, and the proportion of controls who are exposed in a case–control study

$\overline{p}$ = the weighted average of p_1 and p_2, or

$$\overline{p} = \frac{p_1 + rp_2}{1 + r}$$

In trying to make the sample size as small as possible, it is important to have measurements as precise as possible. Let us consider the situation where one is trying to determine if a given exposure is associated with a certain disease, and let us assume that the measurement error is nondifferential, meaning that the magnitude of error for one variable (e.g., exposure) does not vary according to the actual value of the other variable (e.g., disease). The effect of such misclassification on measures of association concerned with two variables is to attenuate the measures towards showing no association, and a larger sample size will usually be needed to show that an association is statistically significant. Suppose that the presence of disease is measured without error but that the measurement of exposure is subject to error. If the true odds ratio is 10.0, and 50% of the population is exposed (as would be the case in many experimental situations), with 90% sensitivity (90% of those who truly have the exposure are correctly classified) and 60% specificity (60% of those who truly do not have the exposure are correctly classified), the observed odds ratio will be 4.79 rather than 10.0.[3] If only 1% of the population is exposed, then the observed odds ratio under these circumstances would be 1.73 rather 10.0. Not only will a larger sample size be needed in the presence of measurement error, but the estimated measure of association will be a poor approximation to the true one.

Other principles of experimental design that help to increase efficiency and reduce sample size in studies that involve random assignment of study subjects (either human or animal groups) can be found in Fleiss.[41]

11.8 Future Directions in Epidemiology

Epidemiologic methods are now being applied to a greater variety of diseases than in past years. Epidemiology has long been applied to the study of causes of infectious diseases, and over the past few decades it has been applied extensively to cancer and cardiovascular diseases. Its application to other conditions, such as aging, neurological diseases, musculoskeletal diseases, reproductive outcomes, and psychiatric disorders, has been growing in recent years. Also, case–control studies of various diseases, especially cancers, have been undertaken in pet animals.

Perhaps the most significant new emphasis for epidemiologic studies is the increasing use of biological markers. Biomarkers can be used as indicators of host susceptibility, internal dose of exposure, biologically effective dose, biologic response, and early disease.[42-44] Biomarkers of exposure and of effects of exposure (e.g., antibodies) have long existed for infectious diseases. For example, in a prospective cohort study of chronic hepatitis B as a cause of primary liver cancer, serum markers of hepatitis B were used to define exposure, since hepatitis B is often asymptomatic.[45] Now biomarkers are being developed for noninfectious diseases as well. By biomarkers of exposure, we mean biological measurements of internal dose or body burden, such as blood lead levels as a marker of environmental lead exposure.[44] Biomarkers of exposure may be more precise and accurate than measurements made by questionnaire, since with questionnaires a person may not know exactly what he/she was exposed to, may forget exposures, or may deliberately misinform the investigator. Biomarkers may also be useful when environmental data are poor approximations of individual dose (because of individual variation in uptake and pharmacokinetics, for instance), when it is desired to document exposure in target tissue, and when one wishes to quantify the biological load from an exposure. Also, such markers can be used to validate in small samples of individuals information obtained from less expensive and more feasible sources such as questionnaires.

Biomarkers of effect may be defined as any biologically measurable response to exposure.[44] If the marker of effect is highly correlated with the subsequent development of disease and can be measured before the disease becomes symptomatic or can be diagnosed, then prospective cohort studies can be conducted in a more timely fashion. Biomarkers of effect can also be useful in suggesting mechanisms of action. For instance, in a study of effects of maternal stress during pregnancy, it was hypothesized that sustained elevations of catecholamines might, because of their vasoconstricting action, interfere with uteroplacental blood flow, which in turn could lead to vascular damage in the placenta and to decreased birthweight and other problems in the offspring.[44] In addition to the traditional method of obtaining data by questionnaire on maternal psychosocial stress and from records on birthweight, the investigators collected maternal urine specimens for the measurement of catecholamine concentrations and placental specimens for identification of placental abnormalities. In this way, it is hoped that a better understanding will be achieved of the biology of psychosocial stress and the role of placental abnormalities in the pathogenesis of low birthweight and other perinatal problems.

As further advances are made, this linking of techniques of molecular biology, biochemistry, and other biological sciences with epidemiology may also provide information about mechanisms of action that is directly applicable to humans.

REFERENCES

1. Last, J. M., Ed. *A Dictionary of Epidemiology*, 2nd ed. (New York: Oxford University Press, 1988).
2. Hennekens, C. and J. Buring. *Epidemiology in Medicine* (Boston: Little, Brown, 1987).
3. Kelsey, J. L., W. D. Thompson, and A. S. Evans. *Methods in Observational Epidemiology* (New York: Oxford University Press, 1986).

4. Rothman, K. J. *Modern Epidemiology* (Boston: Little, Brown, and Co., 1986).

5. Schlesselman, J. J. *Case–control Studies* (New York: Oxford University Press, 1982).

6. Mason, T. J., F. W. McKay, R. Hoover, W. J. Blot, and J. F. Fraumeni, Jr. *Atlas of Cancer Mortality for U.S. Counties: 1950–69,* DHEW Publication No. (NIH)75-780 (Washington, D.C.: U.S. Department of Health, Education, and Welfare, 1975).

7. Doll, R. and A. B. Hill. "A Study of the Aetiology of Carcinoma of the Lungs," *Br. Med. J.* 2:1271–76 (12/13/52).

8. Herbst, A. L., H. Ulfelder, and D. C. Poskanzer. "Adenocarcinoma of the Vagina: Association of Maternal Stilbestrol Therapy with Tumor Appearance in Young Women," *N. Engl. J. Med.* 284(16):878–81 (1971).

9. Centers for Disease Control Cancer and Steroid Hormone Study. "Oral Contraceptive Use and the Risk of Breast Cancer," *JAMA* 249(12):1591–95 (1983).

10. Centers for Disease Control Cancer and Steroid Hormone Study. "Oral Contraceptive Use and the Risk of Endometrial Cancer," *JAMA* 249(12):1600–04 (1983).

11. Centers for Disease Control Cancer and Steroid Hormone Study. "Oral Contraceptive Use and the Risk of Ovarian Cancer," *JAMA* 249(12):1596–99 (1983).

12. Wingo, P. A., H. W. Ory, P. M. Layde, N. C. Lee, and the Cancer and Steroid Hormone Study Group. "The Evaluation of the Data Collection Process for a Multicenter, Population-Based, Case–control Design," *Am. J. Epidemiol.* 128(1):206–17 (1988).

13. MacMahon, B., S. Yen, D. Trichopoulos, et al. "Coffee and Cancer of the Pancreas," *N. Engl. J. Med.* 304(11):630–33 (1981).

14. Sackett, D. L. "Bias in Analytic Research," *J. Chron. Dis.* 32(1–2):51–68 (1979).

15. Doll, R. and A. B. Hill. "Lung Cancer and Other Causes of Death in Relation to Smoking," *Br. Med. J.* 2:1071–81 (11/10/56).

16. Willett, W. C., M. J. Stampfer, G. A. Colditz, B. A. Rosner, C. H. Hennekens, and F. E. Speizer. "Dietary Fat and the Risk of Breast Cancer," *N. Engl. J. Med.* 316(1):22–8 (1987).

17. Prentice, R. L., F. Kakar, S. Hursting, L. Sheppard, R. Klein, and L. H. Kushi. "Aspects of the Rationale for the Women's Health Trial," *J. Natl. Can. Inst.* 80(11):802–14 (1988).

18. Selikoff, I. J., E. C. Hammond, and J. Churg. "Asbestos Exposure, Smoking, and Neoplasia," *JAMA* 204(2):106–12 (1968).

19. Newhouse, M. L. and G. Berry. "Asbestos and Laryngeal Cancer," *Lancet* 2(7829):615 (1973).

20. Jones, D. Y., A. Schatzkin, S. B. Green, G. Black, L. A. Brinton, R. G. Ziegler, R. Hoover, and P. R. Taylor. "Dietary Fat and Breast Cancer in the National Health and Nutrition Examination Survey. I. Epidemiology Follow-up Study," *J. Natl. Cancer Inst.* 79(3):465–71 (1987).

21. Dohrenwend, B. S. and B. P. Dohrenwend, Eds. *Stressful Life Events and Their Contexts* (New York: Prodist, 1981).

22. Rosenman, R. H., R. J. Brand, C. D. Jenkins, M. Friedman, R. Straus, and M. Wurm. "Coronary Heart Disease in the Western Collaborative Study. Final Follow-up Experience of 8½ Years," *JAMA* 233(8):872–77 (1975).

23. Shekelle, R. B., W. J. Raynor, Jr., A. M. Ostfeld, D. C. Garron, L. A. Bieliaukas, S. C. Liu, C. Maliza, and O. Paul. "Psychological Depression and 17-Year Risk of Death From Cancer," *Psychosomatic Med.* 43(2):117–25 (1981).

24. Berkman, L. F. and S. L. Syme. "Social Networks, Host Resistance and Mortality: A Nine-Year Follow-up Study of Alameda County Residents," *Am. J. Epidemiol.* 109(2):186–204 (1979).

25. Kasl, S. V. "When to Welcome a New Measure," *Am. J. Pub. Hlth.* 74(2):106–7 (1984).

26. Syme, S. L. "Social Determinants of Health and Disease," in *Maxcy-Rosenau Public Health and Preventive Medicine*, 13th ed. (Norwalk, CT: Appleton & Lange, 1992).

27. Kamol, M. "Statistical Study on Relation Between Breast Cancer and Lactation Period," *Tohoku J. Exp. Med.* 72(1):59–65 (1960).

28. MacMahon, B., T. W. Lin, C. R. Lowe, A. P. Mirra, B. Ravnihar, E. J. Salber, D. Trichopoulos, V. G. Valaoras, and S. Yuasa. "Age at First Birth and Breast Cancer Risk," *Bull. WHO* 43(2):209–21 (1970).

29. LeMarchand, L., L. N. Kolonel, M. E. Earle, and M. P. Mi. "Body Size at Different Periods of Life and Breast Cancer Risk," *Am. J. Epidemiol.* 128(1):137–52 (1988).

30. Hellberg, D., S. Nilsson, N. J. Haley, D. Hoffman, and E. Wynder. "Smoking and Cervical Intraepithelial Neoplasia: Nicotine and Cotinine in Serum and Cervical Mucus of Smokers and Nonsmokers," *Am. J. Obstet. Gynec.* 158(4):910–13 (1988).

31. Auerbach, O., E. C. Hammond, D. Kirman, L. Garfinkel, and A. P. Stout. "Histo-logic Changes in Bronchial Tubes of Cigarette-Smoking Dogs," *Cancer* 20(12):2055–66 (1967).

32. Hammond, E. C., O. Auerbach, D. Kirman, and L. Garfinkel. "Effects of Cigarette Smoking on Dogs. I. Design of Experiment, Mortality, and Findings in Lung Parenchyma," *Arch. Environ. Hlth.* 21(6):740–53 (1970).

33. Auerbach, O., E. C. Hammond, D. Kirman, and L. Garfinkel. "Effects of Cigarette Smoking on Dogs. II. Pulmonary Neoplasms," *Arch. Environ. Hlth.* 21(6):754–68 (1970).

34. U.S. Public Health Service. Smoking and Health. *Report of the Advisory Committee of the Surgeon General of the Public Health Service,* PHS Publication No. 1103 (Washington, D.C., U.S. Government Printing Office, 1964).

35. U.S. Public Health Service. Smoking and Health. *Report of the Surgeon General,* DHEW Publication No. (PHS)79-50066 (Washington, D.C., U.S. Gov. Printing Office, 1979).

36. Lilienfeld, A. M. "Epidemiological Methods and Inferences in Studies of Noninfec-tious Diseases," *Pub. Hlth. Rep.* 72(1):51–60 (1957).

37. Gardner, M. B. and P. A. Lucius. "Animal Models of AIDS," *Fed. Am. Soc. Exp. Biol. J.* 3(3):2593–606 (1989).

38. Heyward, W. L. and J. W. Curran. "The Epidemiology of AIDS in the U.S.," *Sci. Am.* 259(4):72–81 (1988).

39. Centers for Disease Control. "Pneumocystis Pneumonia—Los Angeles," *MMWR* 30(21):250–51 (1981).

40. Centers for Disease Control. "Kaposi's Sarcoma and Pneumocystis Pneumonia Among Homosexual Men—New York City and California," *MMWR* 30(25):305–8 (1981).

41. Fleiss, J. F. *The Design and Analysis of Clinical Experiments* (New York: J. Wiley & Sons, 1986).

42. Perera, F. P. and I. B. Weinstein. "Molecular Epidemiology and Carcinogen-DNA Adduct Detection: New Approaches to Studies of Human Cancer Causation," *J. Chron. Dis.* 35(7):581–600 (1982).

43. Hulka, B. S. and T. Wilcosky. "Biological Markers in Epidemiologic Research," *Arch. Environ. Hlth.* 43(2):83–9 (1988).

44. Stein, Z. and M. Hatch. "Biological Markers in Reproductive Epidemiology: Prospects and Precautions," *Environ. Hlth. Persp.* 74(1):67–75 (1987).

45. Beasley, R. P., L-Y. Hwang, C-C. Lin, and C-S. Chen. "Hepatocellular Carcinoma and Hepatitis B Virus: a Prospective Study of 22,707 Men in Taiwan," *Lancet* 2(8256):1129–32 (1981).

CHAPTER 12

Alternatives to Animals in Preventive Medicine

John Last

12.0 Introduction

The rise of technology has added greatly to the range and difficulty of the moral dilemmas that occur in every branch of medical practice, and has brought into greater prominence the necessity for all who practice medicine to abide by clearly enunciated ethical principles.

This is as true for the specialist in preventive medicine as for the reproductive biologist, the neonatologist, the palliative care physician, the physiatrist, the psychiatrist, and the transplant surgeon. Moreover, in preventive medicine, ethical problems arise not only in relation to the human populations whose health is to be safeguarded, but also in relation to animals. Preventive medicine increasingly recognizes the interdependence of life forms: the health of humans is dependent upon the health of the earth, on the well-being of all other forms of life with which we share our planet. The specialist in preventive medicine who aspires to show due respect for life and living things other than people, and recognizes that all forms of life on our planet are interdependent, must confront and resolve moral dilemmas that arise at times when human interests clash with the welfare of animals. Technology can help resolve some of these dilemmas while at the same time other aspects of technology may cause new dilemmas.

0-87371-504-7/93/$0.00+$.50
© 1993 by Lewis Publishers

Preventive medicine is defined as the medical specialty that aims to promote and protect the good health of populations and individuals, and to prevent premature death and disability. It makes use of many strategies and tactics. It works mainly by applying a variety of measures and specialized skills that include epidemiologic surveillance, environmental sciences, immunization procedures, health education, nutritional programs, maternal and child care, genetic counseling, special programs for high-risks groups, and much more. It includes a number of more or less self-contained areas of specialization, notably occupational medicine, aerospace medicine, and preventive programs that focus on special groups such as pregnant women, infants, military recruits, persons who are overweight, psychiatric patients. An increasingly important focus of concern is the field called clinical preventive medicine, which means the disease-preventing and health-promoting activities carried out by physicians in their offices with individual patients. This aspect of preventive medicine stands at the opposite extreme from the aspects that are often known as public health practice, i.e., the aspects that are oriented towards populations rather than persons.

12.1 Moral Dilemmas of Public Health and Preventive Medicine

Some of the moral dilemmas of public health and preventive medicine are quite old, others relatively new. Some involve other living creatures as well as humans. While upholding the principle of "live and let live" we inevitably face difficult choices from time to time. These choices can apply to human populations that must be deliberately exposed to certain risks, as well as to animal populations of many kinds.

For example, just after World War II, public health authorities in New York City had to deal with the threat of a smallpox epidemic. If the epidemic had struck New York City, there would have been hundreds, probably thousands of cases, and many hundreds of deaths, to say nothing of disfigurement, blindness, and permanent brain damage among a proportion of the survivors. Over a period of a few weeks, about 5 million people were vaccinated against smallpox, and the epidemic was prevented. The human costs of this were 45 known cases of severe encephalitis and four deaths. The public health authorities knew in advance that there would be some severe adverse reactions of this sort, including a few deaths; they had to balance the risks of these against the benefits, the protection of a city of 8 million people against a devastating epidemic.[1] Another example of balancing risks and benefits to human health is to be found in the early community-wide experiments on fluoridation of drinking water supplies, in which entire populations were deliberately exposed to communal water supplies to which trace amounts of fluoride salts had been added. The empirical basis for this was the observation that in localities where fluoride content was naturally at a level of about 2 to 3 ppm, dental caries was far less prevalent than in communities where fluoride content was lower than 1 ppm. The differing metabolic response of humans and animals to fluoride supplements would have rendered animal studies of fluoridation irrelevant. In these examples, only risks and benefits to human health were involved and had to be balanced. The health of animal populations is often an issue also.

12.2 Disease Control Programs and Animal Diseases

In many disease control programs mounted by specialists in preventive medicine, animal populations suffer and may even face extinction. For example, we control the threat of the most deadly of all epidemic diseases, bubonic plague, by exterminating rats, the natural hosts, who in the past often carried plague epidemics from one country to another on board ships.[2]

In some occupational exposures, animals have been deliberately exposed to risks in order to provide early warning that workers' health and lives could be in jeopardy. The classic example is caged song-birds (canaries) which were taken down into coal mines, where their respiratory distress and death provided early warning to miners that the air was becoming foul, and that the miners would die too unless they got out quickly.[3]

A modern variation on this theme is observation of the health status of wild life populations: departures from good health in free-living wild creatures can sometimes provide early warning of environmental pollution. For instance, there was a reproductive catastrophe among herring-gull colonies on Lake Ontario in the mid-1970s; most of the chicks died in the shell, and the few that hatched were almost all suffering from deformities incompatible with developing to maturity.

Investigation revealed that the cause was a spill of dioxins and PCBs into the Niagara River from a chemical waste disposal site in upstate New York; the chemicals were slowly concentrated in the food chain from microscopic flora and fauna through fish, that had herring-gulls at its terminal point, taking about 5 years to reach the levels that caused this wild-life disaster.[4] Investigation of human reproductive outcomes in this instance failed to reveal evidence of an epidemic of miscarriages or birth defects; the numbers of people affected were too small to reach statistically significant levels.[5]

12.3 Interconnections Between Animal and Human Health

This is a good example of the reality that we often have overlooked in the past: human health and the health of every other living creature on earth are interconnected. This concept is embodied in a useful definition of health: "A state of dynamic balance in which an individual's or a group's capacity to cope with all the circumstances of living is at an optimum level."[6]

In an ideal world, we would like to find alternatives to situations in which the health of animal populations—and for that matter, the health of animals—is jeopardized; and alternatives to situations in which animals are deliberately exposed to pain, suffering, or the risk of death, in order to protect human health with vaccines, or to provide warning that human health is threatened by exposure to environmental or occupational toxins.

Increasingly, this is possible. Nowadays we would not take caged canaries down into coal mines, because air monitoring that is far more accurate can be conducted with special equipment.[7] Similarly, we can use genetic engineering techniques to manufacture sera and vaccines[8] that formerly were produced by various procedures that required animals—sheep, horses, cows, rabbits, whatever—to be confined and made to suffer considerably while they were being used as living factories to make sera and vaccines.

12.4 What Is an Animal?

Challenging philosophical questions persists, however. One concerns the definition of an animal. Classification systems enable us to answer this question several ways, most precisely by placing every living creature in its proper phylum, class, genus, and so forth. Then there is a further classification into species that are feral, free-living or wild, those that are domesticated, those that are household pets, those that are grown and used for food—the source of meat protein—and finally those that we describe as vermin or pests, or those that are venomous.

12.4.1 Venomous and Dangerous Animals

These last two categories, i.e., vermin, pests, and venomous animals, are often a central concern of preventive medicine. In India and Malaysia, one of the leading causes of death, especially among children, is snake-bite.[9] Yet in the complex network of life forms, there is no valid case for seeking to exterminate venomous snakes because they sometimes bite and kill children, any more than there is a case for trying to exterminate so-called "man-eating" sharks. Serious attempts to accomplish this were reported from Australia some years ago.[10] But sharks have a very much longer evolutionary history than humans, and easily withstood the impractical proposal to eradicate them from coastal waters off New South Wales. The lesson to be learned from this experience is the same as that which would be learned were any attempt ever made to eradicate venomous snakes: a more elegant and effective strategy is to study the habits and habitat of the threatening species, and to take appropriate measures to ensure as far as possible that humans do not encounter the species.

This strategy probably will not succeed when we have to control species that convey zoonotic infections such as rabies and bubonic plague, although it can be at least partially effective and the situation is changing as science advances. If rabies is widely prevalent among feral animals such as foxes, there has in the past been a strong argument for using poisoned bait or other measures to reduce the numbers, and therefore the risks of transmission from feral foxes to domesticated animals and humans. The only alternative in this situation until very recently was to vaccinate all humans and animals exposed to the risk of rabies. This was almost always impractical in the case of domesticated animal herds at risk, and needlessly hazardous in the case of humans, especially children who would be at risk if feral foxes transmitted rabies to domesticated cats and dogs. In 1989, it became possible to vaccinate feral foxes heavily infected with rabies, by laying baits containing live attenuated rabies virus vaccine. Early experience with this program suggests that it is a practical alternative to the use of poisoned baits that dealt with the problem of sylvatic rabies by attempting to exterminate the infected wild animals.[11,12] Apart from the inhumanity of this approach, it was ecologically unsound because its "success" led to disruption of the natural balance between predatory and nonpredatory species.

In those parts of Africa where trypanosomiasis is common among both domesticated and wild animals (as well as humans) it has sometimes been the policy to reduce the risks of transmission from wild to domesticated animals by culling the wild animal herds—although in this instance the ecology is far from fully worked out, and until it is, caution rather than wholesale slaughter is obviously indicated. The same approach and the same arguments hold true in similar situations elsewhere in the world. For instance, in northern Alberta, Canada, one of the few surviving herds of bison was infected with brucellosis (contagious abortion). To protect the economically important beef cattle herds on ranches further south, slaughter of the affected bison herd has recently been advocated. Ecologists are resisting this proposal not only because it makes very little epidemiological sense but also because the bison seem to have developed a natural balance with the infecting organism. Far better than destroying the infected herd would be to study them and discover more about the biological basis for their relative resistance to brucellosis.

12.4.2 Vermin

There is less argument—indeed probably none at all—about the proper course of action with rats. These are the hosts not only of bubonic plague, but also of several other deadly or dangerous diseases: typhus, trichinosis, leptospirosis, to name a few. Rational humans who believe in the philosophy of "live and let live" probably for the most part draw the line at rats. Even so, there is no justification for subjecting huge populations of laboratory colonies of rats to inhumane experiments, especially when good use of statistical methods makes it possible to obtain the same results with smaller numbers; and inhumane experiments are virtually never justifiable on any grounds at all.

Taxonomically speaking, fleas, lice, mites, and the many varieties of worms that can afflict humans are all animals. These too we should agree, are vermin, if not outright causes of human disease. They are our enemies, and will destroy us unless we destroy them first. While often so, this may not be a universal truth.

12.5 Alternatives to Animals in the Practice of Preventive Medicine

Aside from consideration of animals that can cause disease and premature death among humans, there remains much to discuss about alternatives to animals in the broad field of preventive medicine. The topic can be systematically discussed in relation to the strategies that we employ to promote good health and prevent untimely death and disabling disease and injury, or in relation to the nosology of disease. An orderly approach that combines these two axes of classification reveals the settings in which animals have been used, are now used, and in the future might be used as a means to the ends of preventive medicine and health promotion.

Animals have been used in the past, and are used now, as models for disease causation, in order to plan preventive strategies, in occupational and environmental health. This has been the basis for many toxicologic investigations. Sometimes huge numbers of animals have been "sacrificed" (using that word both literally and metaphorically!) to this end. This is seldom a good or rational use of animals, and it is to be hoped that in future studies of environmental and occupational exposures, more rational and realistic approaches may prevail. It is not a rational approach in many situations because the animal response to the environmental challenge may be quite different from the human response, both qualitatively and quantitatively. Canines, for instance, have quite different tolerance levels for many drugs from those found in humans, so it may be dangerously misleading to use dogs to test for the adverse or beneficial effects of such drugs before they are used on humans. It is not a good use when unnecessarily large numbers, or the wrong kind of animals, are employed for the purpose.

It is rarely, if ever, necessary to use large numbers, especially if suitable statistical procedures are applied; and it is rarely necessary to use, for instance, primates, simply because primates allegedly resemble humans more closely than, say, rodents do. It is as rational, and often as good, to use tissue or cell cultures as to use animals for many purposes in environmental toxicology. This is especially true in the case of tests for carcinogenicity and teratogenicity. A rather barbaric use of animals was the demonstration that forced smoking of tobacco by dogs (beagles) induced respiratory damage, including cancer. Admittedly there were powerful political arguments for this piece of research—the tobacco industry was asserting that no experimental evidence supported the essentially circumstantial epidemiological evidence that tobacco smoking causes lung cancer—so at the time this work was first done, there was some justification for demonstrating in this way the causal connection and the sequence of pathological changes in respiratory epithelium.

Another former use of animals can be condemned outright. Fortunately it has been superceded. In the early days of research on traffic injury and death, live animals such as pigs were placed in prototype cars that were then crashed, so that the nature of the resulting injuries could be studied.[13] The use of mannikins, fitted with sophisticated electronic recording devices, has made this barbaric practice not only unnecessary but irrational.

Laboratory animals have been extensively used in the past for such purposes as experiments to determine the consequences of dietary deficiencies and exposure to noxious respiratory irritants. We have learned a great deal from such studies, but there is little justification for continuing such work on a large scale in the future. Increasingly, the only relevant results of empirical studies that are really meaningful are those conducted upon humans, usually in the setting of clinical research, sometimes in large-scale preventive trials. A very old but excellent example of such trials is those conducted late in the 19th century by the Japanese physician Kanehiro Takaki;[14] these studies established far better than any animal models ever could have done, that vitamin B is an essential dietary ingredient to prevent the occurrence of scurvy. Indeed, clinical and epidemiological studies are a sine qua non whenever questions arise about essential dietary ingredients. The epidemiological studies that established the relationship between dietary intake of kale and similar green vegetables, which cause goiter (thyroid deficiency) by blocking the uptake of iodine by the thyroid gland,[15] could not have been conducted upon experimental animals. Studies aimed at assessing human nutritional requirements must be conducted upon humans, not upon experimental animals. This is true also for studies aimed at establishing the relationship of dietary intake of fats and coronary artery disease: animals such as rabbits that have been used to study this problem have fundamentally different metabolism from humans, and the findings from animal studies simply are not capable of extrapolation;[16] therefore they are pointless, if not actually misleading, and should not be done.

REFERENCES

1. Greenburg, M. and E. Appelbaum. "Postvaccinal Encephalitis; A Report of 45 Cases in New York City," *Am. J. Med. Sci.* 216(5):565–570 (1948).
2. Poland, J. D. "Plague," in *Maxcy-Rosenau Public Health and Preventive Medicine*, 12th ed., J. M. Last, Ed. (Norwalk, CT: Appleton & Lange, 1986), pp 354–359.
3. Hunter, J. *Diseases of Occupations*, 3rd ed. (Oxford and London: English University Press, 1962), pp. 637.
4. Peakall, D. B., G. A. Fox, A. P. Gilman, et al. "Reproductive Success of Herring Gulls as an Indicator of Great Lakes Water Quality," in *Hydrocarbons in the Aquatic Environment*, B. K. Afgan and D. Mackay, Eds. (New York: Plenum, 1980).
5. Fox, G. A. and J. M. Last. "Analysis of Human Reproductive Outcomes in Ontario Counties Adjacent to Lake Ontario, Erie and Huron," unpublished, University of Ottawa (1980–81).
6. Last, J. M., Ed. *A Dictionary of Epidemiology,* 2nd ed. (New York: Oxford University Press, 1988), pp. 57.
7. Olishifski, J. B. "Industrial Hygiene," in *Occupational Medicine*, 2nd ed., C. Zenz, Ed. (Chicago: Yearbook Publications, 1988), pp. 37–38.
8. Hoffenberg, R. "Modern Medicine; Prospects and Problems," in *New Prospects for Medicine*, J. M. Austyn, Ed. (Oxford: Oxford University Press, 1988), pp. 8–22.
9. Chen, P. C. "Poisonous and Venomous Animals and Plants," in *Textbook of Community Medicine in South-East Asia*, W. O. Phoon and P. C. Chen, Eds. (Chichester: J. Wiley, 1986), pp. 175–80.
10. Coppleson, V. L. *Shark Attack* (Sydney and London: Angus & Robertson, 1965).

11. Brochier, B. M., et al. "Use of Recombinant Vaccinia-Rabies Virus for Oral Vaccination of Fox Cubs Against Rabies," *Vet. Microbiol.* 18(2):103–8 (1988).

12. Perry, D. B., D. H. Johnson, S. R. Jenkins, C. M. Foggin, N. Garner, R. Brooks, and J. Bleakley. "Studies on the Delivery of Oral Rabies Vaccines to Wildlife and Dog Populations," *Acta Vet. Scand. Suppl.* 84(1):303–05 (1988).

13. Haddon, W., E. A. Suchman, and D. Klein, Eds. *Accident Research* (New York: Harper & Row, 1964).

14. Takaki, K. *Sei i Kwai* (Tokyo; Abstract, 1885), pp. 4:29–37.

15. Clements, F. W. "A Thyroid Blocking Agent as a Cause of Epidemic Goitre in Tasmania: Preliminary Communication," *Med. J. Austr.* 2(10):369–76 (1955).

16. Rall, D. P. "Relevance of Results from Laboratory Animal Toxicology Studies," in *Maxcy-Rosenau Public Health and Preventive Medicine*, 11th ed., J. M. Last, Ed. (New York: Appleton-Century-Crofts, 1980), pp. 543–9.

CHAPTER 13

Human Autopsies in Biomedical Research

Michael B. Kapis

13.0 Introduction

Human autopsy is the postmortem examination of the tissues and organs of a body to determine cause of death or pathological conditions. Autopsy, also known as necropsy, is one of the oldest methods of medical investigation. From the earliest human autopsy, between 400 and 300 BC, to the fundamental investigations of Morgagni, Bichat, Baille, Rokitanshy, and Virchow in the 18th and 19th centuries, autopsies contributed to the evolution of anatomical knowledge and later to the comprehension of the organic nature of diseases.[1,2]

Before the 18th century, post-mortem dissection was used to learn about human anatomy. When Morgani began to establish associations between anatomic lesions and disease entities, the discipline of pathologic anatomy emerged. Autopsies had a new purpose; namely, clinical medicine. Later, Rokitansky's autopsy studies involved observing and classifying encyclopedias of diseases. Autopsy pathology and clinical medicine contributed greatly to the progress of scientific medicine. Meanwhile, Virchow brought pathologic physiology and rigorous inquiry to acquiesce on his autopsy studies and introduced scientific medicine to the world.[2]

13.1   The Role of Autopsies in Modern Biomedical Research

Autopsy research has been responsible for the discovery and description of thousands of diseases, numerous classifications of lesions, a great many associations between disease states and anatomical abnormalities, and countless ideas for medical and surgical treatment.[3,4,5-21]

A partial list of diseases discovered or critically clarified through autopsies[2] since 1950 includes the following:

Cardiovascular lesions[22-31]
    Tricuspid valve disease due to metastasizing carcinoid tumor
    Understanding of congenital heart lesions leading to modern surgical
       treatment
    Atheromatous embolism
    Asymmetric cardiac hypertrophy
    Dissecting aneurysm and variations thereon
    Primary cardiomyopathy
    Subaortic muscular stenosis
    Rheumatoid disease of aorta and aortic valve
    Complications of cardiac surgery
    Diseases of conducting system
    Idiopathic hypertrophic subaortic stenosis
    Cardiomyopathies
    Mitral valve prolapse

Bronchopulmonary lesions[32-36]
    Alveolitis (diffuse alveolar damage, shock lung, respiratory distress
       syndrome)
    Oxygen toxicity
    Pneumocystis pneumonia
    Infantile respiratory distress syndrome (hyaline membrane disease)
    Legionnaire's disease
    Pulmonary alveolar proteinosis, desquamative pneumonia
    Diseases due to inhalation of industrial dusts: asbestosis, berylliosis,
       bagassosis, silo-filler's disease
    Lipid pneumonia
    Diffuse interstitial fibrosis

Hepatobiliary lesions[37-39]
    Viral hepatitis
    α-1-antitrypsin disease and cirrhosis
    Jamaican bush-tea disease (veno-occlusive disease of liver)
    Infantile kernicterus
    Neonatal giant cell hepatitis and biliary atresia
    Vinyl chloride and angiosarcoma of liver
    Tumors and hyperplasias due to oral contraceptives
    Afatoxin-induced liver disease and tumors

Renal diseases[40-42]
   Damage due to diethylene glycol as drug vehicle
   Renal effects of potassium deficiency
   Elucidation of various types of glomerulonephritis
   Necrotizing papillitis and interstitial nephritis due to phenacetin abuse
   Renal development malformation in polycystic diseases
   Renal vein thrombosis syndrome
   Scleroderma kidney
   Acute tubular necrosis injury (ATN)
   Atheromatous embolic renal disease

Blood, bone marrow, spleen lesions[43,44]
   Role of spleen in thrombocytopenia purpura; value of splenectomy
   Secondary hemochromatosis
   Syndrome of myeloid metaplasia
   Defibrination syndrome
   Effects of incompatible blood transfusion
   Aplasia anemia, granulocytopenia, thrombocytopenia as a complication of
      drug therapy

Gastrointestinal lesions
   Whipple's disease
   Protein-losing enteropathy
   Congenital intestinal atresia
   Pancreatic cystic fibrosis
   Vascular insufficiency syndromes and hemorrhagic enteropathy
   Protein and potassium loss from villous adenoma

Endocrine lesions
   Complications of diabetes mellitus in vessels, eyes, nerves, kidneys
   Adrenal hypersecretion syndrome: aldosteronism (Conn's disease),
      hypercorticism
   Multiglandular endocrine syndromes, Zollinger-Ellison syndrome
   Hormone-secreting tumors in other organs: paraneoplastic syndromes

Nervous system lesions
   Spongiform encephalopathy (Creutzfeldt-Jakob disease)
   Progressive multifocal leukoencephalopathy
   Adrenoleukodystrophy
   Subacute sclerosing panencephalitis
   Carotid artery insufficiency and thrombosis
   Werdnig-Hoffman disease and amyotonia congenita
   Retrolental fibroplasia
   Shy-Drager disease (hypotension-neuron disease)

Radiation effects
   Radiation syndromes
   Radiation fibrosis of various organs
   Bile duct carcinoma due to use of Thorotrast

Bone and mouth cancer in radium workers
Postradiation malignancy due to X-rays: thyroid, leukemia, skin "Transverse
    myelitis"

Miscellaneous lesions
    Hypervitaminoses
    Toxic shock syndrome
    Consequences of erythroblastosis fetalis
    Causes of perinatal death
    Lipid storage and other storage diseases, phenylketonuria, etc.
    Kwashiorkor
    Amniotic fluid embolism
    Collagen diseases or rheumatic diseases
    Disseminated sarcoid
    Disseminated fungal diseases
    Crush syndrome, endotoxin shock
    Complications of adrenal steroid therapy: ulcer, Cushing's syndrome,
        activation of tuberculosis, osteoporosis, infections
    Prognosis and spread of various cancers[45-51]
    Methyl mercury poisoning
    Fetal alcohol syndrome
    Hospital-acquired infections
    Acquired immunodeficiency syndrome (AIDS)[52-60]
    Sudden infant death syndrome (SIDS)[61-63]

Autopsy microbiology is of increasing importance, but unfortunately is often neglected. Secondary or opportunistic fungal, bacterial, and viral diseases are now more frequent at autopsy because of the use of steroids, and antitumor and immunosupressant drugs in debilitated hospital patients.[3]

Autopsies have provided information resulting in the modification or discontinuance of drugs or other forms of therapy that have negative side effects. From autopsy studies it was revealed that zoxazolamine, a muscle relaxant, caused lethal liver disease in a small number of patients; halothane, an anesthetic agent, caused toxic effects in the liver; phenacetin, an analgesic agent, caused kidney disease in patients who used it in large doses over a prolonged period; diethylene glycol, a solvent and carrier for sulfanilamide, occasionally caused serious kidney damage; and methotrexate, a chemotherapeutic drug, sometimes produced brain toxicity when given intrathecally for certain malignancies.[2]

Autopsies have been vital to transplantation research, and autopsies have provided a source of organs and tissues for many areas of transplantation.[37,42,44,64-68]

13.2 Results of 85 Years of Autopsies in Trieste, Italy

The Institute of Pathological Anatomy at the University of Trieste has been conducting a long-term study involving autopsies. The Institute is unique in that it is one of the few biomedical research centers which utilizes autopsies as a primary method of research. In 1901, 20% of autopsied subjects in Trieste were under the age of 30 and 28.8% were over 70. By 1985, only 0.2% were under 30 years of age and 74.5% were over 70.[1]

At the beginning of this century, more than 40% of people who died were under 35 years of age, and 45% of these were children under the age of five. However, in 1985, only 1.4% of people who died were under 35 and 56.5% were over 74 years of age.

An analysis of autopsy reports for 1901 reveals that infectious diseases accounted for 55% of deaths. The primary cause of death at that time was tuberculosis, 22.4%. In 1985 this figure was reduced to approximately 3%. In recent years, there has been a significant increase in the number of deaths due to heart disease and cancer. This increase is due to declining environmental factors, poor nutrition, alcohol, and smoking.

13.3 The Present-Day Decline of Autopsies

Autopsies are no longer one of the principal means of biomedical research. There are two primary reasons for the decline of autopsy investigations. The first is that each autopsy is no longer a unique event. Millions of autopsies have been catalogued and investigated.

The second reason for the diminishing importance of autopsies is the emergence of new technologies and the improvement of existing methods.[2] Image scanning devices, computer simulation/graphics, physicochemical methods, molecular biology/genetics, improved clinical studies, and epidemiology are the preferred methods of many pathologists. Nevertheless, there is a growing concern on the part of some pathologists that autopsies need not only to be continued, but the number of autopsies should be increased.[2]

13.4 Future of Autopsy Research

While the emergence of new biomedical techniques has had a major impact on advances in medicine, some researchers feel that autopsies will enhance research dealing in environmental and occupational diseases, cancer, heart disease, neurological disorders,[69-100] AIDS, SIDS, and aging. In addition, autopsies will continue to provide discovery and ellucidation of new diseases, unusual expressions of known diseases, and the unanticipated complications of therapy.[2,8,11-13,17,19,49,59,71]

REFERENCES

1. Riboli, E. and M. Delendi, Eds. *Autopsy in Epidemiology & Medical Research,* IARC Scientific Publication #112 (Oxford: Oxford University Press, 1991).
2. Hill, R. B. and R. E. Anderson. *The Autopsy: Medical Practice and Public Policy* (Boston: Butterworths, 1988).

3. Baker, R. D. *Postmortem Examination: Specific Methods and Procedures* (Philadelphia: W. B. Saunders, 1967).

4. Ludwig, J. *Current Methods of Autopsy Practice* (Philadelphia: W. B. Saunders, 1972).

5. Durosinmi, M. A., A. O. Ogunseyinda, P. O. Olatunji, and G. J. Esan. "Prevalence of Cholelithiasis in Nigerians with Sickle Cell Disease," *Afr. J. Med. Med. Sci.* 18(3):223–7 (1989).

6. Rossner, S., L. Lagerstrand, H. E. Persson, and C. Sachs. "The Sleep Apnoea Syndrome in Obesity: Risk of Sudden Death," *J. Intern. Med.* 230(2):135–41 (1991).

7. Silbergeld, D. L., R. C. Rostomily, and E. C. Alvord. "The Cause of Death in Patients with Glioblastoma is Multifactorial: Clinical Factors and Autopsy Findings in 117 Cases of Supratentorial Glioblastoma in Adults," *J. Neuroncol.* 10(2):179–85 (1991).

8. Matturri, L. et al. "A Computer Network-Based System for Local Storage and Nationwide Processing of Autopsy Diagnoses," *Int. J. Epidemiol.* 18(3):720–2 (1989).

9. Hawass, N. E. "Fecal Necrogram: A New Technique. Experience With 12,000 Contrast Examinations," *Invest. Radiol.* 24(9):711–20 (1989).

10. Wackym, P. A., F. H. Linthicum, Jr., P. H. Ward, W. F. House, P. E. Micavych, and D. Bagger-Sjoback. "Re-evaluation of the Role of the Human Endolymphatic Sac in Meniere's Disease," *Otolaryngol. Head Neck Surg.* 102(6):732–44 (1990).

11. Burke, M. C., et al. "Use of Autopsy Results in the Emergency Department Quality Assurance Plan," *Ann. Emerg. Med.* 19(4):363–6 (1990).

12. Kircher, T. "The Autopsy and Vital Statistics," *Human Pathol.* 21(2):166–73 (1990).

13. Vance, R. P. "An Unintentional Irony: The Autopsy in Modern Medicine and Society," *Human Pathol.* 21(2):136–44 (1990).

14. Redline, R. W., D. R. Genest, and B. Tycko. "Detection of Enteroviral Infection in Paraffin-Embedded Tissue by the RNA Polymerase Chain Reaction Technique," *Am. J. Clin. Pathol.* 96(5):568–71 (1991).

15. Chang, Y., D. Soffer, D. S. Horoupian, and L. M. Weiss, "Evolution of Post-Natal Herpes Simplex Virus Encephalitis to Multicystic Encephalopathy," *Acta Neuropathol. Berl.* 80(6):666–70 (1991).

16. Angelico, M., C. Gandin, P. Canuzzi, S. Bertasi, A. Cantafora, A. De-Santis, S. Quattrucci, M. Antonelli. "Gallstones in Cystic Fibrosis: A Critical Reappraisal," *Hepatology* 14(5):768–75 (1991).

17. Favarra, B. E., et al. "Pediatric Pathology and the Autopsy," *Pediatr. Pathol.* 9(2):109–16 (1989).

18. Takayanaqi, T., M. Inoue, K. Tomimasu, C. Shimomura, T. Matsuzaka, Y. Tsuji, and I. Nonaka. "Infantile Cytochrome c Oxidase Deficiency with Neonatal Death," *Pediatr. Neurol.* 5(3):179–81 (1989).

19. Stothert, J. C., et al. "The Role of Autopsy in Death Resulting from Trauma," *J. Trauma* 30(8):1021–5 (1990).

20. Smithers, B. M., B. O'Loughlin, and R. W. Strong. "Diagnosis of Ruptured Diaphragm Following Blunt Trauma: Results from 85 Cases," *Aust. N.Z. J. Surg.* 61(10):737–41 (1991).

21. Spigland, N., M. Di-Lorenzo, S. Youssef, P. Russo, and M. Brandt. "Malignant Thymoma in Children: A 20-Year Review," *J. Pediatr. Surg.* 25(11):1143–6 (1990).

22. Weintraub, W. S. "Cigarette Smoking as a Risk Factor for Coronary Artery Disease," *Adv. Exp. Med. Biol.* 273:27–37 (1990).

23. Fradet, G., W. R. Jamieson, M. T. Janusz, H. Ling, R. T. Miyagishima, and A. I. Munro, "Aortic Dissection: Current Expectations and Treatment. Experience with 258 Patients over 20 Years," *Can. J. Surg.* 33(6):465–9 (1990).

24. Zeien, L. B., et al. "Cardiac Valve Prosthesis at Autopsy," *Arch. Pathol. Lab. Med.* 114(9):933–7 (1990).

25. Janatuinen, M. J., E. A. Vanttinen, V. Rantakokko, J. Nikoskelainen, and M. V. Inberg. "Prosthetic Valve Endocarditis," *Scand. J. Thorac. Cardiovasc. Surg.* 25(2):127–32 (1991).

26. Sawada, K. and K. Kawamura. "Architecture of Myocardial Cells in Human Cardiac Ventricles with Concentric and Eccentric Hypertrophy as Demonstrated by Quantitative Scanning Electron Microscopy," *Heart Vessels* 6(3):129–42 (1991).

27. Brown, B. C., T. E. Mason, W. P. Ballard, C. W. Wickliffe, and D. Bone. "Cardiac Angiosarcoma: A Case Report," *J. Med. Assoc. GA* 80(8):435–8 (1991).

28. Kodali, S., W. R. Jamieson, M. Leia-Stephens, R. T. Miyagishima, M. T. Janusz, and G. F. Tyers, "Traumatic Rupture of the Thoracic Aorta, a 20-Year Review: 1969–1989, *Circulation* 84(5 Suppl):III40–6 (1991).

29. Ursell, P. C., J. M. Byrne, T. R. Fears, B. A. Strobino, and W. M. Gersony. "Growth of the Great Vessels in the Normal Human Fetus and in the Fetus with Cardiac Defects, *Circulation* 84(5):2028–33 (1991).

30. Omokhodion, S. I., T. G. Losekoot, and F. Jaiyesimi. "Serum Creatine Kinase and Creatine Kinase-MB Isoenzyme Activity in Perinatally Asphyxiated Newborns," *Eur. Heart J.* 12(9):980–4 (1991).

31. Russell, G. A. "Postmortem Audit in a Paediatric Cardiology Unit," *J. Clin. Pathol.* 42(9):912–8 (1989).

32. Nicholson, D. "Pulmonary Embolism: An Internist's Perspective," *J. Thorac. Imaging* 4(4):20–2 (1989).

33. Lee, J. K. and T. H. Ng. "Undiagnosed Tuberculosis in Hospitalized Patients: An Autopsy Survey," *J. R. Soc. Health* 110(4):141–3 (1990).

34. Hislop, A. A., J. Wharton, K. M. Allen, J. M. Polak, and S. G. Haworth. "Immunohistochemical Localization of Peptide-Containing Nerves in Human Airways: Age-Related Changes," *Am. J. Respir. Cell. Mol. Biol.* 3(3):191–8 (1990).

35. Genner, J. and O. P. Settnes. "Pathological Characteristics for the Diagnosis of Pneumocystis Carinii Pneumonia: A Retrospective Autopsy Study," *APMIS* 98(12):1098–104 (1990).

36. Burrows, P. E., R. M. Freedom, L. N. Benson, C. A. Moes, G. Wilson, K. Koike, and W. G. Williams. "Coronary Angiography of Pulmonary Atresia, Hypoplastic Right Ventricle, and Ventriculocoronary Communications," *Am. J. Roentganol.* 154(4):789–95 (1990).

37. Hall, W. A. and A. J. Martinez. "Neuropathology of Pediatric Liver Transplantation," *Pediatr. Neurosci.* 15(6):269–75 (1989).

38. Iber, F. L., G. Caruso, C. Polepalle, V. Kuchipudi, and M. Chinoy. "Increasing Prevalence of Gallstones in Male Veterans with Alcoholic Cirrhosis," *Am. J. Gastroenterol.* 85(12):1593–6 (1990).

39. Sartin, J. S. and R. C. Walker. "Granulomatous Hepatitis: A Retrospective Review of 88 Cases at the Mayo Clinic," *Mayo Clin. Proc.* 66(9):914–8 (1991).

40. Tsuji, M., S. Ochiai, T. Taka, Y. Hishitani, T. Nagareda, and H. Mori. "Nonamyloidotic Nephrotic Syndrome in Waldenstrom's Macroglobulinemia," *Nepron* 54(2):176–8 (1990).

41. Obana, M., M. Adachi, Y. Matsuoka, S. Irimajiri, H. Kishimoto, and J. Fukuda. "Clinical Studies on Amyloidosis Complicated with Rheumatoid Arthritis with Particular Reference to Nephropathy," *Jpn. J. Med.* 29(3):274–82 (1990).

42. Bertani, T., P. Ferrazzi, A. Schieppati, P. Ruggenenti, A. Gamba, L. Parenzan, G. Mecca, N. Perico, O. Imberti, and A. Remuzzi. "Nature and Extent of Glomerular Injury Induced by Cyclosporine in Heart Transplant Patients," *Kidney Int.* 40(2):243–50 (1991).

43. Crisco, J. J., M. M. Panjabi, T. Oda, D. Grob, and J. Dvorak. "Bone Graft Translation of Four Upper Cervical Spine Fixation Techniques in a Cadaveric Model," *J. Orthop. Res.* 9(6):835–46 (1991).

44. Levy, J., R. A. Wodell, C. S. August, and E. Bayever. "Adenovirus-Related Hemophagocytic Syndrome after Bone Marrow Transplantation," *Bone Marrow Transplant* 6(5):349–52 (1990).

45. Tomioka T, A. Andren-Sandberg, H. Fujii, H. Egami, Y. Takiyama, and P. M. Pour. "Comparative Histopathological Findings in the Pancreas of Cigarette Smokers and Non-Smokers," *Cancer Lett.* 55(2):121–8 (1990).

46. Caskey, C. I., J. C. Scatarige, and E. K. Fishman. "Distribution of Metastases in Breast Carcinoma: CT Evaluation of the Abdomen," *Clin. Imag.* 15(3):166–71 (1991).

47. Sutton, G. P., J. A. Blessing, H. D. Homesley, M. L. Berman, and J. Malfetano. "Phase II Trial of Ifosfamide and Mesna in Advanced Ovarian Carcinoma: A Gynecologic Oncology Group Study," *J. Clin. Oncol.* 7(11):1672–6 (1989).

48. Scardino, P. T. "Early Detection of Prostate Cancer," *Urol. Clin. N. Am.* 16(4):635–55 (1989).

49. Landefeld, C. S., et al. "The Value of Autopsy in Modern Oncology," *Eur. J. Cancer Clin. Oncol.* 25(4):607–9 (1989).

50. Ihde, J. K. and D. G. Coit. "Melanoma Metastatic to Stomach, Small Bowel, or Colon," *Am. J. Surg.* 162(3):208–11 (1991).

51. McKeown, K. C. "Multiple Primary Malignant Neoplasms," *Eur. J. Surg. Oncol.* 17(5):429–46 (1991).

52. Holland, H. K., R. Saral, J. J. Rossi, A. D. Donnenberg, W. H. Burns, W. E. Baschorner, H. Farzadegan, R. J. Jones, G. V. Quinnan, and G. B. Vogelsang. "Allogeneic Bone Marrow Transplantation, Zidovudine, and Human Immunodeficiency Virus Type 1 (HIV-1) Infection. Studies in a Patient with Non-Hodgkin Lymphoma, *Ann. Int. Med.* 111(12):973–81 (1989).

53. Voelkerding, K. V., L. M. Sandhaus, H. C. Kim, J. Wilson, T. Chittenden, A. J. Levine, and K. Raska. "Plasma Cell Malignancy in the Acquired Immune Deficiency Syndrome: Association with Epstein Barr Virus," *Am. J. Clin. Pathol.* 92(2):222–8 (1989).

54. Wiley, C. A. "Neuromuscular Diseases of AIDS," *FASEB J.* 3(13):2503–11 (1989).

55. Radin, D. R., E. L. Baker, E. C. Klatt, E. J. Balthazar, R. B. Jeffrey, Jr., A. J. Magibow, and P. W. Ralls. "Visceral and Nodal Calcification in Patients with AIDS-Related Pneumocystis Carinii Infection," *AJR Am. J. Roentgenol.* 154(1):27–31 (1990).

56. Gachot, B., M. Wolff, B. Clair, and B. Regnier. "Severe Tuberculosis in Patients with Human Immunodeficiency Virus Infection," *Intensive Care Med.* 16(8):491–3 (1990).

57. Speich, R., R. Jenni, M. Opravil, M. Pfab, E. W. Russi. "Primary Pulmonary Hypertension in HIV Infection," *Chest* 100(5):1268–71 (1991).

58. Beschorner, W. E., K. Baughman, R. P. Turnicky, G. M. Hutchins, S. A. Rowe, A. L. Kavanaugh-McHugh, D. L. Suresch, and A. Herskowitz. "HIV-Associated Myocarditis. Pathology and Immunopathology," *Am. J. Pathol.* 137(6):1365–71 (1990).

59. Geller, S. A. "The Autopsy in Acquired Immunodeficiency Syndrome: How and Why," *Arch. Pathol. Lab. Med.* 114(3):324–9 (1990).

60. Ullrich, R., M. Zeitz, C. Bergs, K. Janitschke, and E. O. Riecken. "Intestinal Microsporidiosis in a German Patient with AIDS," *Klin. Wochenschr.* 69(10):443–5 (1991).

61. Harpey, J. P., C. Charpentier, and M. Jouas-Paturneau. "Sudden Infant Death and Inherited Disorders of Fatty Acid Beta-Oxidation," *Biol. Neonate* 58(Suppl 1):70–80 (1990).

62. Burchfield, D. J. and D. J. Rawlings. "Sudden Deaths and Apparent Life-Threatening Events in Hospitalized Neonates Presumed to Be Healthy," *Am. J. Dis. Child.* 145(11):1319–22 (1991).

63. Becker, L. E. "Neural Maturational Delay As a Link in the Chain of Events Leading to SIDS," *Can. J. Neurol. Sci.* 17(4):361–71 (1990).

64. Gnant, M. F., A. Rosenmayr, P. Wamser, P. Goetzinger, T. Sautner, F. Laengle, R. Steininger, C. Banhegyi, and F. Muehlbacher. "Prenephrectomy Tissue Typing Using Donor Lymph Node Cells: A Reliable and Safe Way of Shortening Cadaver Kidney Ischemia Time," *Transplant Proc.* 23(5):2683–4 (1991).

65. Vincenti, F., P. Weber, G. Kuo, J. Forsell, S. Hunt, J. Melzer, O. Salvatierra, and C. Stempel. "Hepatitis C Virus in Cadaver Organ Donors: Prevalence and Risk of Transmission to Transplant Recipients," *Transplant Proc.* 23(5):2651–2 (1991).

66. Mora, M., H. Wilms, and G. Kirste. "Significance of Bacterial Contamination of Cadaver Donor Renal Allografts before Transplantation," *Transplant Proc.* 23(5):2648 (1991).

67. Oesterwitz, H. E. and K. Lucius. "Transmission of Cancer with Cadaveric Donor Kidneys," *Transplant Proc.* 23(5):2647 (1991).

68. Koselj, M., T. Rott, A. Vizjak, and R. Kveder. "IgA Nephropathy as a Donor-Transmitted Disease in Renal Transplant Recipients," *Transplant Proc.* 23(5):2643–6 (1991).

69. Raffel, C., J. G. McComb, S. Bodner, and F. E. Gilles. "Benign Brain Stem Lesion in Pediatric Patients with Neurofibromatosis: Case Reports," *Neurosurgery* 25(6):959–64 (1989).

70. Lombes, A., J. R. Mendell, H. Nakase, R. J. Barohn, E. Bonilla, M. Zeviani, A. J. Yates, J. Omerza, T. L. Gales, and K. Nakahara. "Myoclonic Epilepsy and Ragged-Red Fibers with Cytochrome Oxidase Deficiency: Neuropathology, Biochemistry, and Molecular Genetics," *Ann. Neurol.* 26(1):20–33 (1989).

71. Grigsby, P. W., D. M. Garcia, and R. Ghiselli. "Analysis of Autopsy Findings in Patients Treated with Irradiation for Thalamic and Brain Stem Tumors," *Am. J. Clin. Oncol.* 12(3):255–8 (1989).

72. Moore, M. R., E. Rossitch, and J. Shillito. "Cushing and Epilepsy Surgery: Two Successfully Treated Cases with Long-Term Follow-Up," *Surg. Neurol.* 32(3):241–5 (1989).

73. Mahler, M. E. and J. L. Cummings. "Alzheimer Disease and the Dementia of Parkinson Disease: Comparative Investigations," *Alzheimer Dis. Assoc. Disord.* 4(3):133–49 (1990).

74. Mizutani, Y., M. Yokochi, and S. Oyanagi. "Juvenile Parkinsonism: A Case with First Clinical Manifestation at the Age of Six Years and with Neuropathological Findings Suggesting a New Pathogenesis," *Clin. Neuropathol.* 10(2):91–7 (1991).

75. Risse, S. C., T. H. Lampe, T. O. Bird, D. Nochlin, S. M. Sumi, T. Keenan, L. Cubberley, E. Peskind, and M. A. Raskind. "Myoclonus, Seizures, And Paratonia in Alzheimer Disease," *Alzheimer Dis. Assoc. Disord.* 4(4):217–25 (1990).

76. Weiler, R., H. Lassmann, P. Fischer, K. Jallinger, and H. Winkler. "A High Ratio of Chromogranin A to Synaptin/Synaptophysin is a Common Feature of Brains in Alzheimer and Pick Disease," *FEBS Lett.* 263(2):337–9 (1990).

77. Itoh, Y., S. Yagishita, N. Amano, and K. Iwabuchi. "An Autopsy Case of Peroneal Muscular Atrophy with Rigidity and Tremor: Ultrastructural and Systematic Morphometrical Studies on Peripheral Nerves," *Acta. Neuropathol. Berl.* 80(6):671–9 (1990).

78. Mirra, S. S., A. Heyman, D. McKeel, S. M. Sumi, B. J. Crain, L. M. Brownlee, F. S. Fogel, J. P. Hughes, G. van Belle, and L. Berg. "The Consortium to Establish a Registry for Alzheimer's Disease (CERAD). Part II. Standardization of the Neuropathologic Assessment of Alzheimer's Disease," *Neurology* 41(4):479–86 (1991).

79. Alberts, M. J., M. A. Pericak-Vance, V. Royal, J. Bebout, P. Gaskell, J. Thomas, W. J. Hung, C. Clark, N. Earl, and A. Roses. "Genetic Linkage Analysis of Nerve Growth Factor (Beta) in Familial Alzheimer's Disease," *Ann. Neurol.* 30(2):216–9 (1991).

80. Nidecker, A., M. Kocher, M. Maeder, O. Gratzl, G. A. Zach, U. F. Benz, and B. Burckhardt. "MR-Imaging of Chronic Spinal Cord Injury. Association with Neurologic Function," *Neurosurg. Rev.* 14(3):169–79 (1991).

81. Petty, G. W., T. K. Tatemichi, R. L. Sacco, J. Owen, and J. P. Mohr. "Fatal or Severely Disabling Cerebral Infarction during Hospitalization for Stroke or Transient Ischemic Attack," *J. Neurol.* 237(5):306–9 (1991).

82. Suzuki, S., M. Kimura, M. Souma, H. Ohkima, T. Shimizu, and T. Iwabuchi. "Cerebral Microthrombosis in Symptomatic Cerebral Vasospasm: A Quantitative Histological Study in Autopsy Cases," *Neurol. Med. Chir. Tokyo* 30(5):309–16 (1991).

83. Vieregge, P., V. Reinhardt, and B. Hoft. "Is Progression in Postencephalitic Parkinson's Disease Late or Age-Related?," *J. Neurol.* 238(5):299–303 (1991).

84. Rajput, A. H., B. Rozilsky, and A. Rajput. "Accuracy of Clinical Diagnosis in Parkinsonian: A Prospective Study," *Can. J. Neurol. Sci.* 18(3):275–8 (1991).

85. Wender, M., Z. Adamczewska-Goncerzewicz, and J. J. Dorszewska. "Myelin Proteins in Aging Human Brain," *Mol. Chem. Neuropathol.* 14(1):1–10 (1991).

86. Scott, S. A., S. T. DeKosky, and S. W. Scheff. "Volumetric Atrophy of the Amygdala in Alzheimer's Disease: Quantitative Serial Reconstruction," *Neurology* 41(3):351–6 (1991).

87. Gautrin, D., J. Nalbantoglu, G. Lacoste-Royal, M. Grenon, S. Gauthier, R. Bouchard, J. Mathieu, Y. Robitaille, L. P. Doyon, and H. Bergman. "Ascertainment of Informative Alzheimer Disease Families from the IMAGE Project Registry for Genetic Linkage Analysis Studies," *Can. J. Neurol. Sci.* 16(4 Suppl):468–72 (1989).

88. Tanzi, R. E. "Molecular Genetics of Alzheimer's Disease and the Amyloid Beta Peptide Precursor Gene," *Ann. Med.* 21(2):91–4 (1989).

89. Sadovnick, A. D., M. E. Irwin, P. A. Baird, and B. L. Beattie. "Genetic Studies on an Alzheimer Clinic Population," *Genet. Epidemiol.* 6(5):633–43 (1989).

90. Mann, D. M., D. Prinja, C. A. Davies, Y. Ihara, A. Delacourte, A. Defossez, R. J. Mayer, and M. Landon. "Immunocytochemical Profile of Neurofibrillary Tangles in Down's Syndrome Patients of Different Ages," *J. Neurol. Sci.* 92(2–3):247–60 (1989).

91. Soustek, Z. "Ultrastructure of Cortical Synapses in the Brain of Schizophrenics," *Zentralbl. Allg. Pathol.* 135(1):25–32 (1989).

92. Kitamura, N., T. Hashimoto, N. Nishino, and C. Tanaka. "Inositol 1,4,5-Triphosphate Binding Sites in the Brain: Regional Distribution, Characterization, and Alterations in Brains of Patients with Parkinson's Disease," *J. Mol. Neurosci.* 1(3):181–7 (1989).

93. Jankovic, J., R. Grossman, C. Goodman, F. Pirozzolo, L. Schneider, Z. Zhu, P. Scardino, A. J. Garber, S. G. Jhingran, and S. Martin. "Clinical, Biochemical, and Neuropathologic Findings Following Transplantation of Adrenal Medulla to the Caudate Nucleus for Treatment of Parkinson's Disease," *Neurology* 39(9):1227–34 (1989).

94. Rich, C. L., M. Sherman, and R. C. Fowler. "San Diego Suicide Study: The Adolescents," *Adolescence* 25(100):855–65 (1990).

95. Marttunen, M. J., H. M. Aro, M. M. Henriksson, and J. K. Lonnqvist. "Mental Disorders in Adolescent Suicide. DSM-III-R Axes I and II Diagnoses in Suicides among 13 To 19-Year-Olds in Finland," *Arch. Gen. Psychiatry* 48(9):834–9 (1991).

CHAPTER 14

Medical Microbiology

Michael B. Kapis

14.0 Introduction

Microbiology is the study of living organisms that are so small as to be visible only through microscopes. Microorganisms may be viruses, bacteria, fungi, algae, and protozoa. They constitute the oldest, most numerous, and the most diverse form of life. Most microorganisms benefit plants and animals, mainly by decomposing dead plant and animal matter, thus fertilizing soils. However, there exist small numbers of microorganisms which pose a significant health risk to many animals, including humans. Research in medical microbiology is a primary reason why the human life expectancy has been increased 50% during this century.[1-9]

Infection is the replication of organisms in the tissue of the host; disease is the overt clinical manifestation of infection. A carrier is a person in whom organisms are present and may be multiplying, but who shows no clinical response to their presence. Dissemination is the movement of an infectious agent from one source individual directly into the environment.[1,3,6]

The occurrence of disease in a defined population includes sporadic (occasional occurrence); endemic (regular, ongoing occurrence); epidemic (significantly increased occurrence); and pandemic (epidemic occurrence in multiple countries).[1,6]

0-87371-504-7/93/$0.00+$.50
© 1993 by Lewis Publishers

14.1 A Brief History of Discoveries in Medical Microbiology

In 1683 a Dutchman, Antony van Leeuwenhoek, was the first person to observe "animalcules" (microorganisms) through a microscope that he had made. His observation was the first reliable evidence of the existence of micro-organisms, although the germ theory of disease had been proposed centuries before his time (Varro—116 to 26 B.C.; Columella—60 B.C.; Fracastoro—1546).[2]

In 1796, Edward Jenner showed that smallpox could be prevented with cowpox. Ignaz Semmelweis used chemical disinfectants to control the spread of disease in hospital maternity wards. Florence Nightingale showed that post-traumatic infection and epidemic diseases in hospitals could be reduced by cleanliness and disinfection. Louis Pasteur proved that living organisms origi-nate from living organisms. Pasteur urged hospital workers to insure that instru-ments and bandages were clean. Robert Koch is primarily responsible for developing methods for isolating bacteria in pure culture. Joseph Lister intro-duced a carbolic spray mist as an aseptic surgical technique. Hans Christian Gram developed the staining procedure that carries his name. Emil von Behring discovered the neutralization of diphtheria toxin by antitoxin. Ronald Ross conclusively demonstrated the role of the anopheline mosquito in the transmis-sion of malaria. Jules Bordet described the lysis of some Gram-negative bacteria by antibody and complement.[1,6]

In the 1900s, August von Wasserman developed the first serologic test for syphilis. Walter Reed reported studies in 1902 which established that yellow fever virus, the first recognized human virus, could be transmitted by mos-quito bites. Frederick Twort and Felix d'Herelle independently discovered bacterial viruses (bacteriophages). Alexander Fleming discovered lysozymes and penicillin, the first antibiotic, later used successfully for antibacterial chemotherapy. E. Ruska and L. Marton developed the electron microscope. S. Waksman discovered streptomycin, the first antibiotic effective against tuber-culosis. Oswald Avery, Colin MacLeod, and Maclyn MacCarty discovered genetic transformation of bacteria by DNA. John Enders, Frederick Robbins, and Thomas Weller grew the poliomyelitis virus in cell culture (*in vitro*) opening the way to vaccine production. James Watson and Francis Crick described the double helical structure of DNA. Jonas Salk developed the inactivated poliomyelitis vaccine. Alick Isaacs discovered interferon. Jacques Monod and Francis Jacob reported their studies on enzyme regulation leading to recognition of promoters, regulatory proteins, and the role of mRNA. Gershon and Konda discovered T suppressor cells. Herbert Boyer, Stanley Cohen developed techniques for *in vitro* splicing of DNA. Luc Montagnier and Robert Gallo independently isolated the virus causing AIDS and defined its activity on human immunocutes.[2,6]

14.2 Microbial Control

Some of the methods used in microbial control are[1,3,5,10,11]

- *Sterilization* involves the killing or removal of all living organisms from a particular location or material. Sterilization methods include incineration, nondestructive heat treatments, certain gases, exposure to ionizing radiation, some liquid chemicals, and filtration.
- *Disinfection* involves the destruction of harmful microbes, especially by means of liquid chemicals (disinfectants). Antiseptics are disinfectant agents that can be used on body surfaces.
- *Sanitization,* similar to disinfection, involves providing an acceptable level of microbial cleanliness.
- *Pasturization* is the use of heat at a temperature sufficient to inactivate certain harmful microorganisms in a liquid, such as milk.
- *Aseptic* involves the prevention of microorganisms from reaching a protected environment, such as a surgical operating room.

14.3 Introduction to Medical Bacteriology

Bacteria are single-celled microorganisms that lack a nuclear membrane but are metabolically active and divide by binary fission. Bacteria are ubiquitous, existing in both parasitic and free-living forms.

In developed countries, 90% of documented infections in hospitalized patients are caused by bacteria.[3,12] Malnutrition, parasitic infections, and poor sanitation are a few of the factors contributing to the increased susceptibility of these individuals to bacterial pathogens. Antibiotics have substantially improved the clinical course of many bacterial infections. Meanwhile, only a few bacterial vaccines have been shown to be highly effective. Improved sanitation and water purification often have a greater effect on the number of bacterial infections than does the availability of antibiotics or bacterial vaccines.

Medically important bacteria are classified into the following general forms: (1) cocci, or spherical cells; (2) bacilli, or cylindrical or rod-shaped cells; and (3) spiral or curved cells.

14.4 A List of Some of the Important Medical Bacteria[13-24]

Streptococci	Scarlet fever, rheumatic fever, meningitis, pneumonia
Straphylococci	Food poisoning, pneumonia, toxic shock syndrome, meningitis
Neisseria	Meinggococcal, gonorrhea
Enterobacteriaceae	Gastrointestinal infections, typhoid fever, Klebsiella pneumonia
Vibrionaceae	Cholera, food poisoning, diarrhea

Pseudomonas	Urinary tract infections, surgical wound infections, lower respiratory tract infections
Yersinia	Bubonic plague
Bordetella	Whooping cough
Legionella	Legionnaires' disease
Bacillus	Anthrax and food poisoning
Clostridium	Tetanus, gas gangrene, botulism
Corynebacterium	Diphtheria
Mycobacterium	Tuberculosis, leprosy
Treponema	Syphilis, yaws
Leptospira	Leptospirosis
Borrelia	Lyme disease
Mycoplasma	Primary atypical pneumonia
Rickettsiae	Typhus and Rocky Mt. Spotted Fever
Chlamydiae	Genital tract infections, infant pneumonia, trachoma, inclusion conjunctivitis
Actinomycoses	Peridontal disease

14.5 Introduction to Medical Mycology

Medical mycology is the study of those fungi (commonly called yeast, mushrooms, and molds) that cause disease in humans and other animals. While over 100,000 species of fungi are recognized, fewer than 50 species are responsible for the majority of the fungal infections (mycoses) of humans.[2]

Human mycotic infections may be grouped into superficial, subcutaneous, and deep (or systemic) mycoses. Superficial fungal infections of skin, hair, and nails may be chronic and resistant to treatment but rarely affect the general health of the patient. Deep mycoses, may produce systemic involvement and are sometimes fatal. Deep mycoses are caused by organisms that live free in nature, in soil, or on decaying material and are frequently limited to certain geographic areas.[4]

Fungal disease is an increasing health problem because of widespread use or misuse of antibacterial antibiotics, radiation, and immunosuppressive agents. Individuals with reduced defense mechanisms are more likely to contract opportunistic fungal infections, such as candidiasis.

Fungi are eukaryotes and as such have a nucleus enclosed by a nuclear membrane. Some aspects of their structure, including their cell walls, endoplasmic reticula, and mitochondria, closely resemble those of plant and animal cells and are substantially different from those of bacteria.

14.6 A List of Some of the Medically Important Mycoses[25,26]

Aspergillosis	Farmer's lung, bronchitis, asthma, tuberculosis
Tinea	Athlete's foot, ringworm
Candida	Infections of the vagina, oral cavity, eye, intestinal, skin, endocarditis thrombophlebitis
Coccidioides	Valley fever

Histoplasma	Lung infections
Balstomyces	Lung infections
Crytococcus	Pulmonary infections

14.7 Introduction to Medical Virology

For years after the discovery of the tobacco mosaic virus (TMV) by Iwanowski in 1892, viruses were known mainly by the diseases they caused. Examples of human viral diseases are AIDS, herpes, hepatitis, poliomyelitis, influenza measles, mumps, warts, chickenpox, and the common cold. More than 1000 viruses are known at present.[1,5]

Viruses range in size from 20 to 300 nm, containing only one kind of nucleic acid (RNA or DNA) as their genome. The nucleic acid is encased in a protein shell known as a capsid. An intact, infectious viral particle is termed a virion. Viruses replicate only in living cells. They are inert in the extracellular environment.

The host range for a given virus may be broad or extremely limited. Viruses are known to infect unicellular organisms such as mycoplasmas, bacteria, and algae as well as all higher plants and animals. Viruses can be clearly separated into major grouping, called families, on the basis of the type of nucleic acid genome and the size, shape, substructure, and mode of replication of the virus particle by physicochemical or serologic properties.

Viral diseases range from the trivial infections to plagues that have altered the course of history. A large variety of viruses is shed from the respiratory tract; indeed this constitutes the main route of excretion for all the viruses. Herpes simplex and chickenpox are exceptions, because the vesicles on the skin contain virus, as are rubella and cytomegalovirus, which may be transmitted transplacentally.[5]

Each virus presents its own set of problems to those seeking solutions. The most spectacular progress so far has involved the concept of immunoprophylaxis. Vector control and sanitation have both contributed greatly. Antiviral drugs hold exciting future promise, but, to date, efficacy has been shown in only a few cases.

14.8 A List of Some of the Medically Important Viruses[27-39]

DNA-Containing Viruses

Parvoviruses	Very small virus infecting, dogs, rodents, and swine
Papovaviruses	Papilloma (wart) virus, multifocal leukoencephalopathy, and BK virus
Adenoviruses	Mucous membranes, lymphoid tissues, respiratory diseases, pharyngitis, and conjunctivitis
Herpesviruses	Herpes simplex types 1 and 2 (oral and genital lesions), varicella-zoster virus (shingles and chickenpox), cytomegalovirus, and EB virus (infectious mononucleosis and association with human neoplasms)

| Poxviruses | Skin lesions, smallpox, vaccinia, molluscum contagiosum; some poxviruses pathogenic for animals can infect humans, e.g., cowpox, monkeypox |
| Hepadnaviruses | Liver lesions |

RNA-Containing Viruses

Piconaviruses	Rhinovirus (common cold), enteroviruses (poliovirus, coxsackievirus, and echovirus
Reoviruses	Infantile gastroenteritis, Colorado tick fever virus
Arboviruses	Yellow fever, dengue, encephalitis virus
Togaviruses	Rubella virus, Sinbis virus
Flaviviruses	Yellow fever virus
Arenaviruses	Lassa fever virus
Coronaviruses	Acute upper respiratory tract illnesses
Retroviruses	AIDS, leukemia and sarcoma viruses
Orthomyoxviruses	Influenza virus
Paramyoxoviruses	Mumps, measles, parainfluenza virus, respiratory syncytial virus
Rhabdoviruses	Rabies virus

14.9 Diagnostic Methods in Medical Microbiology

Diagnostic medical microbiology is the discipline that recognizes and identifies etiologic microbial agents of disease. The identification of a pathogenic microorganism infecting a patient may not help in the selection of appropriate antimicrobial therapy for that patient, but may be of critical important in detecting disease and determining the appropriate isolation procedures to minimize the role of spreading the infection to medical personnel and other patients. Identification of a *Salmonella* isolated from a number of patients may provide the first clue in an epidemiologic study to detect a common source in water or food and present widespread disease in the community.[6-9]

- **Direct examination** involves stained or unstained preparations by light microscopy, dark-field, ultraviolet microscopy, fluorescence microscopy, phase-contrast microscopy, electron microscope, transmission electron microscope, and the scanning electron microscope.
- ***In vitro* methods**[40-43] are the most commonly used method for investigating bacterial, mycotic, and chlamydial agents of disease. *In vitro* methods are second only to immunologic studies for viral agents.
- **Antibody detection**[44,45] is used to determine whether an infection has occurred by testing the blood (or serum, the fluid part of blood after clotting) for distinctive protein substances (types of globulins, especially gamma globulins or immunoglobulins) called antibodies. Usually, each type of infection evokes antibodies that react with the specific infectious agents (antigens) that are stimulated by the tissues.

- **Antigen detection** procedures have the advantage of speed: they can yield results within an hour or two; sometimes within a few minutes.[5-8,46]

Some of the recent techniques currently used that have significantly contributed to the rapid advances in medical microbiology include enzymatic chemistry, immunofluorescence, bioluminescence, mass spectrometry, high performance liquid chromatography, immunoelectrophoresis, radioimmunoassay, enzyme-linked immunosorbent assay, and computers.[5-11]

REFERENCES

1. Frobisher, M. and R. Fuerst. *Microbiology in Health and Disease* (Philadelphia: W. B. Saunders, 1983).
2. Myrvik, Q. N. and R. S. Weiser. *Fundamentals of Medical Bacteriology and Mycology* (Philadelphia: Lea & Febiger, 1988).
3. Volk, W. A., D. C. Benjamin, R. J. Kadner, and J. T. Parsons. *Essentials of Medical Microbiology*, 3rd ed. (Philadelphia: J. P. Lippincott, 1986).
4. Jawetz, E., J. Melnick, and E. Adelberg. *Review of Medical Microbiology*, 17th ed. (Norwalk, CT: Appleton & Lange, 1987).
5. Baron, S., R. Robillard, and D. Weigent, Eds. *Medical Microbiology*, 2nd ed. (Menlo Park, CA: Addison-Wesley, 1986).
6. Sherris, J. C., K. J. Ryan, C. G. Ray, J. J. Plorde, L. Corey, F. C. Neidhardt, and J. J. Champoux, Eds. *Medical Microbiology: An Introduction to Infectious Diseases*, 2nd ed. (New York: Elsevier, 1990).
7. Prier, J. E., J. T. Bartola, and H. Friedman. *Modern Methods in Medical Microbiology: Systems and Trends* (Baltimore: University Park Press, 1976).
8. Boyd, R. F. and B. G. Hoerl. *Basic Medical Microbiology* (Boston: Little & Brown, 1986).
9. Finegold, S. M. and E. J. Baron, Eds. *Diagnostic Microbiology*, 7th ed. (St. Louis: C. V. Mosby, 1986).
10. Wust, J., I. Smid, and M. Salfinger. "Experience of Gas-Liquid Chromatography in Clinical Microbiology," *Ann. Biol. Clin. Paris* 48(6):416–9 (1989).
11. Cash, P. "The Application of Two-Dimensional Polyacrylamide Gel Electrophoresis to Medical Microbiology: Molecular Epidemiology of Viruses and Bacteria," *Electrophoresis* 12(7–8):592–604 (1991).
12. Moller, J. K. "Monitoring Antimicrobial Drug Resistance in Hospital Microorganisms," *Dan. Med. Bull.* 37(3):26,374 (1990).
13. Hancock, I. C. "Encapsulation of Coagulase-Negative *Staphylococci*," *Int. J. Med. Microbiol.* 272(1):11–8 (1989).
14. Anderson, J. D., C. Trombley, and N. Cimolai. "Assessment of the BACTEC NR660 Blood Culture System for the Detection of Bacteremia in Young Children," *J. Clin. Microbiol.* 27(4):721–3 (1989).
15. Faulmann, E. L., J. L. Duvall, and M. D. Boyle. "Protein B: A Versatile Bacterial Fc-Binding Protein Selective for Human IgG," *Biotechniques* 10(6):748–55 (1991).
16. Rutz, J. M., T. Abdullah, S. P. Singh, V. I. Kalve, and P. E. Klebba. "Evolution of the Ferric Enterobactin Receptor in Gram-Negative Bacteria," *J. Bacteriol.* 173(19):5964–74 (1991).

17. Eke, P. I. and V. O. Rotimi. "Rapid Presumptive Identification of Human Black Pigmented *Bacteroides* Species," *Afr. J. Med. Sci.* 20(2):115–21 (1991).

18. Apperloo-Renkema, H. Z., B. D. van-der-Waaij, and D. van-der-Waaij. "Determination of Colonization of the Digestive Tract by Biotyping of Enterobacteriaceae," *Epidemiol. Infect.* 105(2):355–61 (1990).

19. Weel, J. F., C. T. Hopman, and J. P. van-Putten. "Bacterial Entry and Intracellular Processing of *Neisseria gonorrhoeae* in Epithelial Cells: Immunomorphological Evidence for Alterations in the Major Outer Membrane Protein P. IB," *J. Exp. Med.* 174(3):705–15 (1991).

20. Frank, D. W. and B. H. Iglewski. "Cloning and Sequence Analysis of a Trans-Regulatory Locus Required for Exoenzyme S Synthesis in *Pseudomonas aeruginosa*," *J. Bacteriol.* 173(20):6460–8 (1991).

21. Hauser, A. R. and P. M. Schlievert. "Nucleotide Sequence of the *Streptococcal* Pyrogenic Exotoxin Type B Gene and Relationship Between the Toxin and the *Streptococcal* Proteinase Precursor," *J. Bacteriol.* 172(8):4536–42 (1990).

22. Zhanel, G. G., J. A. Karlowsky, D. J. Hoban, and R. J. Davidson. "Antimicrobial Activity of Subinhibitory Concentrations of Aminoglycosides Against *Pseudomonas aeruginosa* as Determined by the Killing-Curve Method and the Postantibiotic Effect," *Chemotherapy* 37(2):114–21 (1991).

23. Pfeffer, K., B. Schoel, H. Gulle, S. H. Kaufmann, and H. Wagner. "Human Gamma/Delta T Cells Responding to Myobacteria," *Behring Inst. Mitt.* 88:36–42 (1991).

24. Michelini-Norris, M. B., D. K. Blanchard, H. Friedman, J. Y. Djeu. "Involvement of HLA- DR⁺ Large Grandular Lymphocytes in the Induction of Tumor Necrosis Factor by *Mycobacterium avium-intracellulare* Complex," *J. Leukoc. Biol.* 50(6):529–38 (1991).

25. Edwards, J. H., M. Alfaham, R. Fifield, C. Philpot, M. J. Clement, and M. C. Goodchild. "Sequential Serological Responses to *Aspergillus fumigatus* in Patients with Cystic Fibrosis. Use of Antigen Stretching to Delineate IgG and IgE Activity," *Clin. Exp. Immunol.* 81(1):101–8 (1990).

26. Davies, B. I., F. P. Maesen, H. L. Gubbelmans, and H. M. Cremers. "Temafloxacin in Acute Purulent Exacerbations of Chronic Bronchitis," *J. Antimicrob. Chemother.* 26(2):237–46 (1989).

27. Booth, J. C., H. O. Kangro, K. M. Liu, L. el-Mohndes, and Y. S. Tryhorn. "Discordant Results Obtained on Testing Sera from Immunocomprised Patients for Cytomegalovirus IgG by Enzyme-Linked Immunosorbent Assay and Radioimmunoassay," *J. Virol. Methods* 26(1):77–89 (1989).

28. Kimpton, C. P., G. Corbitt, and D. J. Morris. "Detection of Cytomegalovirus DNA Using Probes Labelled with Digoxigenin," *J. Virol. Methods* 24(3):335–46 (1989).

29. Tyms, A. S., D. L. Taylor, and J. M. Parkin. "Cytomegalovirus and the Acquired Immunodeficiency Syndrome," *J. Antimicrob. Chemother.* 23(Suppl A):89–105 (1989).

30. Diaz-Mitoma, F., A. Ruiz, G. Flowerdew, S. Houston, B. Romanowski, T. Kovithavongs, J. Preiksaitis, and D. L. Tyrrell. "High Levels of Epstein-Barr Virus in the Oropharynx: A Predictor of Disease Progression in Human Immunodeficiency Virus Infection," *J. Med. Virol.* 31(2):69–75 (1990).

31. Goswami, K. K., R. F. Miller, M. J. Harrison, D. J. Hamel, R. S. Daniels, and R. S. Tedder. "Expression of HIV-1 in the Cerebrospinal Fluid Detected by the Polymerase Chain Reaction and Its Correlation with Central Nervous System Disease," *AIDS* 5(7):797–803 (1991).

32. Goswami, K. K., S. Kaye, R. Miller, R. McAllister, and R. Tedder. "Intrathecal IgG Synthesis and Specificity of Oligoclonal IgG in Patients Infected with HIV-1 do not Correlate with CNS Disease," *J. Med. Virol.* 33(2):106–13 (1991).

33. Sample, M., C. Loveday, I. Weller, and R. Tedder. "Direct Measurement of Viraemia in Patients Infected with HIV-1 and Its Relationship to Disease Progression and Zidovudine Therapy," *J. Med. Virol.* 35(1):38–45 (1991).

34. Hollsberg, P., A. Moller-Larsen, F. Skou-Pedersen, J. Justesen, H. J. Hansen, and S. Haahr. "Search for a Retrovirus in Long-Term Cultured Cerebrospinal Fluid Cells and Peripheral Blood Mononuclear Cells from Patients with Multiple Sclerosis," *Acta Neurol. Scand.* 80(6):603–9 (1989).

35. Williams, M. V., D. V. Ablashi, S. Z. Salahuddin, and R. Glaser. "Demonstration of the Human Herpesvirus 6-Induced DNA Polymerase and DNase," *Virology* 173(1):223–30 (1989).

36. Wu, C. L. and K. W. Wilcox. "Codons 262 to 490 from the Herpes Simplex Virus ICP4 Gene are Sufficient to Encode a Sequence-Specific DNA Binding Protein," *Nucleic Acids Res.* 18(3):531–8 (1990).

37. Sherlock, C. H., J. F. Danegri, and R. L. Ashley. "Serological Responses to Cytomegalovirus during Renal Transplant Rejection," *Transplantation* 52(2):272–5 (1991).

38. Huppertz, H. I., N. P. Niki, and J. K. Chantler. "Susceptibility of Normal Human Joint Tissue to Viruses," *J. Rheumatol.* 18(5):699–704 (1991).

39. Clarke, J. R. and A. S. Tyms. "Polyamine Biosynthesis in Cells Infected with Different Clinical Isolates of Human Cytomegalovirus," *J. Med. Virol.* 34(4):212–6 (1991).

40. Karttunen, R., H. M. Surcel, G. Andersson, H. P. Ekre, and E. Herva. "*Francisella tularensis*-Induced *In Vitro* Gamma Interferon, Tumor Necrosis Factor Alpha, and Interleukin 2 Responses Appear Within 2 Weeks of *Tularemia* Vaccination in Human Beings," *J. Clin. Microbiol.* 29(4):753–6 (1991).

41. Forsgren, A., A. Bredberg, and K. Riesbeck. "Effect of Ciprofloxacin on Human Lymphocytes-Laboratory Study," *Scand. J. Infect. Dis. Suppl.* 60:39–45 (1989).

42. Kosseim, M., A. Ronald, F. A. Plummer, L. D'Costa, and R. C. Brunham. "Treatment of Acute Pelvic Inflammatory Disease in the Ambulatory Setting: Trial of Cefoxitin and Doxycycline Versus Ampicillin-Sulbactam," *Antimicrob. Agents Chemother.* 35(8):1651–6 (1991).

43. Granfors, K., S. Jalkanen, A. A. Lindberg, O. Maki-Ikola, R. von-Essen, R. Lahesmaa-Rantala, H. Isomaki, R. Saario, W. J. Arnold, and A. Toivanen. "*Salmonella* Lipopolysaccharide in Synovial Cells from Patients with Reactive Arthritis," *Lancet* 335(8691):685–8 (1990).

44. van-Kessel, K. P., J. A. van-Strijp, M. E. van-der-Tol, H. J. van-Kats-Renaud, R. M. Thijssen, A. C. Fluit, and J. Verhoef. "Quantitation of Conjugate Formation Between Human Polymorphonuclear Leukocytes and Antibody-Coated Target Cells by Flow Cytometry: The Role of Fc Receptor and LFA-1 Antigen," *J. Leukoc. Biol.* 46(5):467–75 (1989).

45. Ison, C. A., B. Kolator, J. H. Reid, E. Dermott, J. Clark, and C. S. Easmon. "Characterizations of Monoclonal Antibodies for Detection of *Mobiluncus* spp. in Genital Specimens," *J. Med. Microbiol.* 30(2):129–36 (1989).

46. Redlich, P. N. and S. E. Grossberg. "Immunochemical Characterization of Antigenic Domains on Human Interferon-Beta: Spatially Distinct Epitopes Are Associated with Both Antiviral and Antiproliferative Activities," *Eur. J. Immunol.* 20(9):1933–9 (1990).

CHAPTER 15

Physicochemical Techniques in Biological Research and Testing

Michael B. Kapis

15.0 Introduction

A wide variety of physicochemical techniques are utilized to identify and analyze physical and chemical properties of pharmaceuticals, proteins, nucleic acids, amino acids, lipids, enzymes, membranes, environmental toxins,[1-6] microbes,[7-33] and other biological and chemical substances. In the last two decades, the rapid progress in physicochemical techniques has been a revolution rather than an evolution. Advances in physicochemical techniques have enabled researchers to solve analytical problems that they, until recently, could only theorize.

This chapter will briefly discuss examples of two major physicochemical areas: chromatography and spectrometry. Finally, an extensive reference list of recent applications of physicochemical techniques will be presented.

15.1 Chromatography

Chromatographic methods are used to separate components of a mixture. The history of chromatography historically dates back to the early 1900s, when Mikhail Tswett reported the separation of plant pigments on an open column

0-87371-504-7/93/$0.00+$.50
© 1993 by Lewis Publishers

217

containing calcium carbonate. The separated pigments appeared as colored bands on the column, which inspired him to formulate the term "chromatography" (color-write). Martin and Synge were awarded the Nobel Prize in chemistry in 1952 for their work in developing the theory and practice of chromatography. For a comprehensive discussion of the theory and application of chromatography see References 34 through 43.

There are many types of chromatographic methods, including adsorption, exclusion, ion-exchange, affinity, gas–liquid, high-performance liquid, reverse-phase, and supercritical fluid. A wide variety of physical separation methods based upon the sample partitioning between a moving phase, gas or liquid, and a stationary phase, liquid or solid, are used to investigate biological and chemical substances. Chromatographic procedures involve one of four types: liquid–solid, liquid–liquid, gas–solid, and gas–liquid.

Chromatographic methods can be further classified according to the mechanism by which solutes are retained by the stationary phase. Partition is a bulk-phase distribution process in which the solute forms homogeneous solutions in each phase. Absorption involves interactions at a surface or on fixed sites on a normally solid stationary phase. Exclusion relies on the ability of a porous solid stationary phase to discriminate on the basis of size by admitting small molecules to its pores but excluding larger molecules.[38]

The molecular differences upon which the separations are based are quite diverse, as well. Molecules can be separated by their differences in molecular change, molecular size, molecular mass, bond polarities, redox potentials, and ionization constants.[41]

Chromatographic techniques are used to investigate: drug analyses, steroids, lipids, carbohydrates, amino acids, proteins, peptides, enzymes, biogenic amines, nucleotides, nucleosides and bases, environmental toxins, and microorganisms.

Some of the major chromatographic techniques[44] used in biological research and testing are gas chromatography (GC) and high-performance liquid chromatography (HPLC). HPLC has now become the most powerful analytical and preparative techniques, the applications of which appear to be limited only by the dedication and experience of the operator. It has an unsurpassed range of applications particularly in the pharmaceutical and biomedical areas. While HPLC is the preferred method chromatographic analysis, GC is an excellent method for the separation, detection, and quantitation of the components of a complex mixture. However, GC is not a good method for qualitative identification. For detailed qualitative analysis, GC must be combined with other analytical methods. Usually, mass spectrometry is selected, due to its sensitivity, to be coupled with gas chromatography (GC/MS).

15.1.1 Gas Chromatography (GC)[45-49,100-111]

The branch of chromatography in which a gas is the mobile phase. There are several important advantages[38] associated with the use of a gas as the mobile phase in chromatographic separations:

1. The low viscosity of gases permits the use of very long columns, thereby improving the efficiency of separations; and the use of high flow rates, which means that separations can be performed quickly.
2. Gases are considered "inert" in terms of their interactions with the solute, and the equilibrium of solute distribution between the phases is largely independent of the gas.
3. Many simple, sensitive, and fast-responding detectors are available for measuring concentrations of substances in a mobile phase.

Since there is little interaction between the solute and the gas phase, GC is limited to the separation of relatively volatile substances.

15.1.2 Gas Chromatography/Mass Spectroscopy (GC/MS)[50-55,112-129]

A combination of two microanalytical methods: GC, a separation method; and MS, an identification method. GC/MS overcomes certain deficiencies or limitations caused by using each method individually. Before the arrival of GC/MS, complex organic mixtures of 20 or more components could not be qualitatively analyzed. In contrast, the GC/MS enables researchers to qualitatively analyze up to 100 components in a mixture.[54]

The accuracy and precision of this combined technique is further increased by the use of stable isotopes. They are particularly suitable for the location and structural identification of metabolites and for the elucidation of biosynthetic pathways. In addition, GC/MS is gaining acceptance in drug metabolism studies.

The GC/MS techniques are now better developed than those of liquid chromatography-mass spectrometry (LC/MS), partly because it is easier to get rid of excess carrier gas than to eliminate liquid mobile phases. However, the techniques of LC/MS are being developed quickly.[41]

15.1.3 High-Performance Liquid Chromatography (HPLC)[56-66,130-153]

HPLC is the branch of chromatography in which high-efficiency columns filled with fine particles packings of uniform particle size are employed and the liquid mobile phase is usually fed under high pressure. HPLC offers the advantages of speed, resolution, and sensitivity. The columns may be reused. It is especially useful for separating the high-molecular-weight compounds which have either a low vapor pressure or undergo pyrolysis when subjected to the higher required temperatures of GC.[58]

15.2 Spectroscopy

Spectroscopy[67-77] is the measurement and interpretation of the energy spectra (electromagnetic or particle) arising from either emission or absorption of radiant energy or particles from a substance upon bombardment by electromagnetic radiation, electrons, neutrons, protons, ions, or upon heating or exciting an electric or magnetic field.

Spectrometry can be used to determine both the elemental and the molecular content of materials. Each spectrometric method has its own benefits, drawbacks, specificities, and interferences. There are two fundamental variables that are measured in all spectrometric methods: (1) the wavelength of radiation, and (2) the intensity of radiation at that wavelength.[41]

Spectrometric methods are used to investigate: drug analyses, proteins, peptides, nucleic acids, lipids, membranes, microorganisms, environmental toxins, enzymes, and probe techniques. Some of the major spectrometry methods[44] used in biological research and testing are MS, Raman spectroscopy (RS), nuclear magnetic resonance spectroscopy (NMR-S), and fluorescence spectroscopy (FS).

15.2.1 Mass Spectrometry (MS)[78-84,154-172]

MS is the branch of spectroscopy concerned with the production, measurement, and interpretation of the mass spectra of a sample exposed to an ionizing beam of electrons. MS can be applied to molecules in any state of matter, including fragile, thermally labile compounds in the solid state. Mixtures are commonly examined by MS, especially in instruments that combine MS with separations based on GC, LC, or a second stage of MS. Recent advances in MS have made possible the investigations of higher-molecular-weight compounds (above 10,000 and being extended), as well as nonvolatile and unstable samples.

15.2.2 Raman Spectroscopy (RS)[85-88,173-196]

RS is the branch of molecular vibrational spectroscopy dealing with measurement and interpretation of light or ultraviolet radiation. RS and infrared spectroscopy are similar in that they both involve the vibrational levels of molecules. However, molecules studied by Raman spectroscopes need not possess a changeable dipole moment as in infrared spectroscopy. A molecule must be able to undergo a change in polarizability in order to exhibit a Raman spectrum. There are certain disadvantages of RS, namely high costs, weakness of Raman spectra, and fluorescence.[71]

15.2.3 Nuclear Magnetic Resonance Spectroscopy (NMR-S)[89-94,197-220]

NMR-S is the branch of spectroscopy that utilizes NMR in the study of molecular structure, autodiffusion processes, hindered rotation, and for qualitative and quantitative chemical analysis. As in other spectrometries, the energy of the transition is determined by molecular and atomic properties; but in NMR-S, the energy also depends on the magnetic field. The frequency of resonance varies in a manner that depends on the chemical environment of the nuclei. This effect is called "chemical shift". In NMR-S, the integrated peak areas are only relative values, depending on the number of nuclei that contribute to the peak. This is one of the great strengths of the NMR method: every proton, when it absorbs energy, contributes equally to an NMR absorption spectrum.[41]

15.2.4 Fluorescence Spectroscopy (FS)[95-99,221-245]

FS is the branch of spectroscopy dealing with the fluorescence spectra due to de-excitation of atoms and molecules excited by absorption of radiation of higher frequency. Fluorescence[38] in organic molecules is due largely to the presence of the aromatic functional group. Fused-ring compounds are especially fluorescent, their photoluminescence efficiency increasing with the number of rings. Temperature, pH, dissolved oxygen, and solvent commonly affect the fluorescence of molecules. The factors to be considered in developing or evaluating a fluorescence method are very similar to those described for ultraviolet-visible absorption methods. Perhaps the most significant difference is the need to select both an excitation and fluorescence wavelength (or band of wavelengths), which requires familiarity with the emission spectrum of the source and the excitation and fluorescence spectra of the analyte. Fluorescence is an extremely valuable tool in biochemistry and related fields for the determination of a number of drugs, vitamins, proteins, and toxins. With macromolecules, fluorescence measurements can give information about conformation, binding sites, solvent interactions, degree of flexibility, intermolecular distances, and the rotational diffusion coefficient of macromolecules.

REFERENCES

1. Galassi, S., A. Provini, and A. DePaolis. "Organic Micropollutants in Lakes: A Sedimentological Approach," *Ecotoxicol. Environ. Safety* 19(2):150–9 (1990).
2. Harrison, L. M., J. E. Morrison, and P. V. Fennessey. "Microtechnique for Quantifying Phenol in Plasma by Gas Chromatography-Mass Spectrometry," *Clin. Chem.* 37(10 Pt 1):1739–42 (1991).
3. Huysman, K. D. and W. T. Frankenberger. "Evolution of Trimethylarsine by a *Penicillium* spp. Isolated from Agricultural Evaporation Pond Water," *Sci. Total Environ.* 105:13–28 (1991).
4. Nash, R. G. "Solid-Phase Extraction of Carbofuran, Atrazine, Simazine, Alachlor, and Cyanazine from Shallow Water," *J. Assoc. Off. Anal. Chem.* 73(3):438–42 (1990).
5. Park, J. M., D. H. Branson, and S. Burks. "Pesticide Decontamination from Fabric by Laundering and Simulated Weathering," *J. Environ. Sci. Health B* 25(3):281–93 (1990).
6. Pleasance, S., M. Xie, Y. LeBlanc, and M. Quilliam. "Analysis of Domoic Acid and Related Compounds by Mass Spectrometry and Gas Chromatography as *N*-Trifluoroacetyl-*O*-Silyl Derivatives," *Biomed. Environ. Mass Spectrum* 19(7):420–7 (1990).

7. Bamford, D. H., J. K. Bamford, S. A. Towse, and G. J. Thomas. "Structural Study of the Lipid-Containing PRD1 and Its Capsid and DNA Components by Laser Raman Spectroscopy," *Biochemistry* 29(25):5982–7 (1990).

8. Beran-Steed, R. K. and Y. C. Tse-Dinh. "The Carboxyl Terminal Domain of *Escherichia coli* DNA Topoisomerase I Confers Higher Affinity to DNA," *Protein* 6(3):249–58 (1989).

9a. Brondz, I. and I. Olsen. "Multivariate Analyses of Cellular Carbohydrates and Fatty Acids of *Candida albicans, Torulopsis glabrata*, and *Saccharomyces cerevisiae*," *J. Clin. Microbiol.* 28(8):1854–7 (1990).

9b. Brondz, I., I. Olsen, M. Haapasalo, and A. J. Van Winkelhoff. "Multivariate Analysis of Fatty Acid Data from Whole-Cell Methanolysates of *Prevotella, Bacteroids*, and *Porphyromonas* spp.," *J. Gen. Microbiol.* 137(Pt 6):1445–52 (1991).

10. Bussat, B., D. Schulz, F. Arminjon, C. Valentin, and J. Armand. "Molecular Size Characterization of Bacterial Capsular Polysaccharide Vaccines by High Performance Liquid Chromatography," *Biologicals* 18(2):117–21 (1990).

11. Chang, M. C., P. M. Callahan, P. S. Parkes-Loach, T. M. Cotton, and P. A. Loach. "Spectroscopic Characterization of the Light-Harvesting Complex of *Rhodospirillum* and Its Structural Subunit," *Biochemistry* 29(2):421–9 (1990).

12. Chapman, J. S. and N. H. Georgopapadakou. "Fluorometric Assay for Fleroxcin Uptake by Bacterial Cells," *Antimicrob. Agents Chemother.* 33(1):27–9 (1989).

13. Choma, C. T., W. K. Surewicz, P. R. Carey, M. Pozsgay, and H. Kaplan. "Secondary Structure of the Entomocidal Toxin from *Bacillus thuringiensis* subspp. *kurstaki* HD-73," *J. Protein Chem.* 9(1):87–94 (1990).

14. Christensen, G. D., L. P. Barker, T. P. Mawhinney, L. M. Baddour, and W. A. Simpson. "Identification of an Antigenic Marker of Slime Production for *Staphylococcus epidermis*," *Infect. Immunol.* 58(9):2906–11 (1990).

15. Clement, J. M., A. Charbit, P. Martineau, D. Callaghan, S. Szmelcman, C. Leclerc, and M. Hofnung. "Bacterial Vectors to Target and/or Purify Polypeptides: Their Use in Immunological Studies," *Ann. Biol. Clin. Paris* 49(4):249–54 (1991).

16. Glass, T. L., M. H. Saxerud, and H. H. Casper. "Properties of a 4-ene-3-ketosteroid-5-alpha Reductase in Cell Extract of the Intestinal Anaerobe, *Eubacterium* spp. strain 144," *J. Steroid Biochem. Mol. Biol.* 39(3):367–74 (1991).

17. Han, T. J. and T. J. Chai. "Occurrence of 2-keto-3-deoxy-D-manno—octonic Acid in Lipopolysaccharides Isolated from *Vibrio parahaemolyticus*," *J. Bacteriol.* 173(19):6303–6 (1991).

18. Hobbs, D. D., A. Kriauciunas, S. Guner, D. B. Knaff, and M. R. Ondrias. "Resonance Raman Spectroscopy of Cytochrome bc1 Complexes from *Rhodospirillum rubrum*: Initial Characterization and Reductive Titrations," *Biochim. Biophys. Acta* 1018(1):47–54 (1990).

19. Homer, K. A. and O. Beighton. "Fluorometric Determination of Bacterial Protease Activity Using Fluorescein Isothiocyanate-Labeled Proteins as Substrates," *Anal. Biochem.* 191(1):133–7 (1990).

20. Jackson, M. A. and G. A. Bennett. "Production of Fumonisin B1 by *Fusarium moniforme* NRRL 13616 in Submerged Culture," *Appl. Environ. Microbiol.* 56(8):2296–8 (1990).

21. Magee, J. T., J. M. Hindmarch, I. A. Burnett, and A. Pease. "Epidemiological Typing of *Streptococcus pyogenes* by pyrolysis mass spectrometry," *J. Med. Microbiol.* 30(4):273–8 (1989).

22. Mandrell, R. E., J. J. Kim, C. M. John, B. W. Gibson, J. V. Sugai, and M. A. Apicella. "Endogenous Sialylation of the Lipooligosaccharides of *Neisseria meningitidis*," *J. Bacteriol.* 173(9):2823–32 (1991).

23. Picorel, R., T. Lu, R. E. Holt, T. M. Cotton, and M. Seibert. "Surface-Enhanced Resonance Raman Scattering Spectroscopy of Bacterial Photosynthetic Membranes: Orientation of the Carotenoids of *Rhodobacter sphaeroides* 2. 4. 1.," *Biochemistry* 29(3):707–12 (1990).

24. Prevelige, P. E., D. Thomas, J. King, S. A. Towse, and G. J. Thomas. "Conformational States of the Bacteriophage P_{22} Capsid Subunit in Relation to Self-Assembly," *Biochemistry* 29(23):5626–33 (1990).

25. Quinlan, G. J. and M. Gutteridge. "DNA Base Damage by Beta-Lactam, Tetracycline, Bacitracin, and Rifamycin Antibacterial Antibiotics," *Biochem. Pharmacol.* 42(8):1595–9 (1991).

26. Rajagopal, B. S., P. A. Lespinat, G. Fauque, J. LeGall, and Y. M. Berlier. "Mass Spectrometric Studies of the Interrelations among Hydrogenase, Carbon Monoxide Dehydrogenase, and Methane-Forming Activities in Pure and Mixed Cultures of *Desulfovibrio vulgaris, Desulfovibrio desulfuricans*, and *Methanosarcina barkeri*," *Appl. Environ. Microbiol.* 55(9):2123–9 (1989).

27. Rogner, M., P. J. Nixon, and B. A. Diner. "Purification and Characterization of Photosystem I and Photosystem II Core Complexes from Wild-Type and Phycocyanin-Deficient Strains of the Cyanobacterium Synechocystis PCC 6803," *J. Biol. Chem.* 265(11):6189–96 (1990).

28. Schulman, M. D., S. L. Acton, D. L. Valentino, and B. H. Arison. "Purification and Identification of d TDP-Oleandrose, the Precursor of the Oleandrose Units of the Avermectins," *J. Biol. Chem.* 265(28):16,965–70 (1990).

29. Stevens, A. C., H. Greenstone, A. C. Bauer, and R. W. Williams. "The Maturation-Dependent Conformation Change of the Major Capsid Protein of Bacteriophage T4 Involves a Substantial Change in Secondary Structure," *Biochemistry* 29(23):5556–61 (1990).

30. Sutherland, J. B., J. P. Freeman, A. L. Selby, P. P. Fu, D. W. Miller, and C. E. Cerniglia. "Stereoselective Formation of a K-Region Dihydrodiol from Phenanthrene by *Streptomyces flavovirens*," *Arch. Microbiol.* 154(3):260–6 (1990).

31. Vasyurenko, Z. P. and Y. Chernyavskaya. "Conformation of *Morganella* Distinction from *Proteus* and *Providencia* among *Enterobacteriaceae* on the Basis of Cellular and Lipopolysaccharide Fatty Acid Composition," *J. Hyg. Epidemiol. Microbiol. Immunol.* 34(1):8190 (1990).

32. Wust, J., I. Smid, and M. Salfinger. "Experience of Gas-Liquid Chromatography in Clinical Microbiology," *Ann. Biol. Clin. Paris* 48(6):416–9 (1990).

33. Xu, P. L., M. Iwata, S. Leong, and S. Sequerira. "Highly Virulent Strains of *Pseudomonas solanacearum* that Are Defective in Extracellular Polysaccharide Production," *J. Bacteriol.* 172(7):3946–51 (1990).

34. Booth, R. F. and P. J. Quinn. "Principles and Applications of High Performance Liquid Chromatography," in *Biochemical Research Techniques: A Practical Introduction*, J. M. Wrigglesworth, Ed. (New York: John Wiley & Sons, 1983).

35. Colpan, M. and D. Riesner. "High Performance Liquid Chromatography of Nucleic Acids," in *Modern Physical Methods in Biochemistry*, A. Neuberger and L. Van Deenen, Eds. (Amsterdam: Elsevier, 1988).

36. Dryer, R. L. and G. F. Lata. *Experimental Biochemistry* (Oxford: Oxford University Press, 1989).

37. Hancock, W. S. and J. T. Sparrow. *HPLC Analysis of Biochemical Compounds: A Laboratory Guide* (New York: Marcel Dekker, 1984).

38. Hargis, L. G. *Analytical Chemistry: Principles and Techniques* (Englewood Cliffs, NJ: Prentice Hall, 1988).

39. Johns, D. "Columns for HPLC of Macromolecules," in *HPLC of Macromolecules: A Practical Approach*, R. W. A. Oliver, Ed. (Oxford: Oxford University Press, 1989).

40. Kuksus, A., Ed. *Chromatography of Lipids in Biomedical Research and Clinical Diagnosis* (Amsterdam: Elsevier, 1987).

41. Rubinson, K. A. *Chemical Analysis* (Boston: Little, Brown and Company, 1987).

42. Snyder, L. R., J. L. Glajch, and J. J. Kirkland. *Practical HPLC Method Development* (New York: John Wiley & Sons, 1988).

43. Welling, C. W. and S. Welling-Wester. "Size-Exclusion HPLC of Proteins," in *HPLC of Macromolecules: A Practical Approach*, R. W. A. Oliver, Ed. (Oxford: Oxford University Press, 1989).

44. Maludzinska, G., Ed. *Dictionary of Analytical Chemistry* (Amsterdam: Elsevier, 1990).

45. Clement, R. E., Ed. *Gas Chromatography: Biochemical, Biomedical & Clinical Applications* (New York: John Wiley & Sons, 1990).

46. Drucker, D. B. *Microbiological Applications of Gas Chromatography* (Cambridge: Cambridge University Press, 1981).

47. Gudzinowicz, B. J. *Gas Chromatography Analysis of Drugs and Pesticides* (New York: Marcel Dekker, 1967).

48. Jack, D. B. *Drug Analysis by Gas Chromatography* (New York: Academic Press, 1984).

49. Mitruka, B. M. *Gas Chromatography Applications in Microbiology and Medicine* (Melbourne, FL: Krieger, 1975).

50. Adamovics, J. A., Ed. "Chromatographic Analysis of Pharmaceuticals" in *Chromatographic Sciences*, Vol. 49, (New York: Marcel Dekker, 1990).

51. Fox, A. et al. Eds. *Analytical Microbiology Methods: Gas Chromatography-Mass Spectrometry* (New York: Plenum Press, 1990).

52. Karasek, F. W. and R. E. Clement. *Basic GC/MS Principles & Techniques* (Amsterdam: Elsevier, 1988).

53. Lai, S. T. *Gas Chromatography-Mass Spectroscopy Operation* (East Longmeadow, MA: Realistic Systems 1988).

54. McFadden, W. *Techniques of Combined Gas Chromatography-Mass Spectroscopy: Applications in Organic Analysis* (Melbourne, FL: Krieger, 1988).

55. Pleger, K. et al. Eds. Mass Spectra & Gas Chromatography Data of Drugs, Poisons & Their Metabolites, 2 Vols, (New York: VCH, 1985).

56. Brown, P. R. *High Pressure Liquid Chromatography: Biochemical & Biomedical* (New York: Academic Press, 1973).

57. Christie, W. W. *HPLC & Lipids: A Practical Guide* (New York: Pergamon Press, 1987).

58. Pease, B. F. *Basic Instrumental Analysis* (New York: D. Van Nostrand, 1980).

59. Hearns, M. and T. Hearns, et al. Eds. *HPLC of Proteins & Peptides: Proceedings of First International Symposium* (New York: Academic Press, 1983).

60. Horvath, C., Ed. *High Performance Liquid Chromatography: Advances & Perspectives*, Vol. 3, (New York: Academic Press, 1983).

61. Kerlavage, A. R., Ed. *The Use of HPLC in Receptor Biochemistry* (New York: John Wiley & Sons, 1989).

62. Lim, C. K., Ed. *HPLC of Small Molecules: A Practical Approach* (Oxford: Oxford University Press, 1986).
63. Jaeger, H., Ed. *Capillary Gas Chromatography-Mass Spectrometry in Medicine and Pharmacology* (Heidelberg: Huthig, 1987).
64. Reeves, D. S. and U. Ullmann, Eds. *HPLC in Medical Microbiology*, Vol. 2, (New York: VCH, 1986).
65. Regnier, F. *High Performance Liquid Chromatography of Proteins* (New York: John Wiley & Sons, 1988).
66. Rossomando, E. F. *HPLC of Enzymatic Analysis: Applications to the Assay of Enzymatic Activity* (New York: John Wiley & Sons, 1987).
67. Alix, A. J., L. Bernard, and M. Manfait, Eds. *Spectroscopy of Biological Molecules* (New York: John Wiley & Sons, 1985).
68a. Carey, P. R. *Biochemical Applications of Raman and Resonance Raman Spectroscopies* (New York: Academic Press, 1982).
68b. Carey, P. R. "Raman and Resonance Raman Spectroscopy," in *Modern Physical Methods in Biochemistry: Part B*, A. Neuberger and L. Van Deenen, Eds. (Amsterdam: Elsevier, 1988).
69. Gaskell, S., Ed. *Mass Spectrometry in Biomedical Research* (New York: John Wiley & Sons, 1986).
70. Handschumacher, R. E. and I. M. Armitage, Eds. *NMR Spectroscopy in Drug Research* (New York: Pergamon Press, 1990).
71. Lambert, J. B., H. F. Shurvell, D. A. Lightner, and R. G. Cooks. *Introduction To Organic Spectroscopy* (New York: Macmillan, 1987).
72. Oki, M. *Applications of Dynamic NMR Spectroscopy To Organic Chemistry* (New York: VCH, 1985).
73. Robyt, J. F. and B. J. White. *Biochemical Techniques: Theory & Practice* (Monterey, CA: Brooks/Cole, 1987).
74. Sandorfy, C. and T. Theophanides, Eds. *Spectroscopy of Biological Molecules: Theory and Applications—Chemistry, Physics, Biology, and Medicine* (Dordrecht, Holland: D. Reidel, 1983).
75. Tabet, J. C. and M. Fetizon. "Mass Spectroscopy," in *Modern Physical Methods in Biochemistry, Part A*, A. Neuberger and L. Van Deenen, Eds. (Amsterdam: Elsevier, 1985).
76. Watson, J. T. *Introduction To Mass Spectrometry* (New York: Raven Press, 1985).
77. Williams, W. P. "Fluorescence Spectroscopy," in *Biochemical Research Techniques: A Practical Introduction*, J. M. Wrigglesworth, Ed. (New York: John Wiley & Sons, 1983).
78. Burlingame, A. L. and N. Castagnoli, Eds. *Mass Spectroscopy in the Health and Life Sciences: Proceedings of an International Symposium, San Francisco*, (Amsterdam: Elsevier, 1984).
79. Hites, R. *CRC Handbook of Mass Spectra of Environmental Contaminants* (Boca Raton, FL: CRC Press, 1985).
80. Facchetti, S. *Mass Spectrometry of Large Molecules* (Amsterdam: Elsevier, 1985).
81. Kawamura, A. and Y. Aoyama, Eds. *Immunofluorescence in Medical Science* (New York: Springer-Verlag, 1983).
82a. McNeal, C. J., Ed. *Mass Spectrometry in the Analysis of Large Molecules: Proceedings of the Texas Symposium of MS* (New York: John Wiley & Sons, 1986).
82b. McNeal, C. J., Ed. *Analysis of Peptides and Proteins by Mass Spectrometry* (New York: John Wiley & Sons, 1988).

83. Mee, J. M. *Direct Mass Spectrometry of Body Metabolites: Quantitative Methodology & Clinical Applications* (Beltsville, MD: Brandon Lane Press, 1984).

84. Suelter, C. H. and J. T. Watson. *Biomedical Applications of Mass Spectrometry* (New York: John Wiley & Sons, 1990).

85. Banerjee, S. B. and S. S. Jha, Eds. *Recent Trends in Raman Spectroscopy* (Riveredge, NJ: World Scientific, 1989).

86. Lin-Vien, D., et al. *The Handbook of Infrared & Raman Characteristic Frequencies of Organic Molecules* (New York: Academic Press, 1991).

87. Spiro, T. G., Ed. *Biological Applications of Raman Spectroscopy: Resonance Raman Spectra of Heme Proteins & Metalloproteins*, Vol. 3, (New York: John Wiley & Sons, 1988).

88. Tu, A. T. *Raman Spectroscopy in Biology: Principles & Applications* (New York: John Wiley & Sons, 1982).

89. Agrawal, P. K., Ed. *Carbon-13 NMR of Flavonoids* (Amsterdam: Elsevier, 1989).

90. Chien, S. and H. Chien, Eds. *NMR in Biological Medicine* (New York: Raven Press, 1986).

91. Cohen, S. M. *Physiological NMR Spectroscopy: From Isolated Cells to Man* (New York: NY Academic Science, 1987).

92. Gupta, R. K., Eds. *NMR Spectroscopy of Cells and Organisms* (Boca Raton, FL: CRC Press, 1987).

93. Jaroszewski, W. W., et al. Eds. *NMR Spectroscopy in Drug Research* (Chicago: Munksgaard, 1988).

94. Live, D., et al. Eds. *Frontiers of NMR in Molecular Biology* (New York: John Wiley & Sons, 1990).

95. Hemmila, I. *Applications of Fluorescence in Immunoassays* (New York: John Wiley & Sons, 1991).

96. Pesce, A. J., et al. Eds. *Fluorescence Spectroscopy: An Introduction for Biology & Medicine* (New York: Marcel Dekker, 1971).

97. Taylor, L. D. and A. S. Waggoner, Eds. *Applications of Fluorescence in the Biomedical Sciences* (New York: John Wiley & Sons, 1988).

98. Valenzuela, R., et al. *Interpretation of Immunofluorescence Patterns in Skin Disease* (Chicago: American Soc. Clinical, 1984).

99. Willingham, M. and I. Pastan. *An Atlas of Immunofluorescence in Cultured Cells* (New York: Academic Press, 1985).

100. Nyyssonen, K. and M. T. Parianes. "Plasma Catecholamines: Laboratory Aspects," *Crit. Rev. Clin. Lab. Sci.* 27(3):211–36 (1989).

101. Brorson,T., G. Skarping, and J. Nielsen. "Biological Monitoring of Isocyanates and Related Amines. II. Test Chamber Exposure of Humans to 1,6-Hexamethylene Diisocyanate (HDI)," *Int. Arch. Occup. Environ. Health* 62(5):385–9 (1990).

102. Skarping, G. and T. Brorson, and C. Sango. "Biological Monitoring of Isocyanates and Related Amines. III. Test Chamber Exposure of Humans To Toluene Diisocyanate," *Int. Arch. Occup. Environ. Health* 63(2):83–8 (1991).

103. Nakamura, K., M. F. Refojo, D. V. Crabtree, and F. L. Leong. "Analysis and Fractionation of Silicons and Fluorosilicone Oils for Intraocular Use," *Invest. Opthalmol. Vis. Sci.* 31(10):2059–69 (1990).

104. Gheuens, E., P. H. Slee, and E. A. de-Bruijn. "Bioavailability of Cyclophosphamide in the CMF Regimen," *Onkologie* 13(3):203–6 (1990).

105. Kersten, H. W. and W. R. Moorer. "Particles and Molecules in Endodontic Leakage," *Int. Endod. J.* 22(3):118–24 (1989).
106. Fedtke, N., J. A. Boucheron, M. J. Turner, and J. A. Swenberg. "Vinyl Chloride-Induced DNA Adducts. I: Quantitative Determination of N2 3-Ethenoguanine Based on Electrophore Labeling," *Carcinogenesis* 11(8):1279–85 (1990).
107. Muranishi, H., M. Nakashima, R. Isobe, T. Ando, and N. Shigematsu. "Measurement of Tuberculostearic Acid in Sputa, Pleural Effusions, and Bronchial Washings. A Clinical Evaluation for Diagnosis of Pulmonary Tuberculosis," *Diag. Microbiol. Infect. Dis.* 13(3):235–40 (1990).
108. Vajreswari, A., K. Narayanareddy, and P. S. Rao. "Fatty Acid Composition of Erythrocyte Membrane Lipid Obtained from Children Suffering from Kwashiorkor and Marasmus," *Metabolism* 39(8):779–82 (1990).
109. Piper, C., C. Staiger, Y. Jumeau-Ziemendorff, V. Uebis, B. Kaufman, and K. Stein. "Pharmacokinetics of the Thromboxane A2 Receptor Antagonist Sulotroban (BM 13. 177) in Renal Failure," *Br. J. Clin. Pharmacol.* 28(3):281–8 (1989).
110. Koletzko, B. and H. J. Bremer. "Fat Content and Fatty Acid Composition of Infant Formulas," *Acta Paediatr. Scand.* 78(4):513–21 (1989).
111. Massey, W. A., C. B. Guo, A. M. Dvorak, W. C. Hubbard, B. S. Bhagavan, V. L. Cohan, J. A. Warner, A. Kagey-Sobotka, and L. M. Lichtenstein. Human Uterine Mast Cells: Isolation, Purification, Characterization, Ultrastructure, and Pharmacology," *J. Immunol.* 147(5):1621–7 (1991).
112. Stentz, F. B., A. E. Kitabchi, J. W. Schilling, L. R. Schronk, and J. M. Seyer. "Identification of Insulin Intermediates and Sites of Cleavage of Native Insulin by Insulin Protease from Human Fibroblasts," *J. Biol. Chem.* 264(34):20,275–82 (1989).
113. Shuker, D. E. "Detection of Adducts Arising from Human Exposure to N-Nitroso Compounds," *Cancer Surv.* 8(2):475–87 (1989).
114. Nagata, O., T. Sakashita, E. Takahara, H. Kato, and N. Kiriyama. "Determination of a New Muscle Relaxant (HY-770) in Human Serum by Gas Chromatography-Mass Spectrometry," *J. Chromatography* 496(2):456–62 (1989).
115. Jackson, J. H., E. Gajewski, I. U. Schraufstatter, P. A. Hyslop, and A. F. Fuciarelli. "Damage to the Bases in DNA Induced by Stimulated Human Neutrophils," *J. Clin. Invest.* 84(5):1644–9 (1989).
116. Bigby, T. D., D. M. Lee, N. Meslier, and D. C. Gruenert. "Leukotriene A4 Hydrolase Activity of Human Airway Epithelial Cells," *Biochem. Biophys. Res. Commun.* 164(1):1–7 (1989).
117. Ferretti, A., J. T. Judd, R. R. Taylor, A. Schtzkin, and C. Brown. "Modulating Influences of Dietary Lipid Intake on the Prostaglandin System in Adult Men," *Lipids* 24(5):419–22 (1989).
118. Axelson, M., B. Mork, and G. T. Everson. "Bile Acid Synthesis in Cultured Human Hepatoblastoma Cells," *J. Biol. Chem.* 266(27):17,770–7 (1991).
119. O'Reilly, R., B. A. Davis, D. A. Durden, L. Thorpe, H. Machnee, and A. A. Boulton. "Plasma Phenylethylamine in Schizophrenic Patients," *Biol. Psychiatry* 30(2):145–50 (1991).
120. Van Rollins, M. "Synthesis and Characterization of Cytochrome P-450 Epoxygenase Metabolites of Eicosapentaenoic Acid," *Lipids* 25(8):481–90 (1990).
121. Kintz, P., A. Tracqui, and P. Mangin. "Codeine Concentration in Human Samples in a Case of Fatal Ingestion," *Int. J. Legal Med.* 104(3):177–8 (1991).

122. Sera, N., H. Tokiwa, and T. Hirohata. "Induction of Nitroarsenes in Cigarette Smoke Condensate Treated with Nitrate," *Toxicol. Lett.* 50(2–3):289–98 (1990).

123. Rohwedder, W. K., S. M. Duval, D. J. Wolf, and E. A. Emken. "Measurement of the Metabolic Interconversion of Deuterium-Labeled Fatty Acids by Gas Chromatography- Mass Spectrometry," *Lipids* 25(7):401–5 (1990).

124. Bennett, G. A. and O. L. Shotwell. "Criteria for Determining Purity of *Fusarium mycotoxins*," *J. Assoc. Off. Anal. Chem.* 73(2):270–5 (1990).

125. Lindemann, C. J., M. M. Singh, H. G. Ramjit, and C. Bell. "Determination of Mevalonolactone in Capsules by Capillary Gas-Liquid Chromatography," *J. Pharm. Biomed. Anal.* 9(4):311–6 (1991).

126. Thomas, M. R., C. S. Irving, P. J. Reeds, E. W. Malphus, W. W. Wong, T. W. Boutton, and P. D. Klein. "Lysine and Protein Metabolism in the Young Lactating Woman," *Eur. J. Clin. Nutr.* 45(5):227–42 (1991).

127. Malins, D. C. and R. Haimanot. "Major Alterations in the Nucleotide Structure of DNA in Cancer of the Female Breast," *Cancer Res.* 51(19):5430–2 (1991).

128. Guengerich, F. P. and D. H. Kim. "Enzymatic Oxidation of Ethyl Carbamate to Vinyl "Carbamate and Its Role as an Intermediate in the Formation of 1, N6-ethenoadenosine," *Chem. Res. Toxicol.* 4(4):413–21 (1991).

129. Faughnan, K. T. and M. A. Woodruff. "Modified Gas Chromatography-Mass Spectrometric Method for Determination of Daminozide in High Protein Food Products," *J. Assoc. Off. Anal. Chem.* 74(4):682–92 (1991).

130. Cook, J. A., M. H., Silverman, D. J. Schelling, D. E. Nix, J. J. Schentag, and R. R. Brown. "Multiple-Dose Pharmacokinetics and Safety of Oral Amifloxacin in Healthy Volunteers," *Antimicrob. Agents Chemother.* 34(6):974–9 (1990).

131. Stevens, F. J. "Size-Exclusion High-Performance Liquid Chromatography in Analysis of Protein and Peptide Epitopes," *Methods Enzymol.* 178:107–30 (1989).

132. Bergeron, M., T. A. Reader, G. P. Layrargues, and R. F. Butterworth. "Monoamines and Metabolites in Autopsied Brain Tissue from Cirrhotic Patients with Hepatic Encephalopathy," *Neurochem. Res.* 14(9):853–9 (1989).

133. Furuya, M., S. Akashi, and K. Hirayama. "The Primary Structure of Human EGF Produced by Genetic Engineering, Studied by High Performance Tandem Mass Spectrometry," *Biochem. Biophys. Res. Commun.* 163(2):1100–6 (1989).

134. Yoshizuka, N., M. Yoshimura, S. Tsuchiya, K. Okamoto, Y. Kobayashi, and T. Osawa. "Macrophage Chemotactic Factor (MCF) Produced by a Human T Cell Hybridoma Clone," *Cell Immunol.* 123(1):212–25 (1989).

135. Schilsky, R. L., K. E. Choi, E. E. Vokes, A. Guaspari, C. Guarnier, S. Whaling. "Clinical Pharmacology of the Stereoisomers of Leucovorin during Repeated Oral Dosing," *Cancer* 63(6 Suppl):1018–21 (1989).

136. Black, D., M. Marabani, R. D. Sturrock, and S. P. Robins. *Ann. Rheum. Dis.* 48(8):641–4 (1989).

137. Posner, J., A. F. Cohen, G. Lang, C. Winton, and A. W. Peck. "The Pharmacokinetics of Lamotrigine (BW430C) in Healthy Subjects with Unconjugated Hyperbilirubinae (Gilberi's Syndrome)," *Br. J. Clin. Pharmacol.* 28(1):117–20 (1989).

138. Wass, U., L. Belin, and N. E. Eriksson. "Immunological Specificity of Chloramine-T- Induced IgE Antibodies in Serum from a Sensitized Worker," *Clin. Exp. Allergy* 19(4):463–71 (1989).

139. Kuhn, T. A., W. R. Garnett, B. K. Wells, and H. T. Karnes. "Recovery of Warfarin from an Enteral Nutrient Formula," *Am. J. Hosp. Pharm.* 46(7):1395–9 (1989).

140. Erni, F. "Use of High-Performance Liquid Chromatography in the Pharmaceutical Industry," *J. Chromatography* 507:141–9 (1990).
141. Konishi, M. and H. Hashimoto. "On-Line Clean-Up System of Plasma Sample for Simultaneous Determination of Morphine and Its Metabolites in Cancer Patients by High-Performance Liquid Chromatography," *J. Pharm. Sci.* 79(5):379–83 (1990).
142. Oda, Y., N. Asakawa, T. Kajima, Y. Yoshida, and T. Sato. "Column-Switching High Performance Liquid Chromatography for On-Line Simultaneous Determination and Resolution of Enantiomers of Verapamil and Its Metabolites," *Pharm. Res.* 8(8):997–1001 (1991).
143. Rotsch, T. D., M. Spanton, P. Cugier, and A. C. Plasz. "Determination of Clarithromycin as a Contaminant on Surface by High Performance Liquid Chromatography Using Electrochemical Detection," *Pharm. Res.* 8(8):989–91 (1991).
144. Jaen, J. C., B. W. Caprathe, S. Priebe, and L. D. Wise. "Synthesis of the Enantiomers of Reduced Haloperidol," *Pharm. Res.* 8(8):1002–5 (1991).
145. Colthup, P. V. and J. L. Palmer. "The Determination in Plasma and Pharmacokinetics of Ondansetron," *Eur. J. Cancer. Clin. Oncol.* 25(Suppl 1):571–4 (1989).
146. Fedarko, N. S., J. D. Termine, and P. G. Robey. "High Performance Liquid Chromatographic Separation of Hyaluronan and Four Proteoglycans Produced by Human Bone Cell Cultures," *Anal. Biochem.* 188(2):398–407 (1990).
147. Voyksner, R. D., D. C. Chen, H. E. Swaisgood. "Optimization of Immobilized Enzyme Hydrolysis Combined with High Performance Liquid Chromatography-Thermospray Mass Spectrometry for the Determination of Neuropeptides," *Anal. Biochem.* 188(1):72–81 (1990).
148. Vlasuk, G. P., L. Waxman, L. J. Davis, R. A. Dixon, L. D. Schultz, K. J. Hofmann, J. S. Tung, C. A. Schulman, R. W. Ellis, and G. H. Bencen. "Purification and Characterization of Human Immunodeficiency Virus (HIV) Core Precursor (p55) Expressed in *Saccharomyces cerevisiae*," *J. Biol. Chem.* 264(20):12,106–12 (1989).
149. Gaspar, L., J. S. Chang, N. G. Seidah, and M. Chretien. "Peptides Related to the N-Terminus of Pro-Opiomelanocortin in the Human Adrenal Medulla," *Clin. Invest. Med.* 12(2):90–8 (1989).
150. Adithan, C., D. Danda, C. H. Shashindran, J. S. Bapna, R. P. Swaminathan, and S. Chandrasekar. "Differential Effect of Type I and Type II Diabetes Mellitus on Antipyrine Elimination," *Methods Find. Exp. Clin. Pharmacol.* 11(12):755–8 (1989).
151. Vandenbrom, R. H., J. M. Wierda, and S. Agoston. "Pharmacokinetics and Neuromuscular Blocking Effects of Atracurium Besylate and Two of Its Metabolites in Patients with Normal and Impaired Renal Function," *Clin. Pharmacokinetic* 19(3):230–40 (1990).
152. Everett, D. W., T. J. Chando, G. C. Didonato, H. Y. Pan, and S. H. Weinstein. "Biotransformation of Pravastatin Sodium in Humans," *Drug Metab. Dispos.* 19(4):740–8 (1991).
153. Sobel, D. D. and V. Abbassi. "Use of Frutosamine Test in Diabetic Children," *Diabetes Care* 14(7):578–83 (1991).
154. Lindback, B. and A. Bergman. "A New Commercial Method for the Enzymatic Determination of Creatinine in Serum and Urine Evaluated: Comparison with a Kinetic Jaffe Method and Isotope Dilution-Mass Spectrometry," *Clin. Chem.* 35(5):835–7 (1989).
155. Heine, C. E., J. F. Holland, and J. T. Watson. "Influence of the Ratio of Matrix To Analyte on the Fast Atom Bombardment Mass Spectrometric Response of Peptides Sampled from Aqueous Glycerol," *Anal. Chem.* 61(23):2674–82 (1989).

156. Emmett, S. E. "ICP-MS: A New Look at Trace Elements in Alzheimer's Disease," *Prog. Clin. Biol. Res.* 317:1077–86 (1989).

157. Ziegler, E. E., R. E. Serfass, S. E. Nelson, R. Figueroa-Colon, B. B. Edwards, R. S. Houk, and J. J. Thompson. "Effect of Low Zinc Intake on Absorption and Excretion of Zinc By Infants Studied with 70 Zn as Extrinsic Tag," *J. Nutr.* 119(11):1647–53 (1989).

158. Fink, S. W. and R. B. Freas. "Enhanced Analysis of Poly(Ethylene Glycols) and Peptides Using Thermospray Mass Spectrometry," *Anal. Chem.* 61(18):2050–4 (1989).

159. Capon, C., Y. Leroy, J. M. Wieruszeski, G. Ricart, G. Strecker, J. Montreuil, and B. Fournet. "Structures of O-Glycosidically Linked Oligosaccharides Isolated from Human Meconium Glycoproteins," *Eur. J. Biochem.* 182(1):139–52 (1989).

160. Madden, S., D. J. Back, C. A. Martin, and M. L. Orme. "Metabolism of the Contraceptive Steroid Desogestrel by the Intestinal Mucosa," *Br. J. Clin. Pharmacol.* 27(3):295–9 (1989).

161. Jones, P. J. "Use of Deuterated Water for Measurement of Short-Term Cholesterol Synthesis in Humans," *Can. J. Physiol. Pharmacol.* 68(7):955–9 (1990).

162. Smith, R. D., J. A. Loo, C. G. Edmonds, C. J. Barinaga, and H. R. Udseth. "New Developments in Biochemical Mass Spectrometry: Electrospray Ionization," *Anal. Chem.* 62(9):882–99 (1990).

163. Electricwala, A., L. Irons, R. Wait, R. J. Carr, R. J. Ling, H. Grossenbacher, and T. Atkinson. "Physicochemical Properties of Recombinant Desulphatohirudin," *Thromb. Haemost.* 63(3):499–504 (1990).

164. Takemoto, L. J., T. Emmons, D. Granstrom, P. R. Griffin, J. Shabanowitz, D. F. Hunt. "Analysis of Tryptic Peptides from the C-Terminal Region of Alpha-Crystallin from Cataractous and Normal Human Lenses," *Exp. Eye. Res.* 50(6):695–702 (1990).

165. Beckman, J. K., M. J. Howard, and H. L. Greene. "Identification of Hydroxyalkenals Formed from Omega-3 Fatty Acids," *Biochem. Biophys. Res. Commun.* 169(1):75–80 (1990).

166. Schuette, S. A., E. E. Ziegler, S. E. Nelson, and M. Janghorbani. "Feasibility of Using the Stable Isotope 25Mg to Study Mg Metabolism in Infants," *Pediatr. Res.* 27(1):36–40 (1990).

167. Clay, K. L., C. Johnson, and G. S. Worthen. "Biosynthesis of Platelet Activating Factor and 1-0-Acyl Analogues by Endothelial Cells," *Biochim. Biophys. Acta* 1094(1):43–50 (1991).

168. van der Kooij, A. M. and S. C. Luijendijk. "Longitudinal Dispersion in Model of Central Airways During High-Frequency Ventilation," *Respir. Physiol.* 84(1):13–29 (1991).

169. Petrilli, P., C. Sepe, and P. Pucci. "A New Procedure for Peptide Alignment in Protein Sequence Determination Using Fast Atom Bombardment Mass Spectral Data," *Biol. Mass Spectrum* 20(3):115–20 (1991).

170. Silberring, J. and F. Nyberg. "Analysis of Tyrosine- and Methionine-Containing Neuropeptides by Fast Atom Bombardment Mass Spectrometry," *J. Chromatography* 562(1–2):459–67 (1991).

171. Sinz, M. W. and R. P. Remmel. "Isolation and Characterization of a Novel Quaternary Ammonium-Linked Glucuronide of Lamotrigine," *Drug Metab. Dispos.* 19(1):149–53 (1991).

172. Tunn, S., G. Pappert, P. Willnow, and M. Krieg. "Multicentre Evaluation of an Enzyme- Immunoassay for Cortisol Determination," *J. Clin. Chem. Clin. Biochem.* 28(12):929–35 (1991).

173. Heremans, L. and K. Heremans. "Raman Spectroscopic Study of the Changes in Secondary Structure of Chymotrypsin: Effect of pH and Pressure on the Salt Bridge," *Biochim. Biophys. Acta* 999(2):192–7 (1989).

174. Fodor, S. P., R. Gebhard, J. Lugtenburg, R. A. Bogomolni, and R. A. Mathies. "Structure of the Retinal Chromophore in Sensory Rhodopsin I from Resonance Raman Spectroscopy," *J. Biol. Chem.* 264(31):18,280–3 (1989).

175. Nagai, M., Y. Yoneyama, and T. Kitagawa. "Characteristics in Tyrosine Coordinations of Four Hemoglobins M Probed by Resonance Raman Spectroscopy," *Biochemistry* 28(6):2418–22 (1989).

176. Ni, F., L. Thomas, and T. M. Cotton. "Surface-Enhanced Resonance Raman Spectroscopy as an Ancillary HPLC Detector for Nitrophenol Compounds," *Anal. Chem.* 61(8):888–94 (1989).

177. Laigle, A., L. Chinsky, P. Y. Turpin, and B. Jolles. "Kinetics of Exchangeable Protons in Z DNA: A UV Resonance Raman Study," *Nucleic Acids Res.* 17(7):2493–502 (1989).

178. Pande, C., R. Callender, J. Baribeau, F. Boucher, and A. Pande. "Effect of Lipid-Protein Interaction on the Color of Bacteriorhodopsin," *Biochim-Biophys. Acta* 973(2):257–62 (1989).

179. Ames, J. B. and R. A. Mathies. "The Role of Back-Reactions and Proton Uptake During the N–O Transition in Bacteriorhodopsin's Photocycle: A Kinetic Resonance Raman Study," *Biochemistry* 29(31):7181–90 (1990).

180. Spiro, T. G., G. Smulevich, and C. Su. "Probing Protein Structure and Dynamics with Raman Spectroscopy: Cytochrome-c Peroxidase and Hemoglobin," *Biochemistry* 29(19):4497–508 (1990).

181. Ghomi, M., R. Letellier, J. Liquier, and E. Taillandier. "Interpretation of DNA Vibrational Spectra by Normal Coordinate Analysis," *Int. J. Biochem.* 22(7):691–9 (1990).

182. Brahms, S. and J. G. Brahms. "DNA with Adenine Tracts Contain Poly(da)*Poly(dt) Conformational Features in Solution," *Nucleic Acids Res.* 18(6):1559–64 (1990).

183. Weidlich, T., S. M. Lindsay, W. L. Peticolas, and G. A. Thomas. "Low Frequency Raman Spectra of Z-DNA," *J. Biomed. Struct. Dyn.* 7(4):849–58 (1990).

184. Erand, M., F. Lakhda-Ghazal, and F. Amalric. "Repeat Peptide Motifs which Contain Beta-Turns and Modulate DNA Condensation in Chromatin," *Eur. J. Biochem.* 191(1):19–26 (1990).

185. Bruzzese, F. E., J. A. Dix, R. P. Rava, and L. C. Cerny. "Resonance Raman Spectroscopy of Chemically Modified Hemoglobins," *Biomat. Artif. Cells Artif. Organs* 18(2):143–56 (1990).

186. Takeuchi, H., Y. Nemoto, and I. Harada. "Environments and Conformations of Tryptophan Side Chains of Gramicidin A in Phospholipid Bilayers Studied by Raman Spectroscopy," *Biochemistry* 29(6):1572–9 (1990).

187. DeGrazia, H., J. G. Harmon, G. S. Tan, and R. M. Wartell. "Investigation of the cAMP Receptor Protein Secondary Structure by Raman Spectroscopy," *Biochemistry* 29(14):3557–62 (1990).

188. Nagai, M., T. Kitagawa, and Y. Yoneyama. "Molecular Pathology of Hemoglobin M Saskatoon Disease," *Biomed. Biochim. Acta* 49(2–3):5317–22 (1990).

189. Siebinga, I., G. F. Vrensen, F. F. De-Mul, and J. Greve. "Age-Related Changes in Local Water and Protein Content of Human Eye Lenses Measured by Raman Microspectroscopy," *Exp. Eye. Res.* 53(2):233–9 (1991).

190. Nabiev, I. R., H. Morjani, and M. Manfait. "Selective Analysis of Antitumor Drug Interaction with Living Cancer Cells As Probed by Surface-Enhanced Raman Spectroscopy," *Eur. Biophys. J.* 19(6):311–6 (1991).

191. Litman, B. J., E. N. Lewis, and I. W. Levin. "Packing Characteristics of Highly Unsaturated Bilayer Lipids: Raman Spectroscopic Studies of Multilameliar Phosphatidylchloline Dispersion," *Biochemistry* 30(2):313–9 (1991).

192. Vincent, J. S., S. D. Revak, C. G. Cochrane, and I. W. Levin. "Raman Spectroscopic Studies of Model Human Pulmonary Surfactant Systems: Phospholipid Interactions with Peptide Paradigms for the Surfactant Protein SP-8," *Biochemistry* 30(34):8395–401 (1991).

193. Rosenberg-Nicolson, N. L. "Probing Nucleosome Core Secondary Structure Before and After Alpha-Chymotrypsin Treatment by Raman Spectroscopy and Thermal Denaturation," *J. Cell. Biochem.* 47(1):11–7 (1991).

194. Manor, D., G. Z. Weng, H. Deng, S. Cosloy, C. X. Chen, V. Balogh-Nair, K. Delaria, F. Jurnak, and R. Callender. "An Isotope Edited Classical Raman Difference Spectroscopic Study of the Interactions of Guanine Nucleotides with Elongation Factors Tu and H-ras p21," *Biochemistry* 30(45):10,914–20 (1991).

195. Coulombeau, C., Z. Dhaouadi, M. Ghomi, H. Jobic, and J. Tomkinson. "Vibrational Mode Analysis of Guanine by Neutron Inelastic Scattering," *Eur. Biophys. J.* 19(9):323–9 (1991).

196. Reginato, A. J. "Calcium Pyrophosphate Dihydrate Gout and Other Crystal Deposition Diseases," *Curr. Opin. Rheumatol.* 3(4):676–83 (1991).

197. Xue, C. B., E. Eriotou, D. Miller, J. M. Becker, and F. Naider. "A Covalently Constrained Congener of the *Saccharomyces cerevisiae* Tridecapeptide Mating Phermone is an Agonist," *J. Biol. Chem.* 264(32):19,161–8 (1989).

198. Bottomley, P. A. "Human *In Vivo* NMR Spectroscopy in Diagnostic Medicine: Clinical Tool or Research Probe," *Radiology* 170(1 Pt 1):1–15 (1989).

199. Bennett, R. M. "Physical Fitness and Muscle Metabolism in the Fibromyalgia Syndrome: An Overview," *J. Rheumatol. Suppl.* 19:28–9 November (1989).

200. Hounsell, E. F., A. M. Lawson, M. S. Stoll, D. P. Kane, G. C. Cashmore, R. A. Carruthers, J. Feeney, and T. Feizi. "Characterization by Mass Spectrometry and 500-MHz Proton Magnetic Resonance Spectroscopy of Penta- and Hexasaccharide Chains of Human Foetal Gastrointestinal Mucins (Meconium Glycoproteins)," *Eur. J. Biochem.* 186(3):597–610 (1989).

201. Nakamura, A., S. Nagai, T. Ueda, J. Sakakibara, Y. Hotta, and K. Takeya. "Studies on the Chemical Modification of Monensin. II. Measurement of Sodium Ion Permeability of Monensylamino Acids Using Sodium-23 Nuclear Magnetic Resonance Spectroscopy," *Chem. Pharm. Bull. Tokyo* 37(9):2330–3 (1989).

202. Deslauriers, R., W. J. Keon, S. Lareau, D. Moir, J. K. Saunders, I. C. Smith, K. Whitehead, and G. W. Mainwood. "Preservation of High-Energy Phosphates in Human Myocardium. A Phosphorus 31-Nuclear Magnetic Resonance Study of the Effect of Temperature on Atrial Appendages," *J. Thorac. Cardiovasc. Surg.* 98(3):402–12 (1989).

203. Fujisawa, S., Y. Kadoma, and Y. Komoda. "Nuclear Magnetic Resonance Spectroscopic Studies of Interaction of bis-GMA Analogues with Phosphatidylcholine Liposomes as a Model for Biomembranes," *Biomaterials* 10(4):269–72 (1989).

204. Lerman, S., M. Moran and N. Matthews. "Photographic and Spectroscopic Correlations of Human Cataracts," *Ophthalmic Res.* 21(1):18–26 (1989).

205. Bottomley, P. A. and C. J. Hardy. "Rapid, Reliable *In Vivo* Assays of Human Phosphate Metabolites by Nuclear Magnetic Resonance," *Clin. Chem.* 35(3):392–5 (1989).

206. Neeman, M. and H. Dagani. "Metabolic Studies of Estrogen- and Tamoxifen-Treated Human Breast Cancer Cells by Nuclear Magnetic Resonance Spectroscopy," *Cancer Res.* 49(3):589–94 (1989).

207. Henry, G. D. and B. D. Sykes. "Structure and Dynamics of Detergent-Solubilized M13 Coat Protein (an Integral Membrane Protein) Determined by 13C and 15N Nuclear Magnetic Resonance Spectroscopy," *Biochem. Cell Biol.* 68(1):318–29 (1990).

208. Shulman, G. I., D. L. Rothman, T. Jue, P. Stein, R. A. DeFronzo, and R. G. Shulman. "Quantitation of Muscle Glycogen Synthesis in Normal Subjects and Subjects with Non-Insulin-Dependent Diabetes by 13C Nuclear Magnetic Resonance Spectroscopy," *NEJM* 322(4):223–8 (1990).

209. Robinson, H., Y. C. Liaw, G. A. van-der-Marel, J. H. van Boom, and A. H. Wang. "NMR Studies on the Binding of Antitumor Drug Nogalamycin to DNA Hexamer d(CGTACG)," *Nucleic Acids Res.* 18(6):4851–8 (199).

210. Merlini, G., R. Bruening, R. A. Kyle, and E. F. Ossereman. "The Second Riboflavin-Binding Myeloma IgG Lambda DOT. I. Biochemical and Functional Characterization," *Mol. Immunol.* 27(5):385–94 (1990).

211. Skelton, N. J., J. Kordel, S. Forsen, and W. J. Chazin. "Comparative Structural Analysis of the Calcium Free and Bound States of the Calcium Regulatory Protein Calbindin D9K," *J. Mol. Biol.* 213(4):593–8 (1990).

212. Schaefer, S., J. R. Gober, G. G. Schwartz, D. B. Twieg, M. W. Weiner, and B. Massie. "*In Vivo* Phosphorus-31 Spectroscopic Imaging in Patients with Global Myocardial Disease," *Am. J. Cardiol.* 65(16):1154–61 (1990).

213. Buck, H. M., L. H. Koole, M. H. van-Genderen, L. Smit, J. L. Geelen, S. Jurriaans, and J. Goudsmit. "Phosphate-Methylated DNA Aimed at HIV-1 RNA Loops and Integrated DNA Inhibits Viral Activity," *Science* 248(4952):208–12 (1990).

214. Mager, P. P. "Linear Free Energy-Related and Quantitative Structure-Activity," *Drug Des. Deliv.* 7(3):203–18 (1991).

215. Xu, G. Y. and C. M. Deber. "Conformations of Neurotensin in Solution and in Membrane Environments Studied by 2-D NMR Spectroscopy," *Int. J. Pept. Protein Res.* 37(6):528–35 (1991).

216. Ishimura, M., N. Nishi, and H. Uedaira. "Hydration of Clupeine in Solution," *Int. J. Pept. Protein Res.* 37(5):399–401 (1991).

217. Fossel, E. T., F. M. Hall, and J. McDonagh. "C-13 NMR Spectroscopy of Plasma Reduces Interference of Hypertriglyceridemia in the H-1 NMR Detection of Malignancy. Application in Patients with Breast Lesions," *Breast Cancer Res. Treat.* 18(2):99–110 (1991).

218. Molyneux, R. J., Y. T. Pan, J. E. Tropea, M. Benson, G. P. Kaushal, and A. D. Elbein. "6, 7-Diepicastanospermine, a Tetrahydroxyindolizidine Alkaloid Inhibitor of Amyloglucosidase," *Biochemistry* 30(41):9981–7 (1991).

219. Pelton, J. G., D. A. Torchia, N. D. Meadow, C. Y. Wong, and S. Roseman. "1H, 15N, and 13C NMR Signal Assignments of IIIG1c, A Signal-Transducing Protein of *Escherichia coli*, Using Three-Dimensional Triple-Resonance Techniques," *Biochemistry* 30(41):10,043–57 (1991).

220. Peltonen, K., B. D. Hilton, J. Pataki, H. Lee, R. G. Harvey, and A. Dipple. "Spectroscopic Characterization of Syn-5-Methylchrysene 1,2-Dihydrodiol-3,4-Epoxide-Deoxyribonucleoside Adducts," *Chem. Res. Toxicol.* 4(3):305–10 (1991).

221. Epps, D. E., H. Schostarez, C. V. Argoudelis, R. Poorman, J. Hinzmann, T. K. Sawyer, and F. Mandel. "An Experimental Method for the Determination of Enzyme-Competitive Inhibitor Dissociation Constants from Displacement Curves: Application to Human Renin Using Fluorescence Energy Transfer to a Synthetic Dansylated Inhibitor Peptide," *Anal. Biochem.* 181(1):172–81 (1989).

222. Tasneem, R. and V. Prakash. "Resistance of Alpha-Globulin from *Sesanum indicum* L. to Protease in Relationship to Its Structure," *J. Protein Chem.* 8(2):251–61 (1989).

223. Surewicz, W. K., K. Surewicz, H. H. Mantsch, and F. Auclair. "Interaction of *Shigella* Toxin with Globotriaosyl Ceramide Receptor-Containing Membranes: A Fluorescence Study," *Biochem. Biophys. Res. Commun.* 160(1):126–32 (1989).

224. Bray, J. T., R. H. Maier, and W. J. Pories. "Screening for Selected Trace Elements in Single Cell Populations by Energy Dispersion X-Ray Fluorescence Spectrometry," *Biol. Trace. Elem. Res.* 23:65–75 Winter (1989–90).

225. Daniels, A. J., E. R. Lazarowski, J. E. Matthews, and E. G. Lapetina. "Neuropeptide Y Mobilizes Intracellular Ca^{2+} and Increases Inositol Phosphate Production in Human Erythroleukemia Cells," *Biochem. Biophys. Res. Commun.* 165(3):1138–44 (1989).

226. Chehab, F. F. and Y. W. Kan. "Detection of Specific DNA Sequences by Fluorescence Amplification: A Colar Complementation Assay," *Proc. Natl. Acad. Sci. U.S.A.* 86(23):9178–82 (1989).

227. Borchman, D., M. C. Yappert, R. Q. Rubini, and C. A. Patwerson. "Distribution of Phospholipid-Malondialdehyde-Adduct in the Human Lens," *Curr. Eye Res.* 8(9):939–46 (1989).

228. Carson, J. J., F. S. Prato, D. J. Drost, L. D. Diesbourg, and S. J. Dixon. "Time-Varying Magnetic Fields Increase Cytosolic Free Ca^{2+} in HL-60 Cells," *Am. J. Physiol.* 259(4 Pt 1):C687–92 (1990).

229. Nalin, C. M., R. D. Purcell, D. Antelman, D. Mueller, L. Tomchak, B. Wegrzynski, E. McCarney, V. Toome, R. Kramer, and M. C. Hsu. "Purification and Characterization of Recombinant Rev Protein of Human Immunodeficiency Virus Type 1," *Proc. Natl. Acad. Sci. U.S.A.* 87(19):7593–7 (1990).

230. Brems, D. N., P. L. Brown, and G. W. Becker. "Equilibrium Denaturation of Human Growth Hormone and Its Cysteine-Modified Forms," *J. Biol. Chem.* 265(10):5504–11 (1990).

231. Menezes, M. E., P. D. Roepe, and H. R. Kaback. "Design of a Membrane Transport Protein for Fluorescence Spectroscopy," *Proc. Natl. Acad. Sci. U.S.A.* 87(5):1638–42 (1990).

232. Lester, D. S., N. Orr, and V. Brumfeld. "Structural Distinction Between Soluble and Particulate Protein Kinase C Species," *J. Protein Chem.* 9(2):209–20 (1990).

233. Ueno, N. and B. Chakrabarti. "Liquefaction of Human Vitreous in Model Aphakic Eyes by 300-nm UV Photolysis: Monitoring Liquefaction by Fluorescence," *Curr. Eye Res.* 9(5):487–92 (1990).

234. Garrett, L. R., D. M. Coder, and J. K. McDougall. "Increased Intracellular Calcium is Associated with Progression of HPV-18 Immortalized Human Keratinocytes to Tumorigenicity," *Cell. Calcium* 12(5):343–9 (1991).

235. Giron-Forest, D., C. Goldbronn, and P. Piechon. "Thermal Analysis Methods for Pharmacopoeial Materials," *J. Pharm. Biomed. Anal.* 7(12):1421–33 (1989).
236. Uesugi, M., T. Sekida, S. Matsuki, and Y. Sugiura. "Selective DNA Cleavage by Elsamicin A and Switch Function of Its Amino Sugar Group," *Biochemistry* 30(27):6711–5 (1991).
237. Sasaki, M., I. Matsuo, and H. Fujita. "Hydrophobicity-Dependent Fluorescence Properties and Intracellular Fluorospectroscopic Behavior of Phototoxic Drugs," *Photochem. Photobiol.* 53(3):385–9 (1991).
238. Singh, B. R. and B. R. DasGupta. "Conformational Changes Associated with the Nicking and Activation of Botulinum Neurotoxin Type E," *Biophys. Chem.* 38(1–2):123–30 (1990).
239. Sourander, P. "Pathology of the Central Nervous System with Special Reference to the Lipids," *Ups J. Med. Sci. Suppl.* 48:145–72 (1990).
240. Javors, M. A., M. Liu, B. S. Cuvelier, C. L. Bowden. "Characterization of the Effect of the Adenosine Agonist Cyclohexyladenosine on Platelet Activating Factor-Induced Increases in [Ca^{2+}] i in Human Platelets *In Vitro*," *Cell. Calcium* 11(10):647–53 (1990).
241. Milner, T. G., K. W. Ko, T. Ohnishi, and S. Tokoyama. "Enhancement of the Human Plasma Lipid Transfer Protein Reaction by Apolipoproteins," *Biochim. Biophys. Acta* 1082(1):71–8 (1991).
242. Guest, C. R., R. A. Hochstrasser, L. C. Sowers, and D. P. Millar. "Dynamics of Mismatched Base Pairs in DNA," *Biochemistry* 30(13):3271–9 (1991).
243. Lewis, C., T. Kramer, S. Robinson, and D. Hilvert. "Medium Effects in Antibody-Catalyzed Reaction," *Science* 253(5023):1019–22 (1991).
244. Deacon, J. K., A. M. Thomson, A. L. Page, J. E. Stops, P. R. Roberts, S. C. Whiteley, J. W. Attridge, C. A. Love, G. A. Robinson, and G. P. Davidson. "An Assay for Human Chorionic Gonadotrophin Using the Capillary Fill Immunosensor," *Biosen. Bioeletron.* 6(3):193–9 (1991).
245. Korbelik, M. and J. Hung. "Cellular Delivery and Retention of Photofrin II: The Effects of Interaction with Human Plasma Proteins," *Photochem. Photobiol.* 53(4):501–10 (1991).

CHAPTER 16

Magnetic Resonance and the Use of Animals

Peter G. Morris

16.0 Imaging Methods

The primary justification for animal experiments is, ultimately, their benefit to mankind. The connection may be obvious—animal models of human disease, or it may be less direct—"pure research" directed towards an understanding of fundamental biological processes. Medical scientists have been forced to use animal models for two main reasons: first, because it is possible to establish well-defined (though not necessarily relevant) models from which reproducible results can be obtained, and second, because direct study of humans has not generally been possible.

The heterogeneity of normal human physiology and particularly of its response to disease will remain problematic: the challenge is to find, among the diverse responses, common causes. However, our previous inability to study disease *in situ* is fast being overcome. Prior to the advent of modern imaging techniques in the early 1970s, indirect information could be gleaned from the analysis of body fluids, but direct information only from limited biopsy material or on surgery or autopsy. It is now possible to monitor the progress of disease and the response to therapy using a variety of imaging techniques, including ultrasound, nuclear imaging, X-ray computerized tomography (CT), positron emission tomography

0-87371-504-7/93/$0.00+$.50
© 1993 by Lewis Publishers

(PET), and magnetic resonance imaging (MRI). X-ray CT and MRI have in turn revolutionized diagnostic radiology, yielding human cross-sectional images in exquisite detail at submillimeter resolution. These techniques yield primarily anatomical information, allowing the radiologist to search for lesions, to identify them according to their image parameters (attenuation coefficient in the case of X-ray CT or nuclear spin relaxation times in the case of MRI) and to monitor their response to possible therapy. Increasingly, these techniques are also used to provide physiological information, such as the patency of the vascular system (angiography), blood flow, cardiac output, etc. Recently, it has also been demonstrated that high-speed MRI techniques can be used, to show changes in regional cerebral blood flow on task activation.

Of potentially even greater future importance are the development of those techniques that allow localized chemical information to be obtained. Noninvasive, *in situ* biochemical analysis is (or should be) every medical scientists dream. Techniques such as nuclear imaging, single photon emission CT (SPECT) and especially PET have started to make this a reality. They require that the substance to be imaged (or one of its precursors) be labeled with a radioactive isotope. In the case of nuclear imaging or SPECT, this is often technecium ($^{99}Tc^m$). In the case of PET, a range of low-atomic-weight positron emitters are available that can be readily incorporated into markers or substrates. Because the annihilation of a positron (through collision with an electron) results in the generation of two γ-ray photons emitted in opposite directions, coincidence detection eliminates noise due to background radiation, making PET an extremely sensitive and versatile technique. It can, for example, be used to measure regional blood flow and metabolic rate, or the distribution of a particular receptor subtype. Because the positron emitters have rather short half-lives (typically only a few hours), it is usual to generate them in a cyclotron on the premises. The radiochemistry is also carried out locally. This makes the method extremely expensive. Despite its high sensitivity, the method also has an inherently limited resolution due to the distance traveled by the positron before its annihilation. None of these radioisotope techniques has any inherent chemical selectivity: the radiolabel is detected regardless of the compound in which it is located.

Magnetic resonance spectroscopy (MRS) retains the analytical advantages of the parent technique, nuclear magnetic resonance (NMR), permitting the levels of metabolites to be simultaneously determined provided they are present above the detection threshold. The sensitivity of this technique is determined primarily by the number of nuclear spins that contribute to the signal. This means that, in principle, spectroscopic studies are better undertaken in man. Of course the high cost of instrumentation involved mitigates against this to some extent.

16.1 Magnetic Resonance Imaging—Basic Principles

The phenomenon of NMR was first observed in the immediate post second-world-war period by two American physicists, working independently: Bloch at

Stanford and Purcell at Harvard. Their observations were reported in 1946 in the same volume of *Physical Review* and led to the joint award of the 1952 Nobel Prize for Physics. Once the details of the interaction had been worked out, and the chemical specificity had been appreciated, a period of instrumentational refinement followed before NMR took its place as arguably the most powerful analytical technique available to the organic chemist.

The first experiments on MRI were conducted in 1972 by Paul Lauterbur at the State University of New York at Stonybrook and, independently, by Peter Mansfield and colleagues at Nottingham.[1,2] These demonstrative experiments were met with considerable scepticism both from radiologists, for whom the introduction of the EMI (now X-ray CT) scanner[3] had recently advanced their subject more than any invention since the discovery of X-rays in 1895, and also from the NMR community. After all, how could radiowaves, with wavelengths of several tens of meters, generate high-resolution images of human anatomy? Images of the human finger[4] and wrist[5] paved the way for widespread acceptance of the technique. From the outset, the primary goal was clinical imaging, and this was hotly pursued, initially in academic institutions—notably at Aberdeen, Nottingham, and Stonybrook—and later in industry too. The problem was one of scale—NMR had hitherto been used principally for the analysis of chemical structures, and so NMR spectrometers were designed for samples of test-tube proportions. The two orders of magnitude increase in linear dimension necessary to accommodate a human torso represented a considerable act of faith on the part both of the development teams and the magnet manufacturers. The first crude images of the human chest[6] and abdomen[7] were published in 1977 and 1978, respectively, and commercial systems became available in the early 1980s.

16.1.1 Spatial Localization

When nuclei with spin I are placed in a magnetic field they can adopt one of $2I + 1$ possible orientations with respect to the field direction. In the case of the proton, $I = 1/2$, and there are two possibilities—parallel or antiparallel to the field. The parallel state has a lower energy than the antiparallel state, the difference (Zeeman splitting) being proportional to the field strength B. Transitions can be induced by electromagnetic radiation at a frequency which exactly matches the energy splitting. The resonance frequency ω is given by the Larmor equation:

$$\omega = \gamma \, B$$

where γ = the magnetogyric ratio, a constant for a particular nucleus.

For normal "high-resolution" NMR where the (small) chemical shifts are observed between nuclei in different chemical environments, B must be very homogeneous (up to a few parts in 10^{10}). In contrast, for MRI, B is made to vary with position, so that nuclei in different locations have different resonance frequencies.

Usually, a linear field variation is employed, and the field gradients are generated by separate gradient coils, distinct from the main magnet windings. For an "x-gradient":

$$B = B_0 + G_x x$$

where $G_x = \dfrac{d\,B_z}{dx}$ and the main magnetic field B_0 is applied along the z-direction.

The corresponding dependence of resonance frequency on position is:

$$\omega = f(x) = \gamma (B_0 + G_x x)$$

The effect of such a gradient on the NMR spectrum recorded from a water-filled test tube is illustrated in Figure 1. In the absence of a gradient, all spins are located in the same field (B_0) and resonate at the same frequency ($\omega = \gamma B_0$). With the gradient applied, spins located on the left-hand edge of the test tube lie in a relatively lower magnetic field and so resonate at a proportionally lower frequency than those on the right-hand edge. Spins located along a vertical strip lie in the same magnetic field and will all contribute to the signal at the corresponding frequency.

In the case of simple objects with uniform spin density, these one-dimensional projections can reveal much about the object. For "real" subjects, an image can be reconstructed by combining a number of such projections, recorded in gradients of different strength and orientation. The mathematical foundation was laid in connection with gravitational theory by Radon in 1917,[9] although the first image-reconstruction techniques were not developed until 1956, when Bracewell[10] used them to map the distribution of microwave emissions from the solar surface. These techniques were independently redeveloped for the determination of molecular structure from transmission electronmicrographs, for optical applications, and, finally, for NMR by Paul Lauterbur.[1] For the reconstruction of NMR images, many different approaches are in fact possible, and these account for the diversity of the early MRI literature.[11]

16.1.2 Image Contrast

The signal in (^{1}H) MRI is derived from mobile protons. We are composed of approximately 70% water and each water molecule has two protons. The images therefore primarily reflect the water distribution, with lesser contributions from the more mobile lipids, for example, the triglycerides in adipose tissue. There is about a 15% variation in water content amongst the different soft tissues, providing a limited degree of spin density contrast. However, other, potentially more important sources of image contrast can be exploited in MRI experiments.

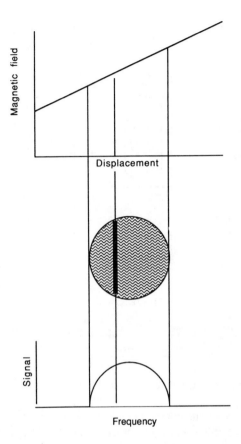

Figure 1.   Application of a linear field gradient to a test-tube sample.

When the nuclear spins are excited in an NMR experiment, the Boltzman distribution between the two spin states is disturbed and takes some time to recover. This process involves an interchange of energy with "the lattice" and the time constant is known as the spin lattice relaxation time T_1. The variation in T_1 between different soft tissues is much greater than the variation in water content and, at low operating frequencies, can be as much as a factor of three to four. The NMR signal is detected by the EMF induced in a radiofrequency receiver coil oriented orthogonal to the direction of the magnetic field. This signal decays by non-energy-dependent processes with a time constant T_2 which shows a similar tissue variation to T_1. The sequences developed by high-resolution spectroscopists for measurement of T_1 and T_2 have been taken over by the imaging community to generate images which show relaxation time, rather than spin density contrast. The contrast in T_1 images is the reverse of that observed in T_2 images: a long T_2 means that the NMR signal decays more slowly, whereas a long T_1 means that it

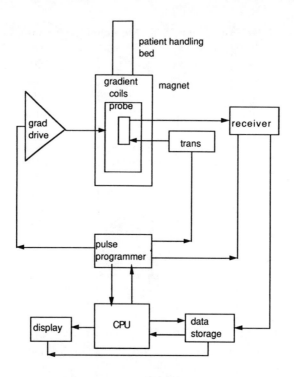

Figure 2.   Schematic diagram of apparatus for MRI.

takes longer to recover. Inevitably, both T_1 and T_2 effects will be present to some degree in all images. Since the effects tend to cancel, it is important to ensure that one relaxation time or the other should dominate and one speaks of T_1- or T_2-weighted images.

16.1.3 MRI Instrumentation

The rapid development in NMR instrumentation, which has taken place over the last two decades, reflects, in part, an increasing demand from the scientific community. Equally significant has been the availability of minicomputers, which are now an essential feature of all NMR spectrometers, and which permit the full multiplex advantages of a Fourier transform approach to be realized. The importance of cheap computing power should not be underestimated: certainly it would not have been possible to have developed MRI techniques without it.

The instrumentation requirements for MRI are broadly similar to those for conventional NMR spectrometers with the following additions: x, y, and z gradient coils and drivers, image display, and a radiofrequency transmitter capable of generating shaped pulses. The apparatus is illustrated schematically in Figure 2.

Most of the early developed MRI systems and many of the first commercial systems employed resistive magnets. These are unstable and cannot easily generate magnetic fields in excess of about 0.25 T. (Most clinical systems now operate in the range 0.3 to 1.5 T). Since 1982 the world MRI market has been dominated by superconducting systems to the extent that, of the 3000 or so MRI installations to date, some 85% have superconducting magnets.[14] Superconducting magnets are inherently stable, and high-field whole-body systems (currently up to 4 T) are readily available from a relatively small number of manufacturers of which the market leader is (and has been from the outset) Oxford Magnet Technology. The drawback with superconducting systems is their cost—both capital and running. Typically, the magnet for a clinical MRI system accounts for about one third of the total system cost of upwards of $1.5M, and the annual cryogen (liquid nitrogen and helium) expenses, which arise from the need to maintain the magnet windings below the critical temperature (T_c) for superconductivity, amount to some tens of thousands of dollars. Siting can also be problematic and expensive, particularly for very high field (>1.5 T) unshielded magnets.

16.2 Magnetic Resonance Imaging—Clinical Applications

Although the first clinical images were of high quality compared to those obtained by nuclear imaging or crude X-ray tomograms, they did not compare favorably with the images obtained by X-ray computerized tomography. However, the pioneering clinical studies at the Hammersmith Hospital in the U.K. and other centers soon established that MRI was capable of exquisite soft-tissue contrast, which could be manipulated, and the images were free from the "streak artefacts", characteristic of the X-ray images, at the level of the posterior fossa, for example. The contrast in MRI head images between white and grey matter was particularly exciting and rapidly lead to important applications in a range of demyelinating diseases, such as multiple sclerosis.[8] In a national survey conducted in 1986/7, the U.K. Medical Research Council identified ten key areas in which MRI had already become established as the investigative method of choice, and a further four in which it was comparable or complementary to X-ray CT. These are listed in Table 1.

The majority of these applications are associated with common focal diseases, particularly in the head. Recent developments in MRI, which permit real-time imaging, measurement of flow velocity, diffusion and perfusion (see below), and increased opportunity to study a wider spectrum of patients, promise to greatly extend the range of method-of-choice applications. This is reflected in the establishment by charitable research foundations and others of many MRI centers dedicated to the study of specific diseases.

In conventional MRI sequences, the signal from fast moving blood becomes "scrambled" and lost so that major vessels are seen as structures with apparently hollow lumens, sometimes referred to as "flow voids". However, it is possible to preserve the signal from the moving blood, and difference images (angiograms) showing the vascular network can be constructed.[15,16] These are finding important clinical applications in the head and neck, and also, more recently, in the peripheral

Table 1.   Clinical Applications of MRI in the UK as of 1988

Areas in which MRI has been established as diagnostic method of choice

- Cerebral palsy (as research tool)
- Posterior fossa lesions
- Foramen magnum lesions
- Multiple sclerosis
- Syringomyelia
- Acoustic neuromas
- Lumbar spine and disc disease
- Great vessels (in context of cardiovascular disease)
- Parotid gland tumours
- Bone tumours

Areas in which MRI is comparable or complementary to X-ray CT

- Tumors of the rectum, prostate, cervix, uterus, bladder, breast, cerebrum, meninges, pituitary gland
- Stroke
- Congenital heart disease
- Dementia

vasculature. Using similar techniques, employing pulsed magnetic field gradients, it is also possible to quantify flow.[17,18] Measurements of flow velocities through defects in the cardiac wall have proved clinically useful but the "Holy Grail" of the measurement of flow through the coronary arteries has proved elusive.

As well as macroscopic flow, there is growing interest in the measurement of tissue perfusion and diffusion.[19] A clean separation of these processes is difficult to achieve, but it is certainly possible to generate images reflecting these properties. It would appear that MRI perfusion/diffusion measurements are the most sensitive to developing pathology. For example, they reveal the earliest signs of ischemic injury in stroke. Also of great interest is the anisotropic diffusion readily observed in the brain in regions where the myelinated nerve bundles run unidirectionally. Freedom from motional artefact, to which diffusion measurements are prone, is greatly assisted by fast imaging methods such as echo-planar imaging (EPI)[13,20,21] which continue to evolve. At the present state-of-the-art, it is possible to generate 256×256 images using this technique. Single-shot volume imaging (echo-volume imaging) is also possible through a straightforward extension of the two-dimensional EPI experiment.[22] Echo-planar and echo-volume imaging methodologies can also be used to generate real time maps of cerebral blood volume and tissue oxygenation, showing differences on task activation (e.g., by photic stimulation).[23] Such studies could well revolutionize the assessment of cerebral deficit in a wide range of neurological disorders.

Echo-volume imaging is capable of generating images at an astonishing rate—potentially a set of 64 every few tens of milliseconds. This presents a storage problem, and, more importantly, a major problem of assessment. It is simply not practicable for a radiologist to search through several thousand conventional images for a single patient. Interactive displays, data-reduction methods and eventually auto-analytical procedures will become essential in the relatively near future.

16.3 Magnetic Resonance Imaging—Animal Studies

16.3.1 Training of Medical Personnel

The need for animal experiments to demonstrate basic anatomy and physiology to medical students could be greatly reduced through the use of MRI. Surgery, solely for the purpose of visibility, could be eliminated, and, because the technique is noninvasive, multiple demonstrations could be conducted using a single animal. Better still, paid human volunteers or patients could take the place of the animals. Apart from being ethically more acceptable, it would also be more realistic from the training point of view.

The principal barrier to this is, of course, cost; few institutions find themselves in the fortunate position of being able to dedicate $2 million worth of equipment to the training of medical personnel. Although there is some prospect that much cheaper MRI systems may become available (see Section 16.5.2), in most cases, it would still mean students attending special sessions at the clinical scanning facility, or watching videotapes of top quality clinical demonstrations.

As far as the training of instument operators, radiographers, and radiologists is concerned, the genuinely noninvasive nature of MRI means that there is no objection to the repeated use of a group of volunteers, or even, of the trainees themselves. Indeed, this is to be preferred, as the group can be properly monitored by the occupational therapist. A range of acceptable tissue-mimicking phantoms is available which permit accurate assessment of machine (and possibly operator!) function.

16.3.2 Clinical Models

In the short-to-medium term, a diminishing need for animal models of disease is likely to persist. The arguments generally advanced in the favor of such animal experimentation center on reproducibility and ease of study. Of course, everyone appreciates that different species may respond differently to insult, and that there may be little relationship with the human response. Indeed, many models rely on anatomical or genetic abnormalities of some particular species, e.g., the gerbil model of stroke. Although it may be widely accepted that there will be differences in the levels of human and animal responses, nevertheless there is an implicit assumption that the models really do mimic the disease in question. As it becomes increasingly possible to study the disease *in situ* in man, so it becomes evident that many of these models are inappropriate, and, if viewed in isolation, can be positively damaging to furthering our understanding of certain diseases.

We take stroke as an example. Stroke is the third commonest cause of death in the western world (after heart disease and cancer) and is the leading cause of disability. The average incidence is a little over 2 per 1000 population per year. In the U.K., a typical general practitioner might expect to see about five new cases each year, and, at any one time, some 10,000 beds are likely to be occupied by stroke patients. The socioeconomic implications of this disease are staggering, and few would argue that research directed at the development of neuroprotective agents to prevent stroke, or ameliorate its effects, was not a worthwhile pursuit. Yet we read in a recent editorial in *Neuroscience Facts,* discussing strategies for neuroprotection in stroke, that: "Progress has probably been hampered by the belief that models for cardiac arrest or for forebrain ischemia in rats and gerbils mimic the brain lesions caused by stroke." *N*-Methyl-D-aspartate(NMDA) antagonists (a particularly promising class of potential neuroprotectives) fail to ameliorate brain lesions in these cases,[24,25] whereas they have been shown to be effective in reducing the infarct size after middle cerebral artery occlusion in rats.[26] MRI studies have also demonstrated long-term differences in the NMR relaxation parameters in the different models. Which, if any, is the appropriate model for the human condition?

The widespread availability of MRI systems now makes it possible to study stroke victims in a noninvasive manner. Until very recently, most imaging techniques, including conventional MRI, failed to show the region affected by the stroke until well after the primary event. However, diffusion-weighted studies have clearly shown that the (water) diffusion constant is affected early on in stroke,[27,28] enabling the primary lesion to be imaged. Of course, stroke victims do not form a homogneous patient population—there are probably as many different stroke types as there are victims. However, the success of diffusion-weighted MRI in imaging these lesions, opens up the possibility of study in sufficient numbers to permit meaningful classification and development of treatment for each subclass. It also permits the proper evaluation of animal models and the rejection of those that bear no relation to the human condition.

As has been repeatedly stated, MRI is an inherently noninvasive method. This means that serial human studies are possible, with a frequency that could never be countenanced with X-ray or radioisotopic methods, where cumulative dose of ionizing radiation is the overriding consideration. Similarly, if animal models must be used, serial studies greatly reduce the total numbers required. This is a potentially very significant advantage, given the amount of animal testing that currently goes on, and will continue to do so for the forseeable future. The advantage is not simply due to the fact that multiple time points can be obtained from a single animal, but also that the (potentially different) responses in different animals can be followed, rather than average responses being calculated. In a sense, each animal acts as its own control. The other advantage of the noninvasive nature of MRI is that multiple imaging measurements (relaxation time, diffusion, flow, etc.) can be conducted at each time point, and, possibly, combined with *in vivo* magnetic resonance spectroscopy of multiple organs.

16.3.3 Veterinary

The emphasis in this section has been on the study of animals as models of humans. Of course, there is considerable interest too, in veterinary applications. The high cost of conventional MRI/S systems puts them beyond the means of the average veterinary practice and applications have so far been rather limited, covering, for example, research into animal husbandry. There are also strong financial incentives to develop specialized systems suitable for examination of highly prized animals, such as racehorses. The likely future development of genuinely low-cost systems could, however, bring MRI within the reach of the larger veterinary centers.

16.4 Magnetic Resonance Spectroscopy

The sister technique to MRI, MRS is less well-developed clinically. It is a very powerful research tool which is advancing our understanding of human biochemistry but has yet to make its mark in the diagnosis of major diseases.[29] This is an essential goal in the eyes of the technologists and industrialists, who have to sell instruments in substantial numbers if they are to recoup their enormous development investment. Their voice is often heard loudest, and there is, therefore, a tendency to measure the effectiveness of MRS in clinical instruments sold, rather than in terms of the scientific advances made through its use.

Atomic nuclei, unless they have even atomic and mass numbers (for example, ^{12}C, ^{16}O, and ^{32}S), will have a net spin by virtue of the spins of the protons and neutrons which constitute them. As nuclei are positively charged, there will be a magnetic moment associated with the spin. This combination of spin angular momentum and magnetic moment causes the nuclei to precess in a magnetic field in much the same way that a gyroscope precesses in the earth's gravitational field. The frequency of precession is the Larmor or resonance frequency. It is directly proportional to the magnetic field B. Thus, as we have previously seen for MRI:

$$\omega = \gamma B$$

The proportionality constant γ differs widely for the different nuclei, ensuring that there is little chance of heteronuclear spectral overlap. For ^1H it is such that, in the earth's magnetic field of 0.5 G, protons precess at an audio frequency of about 2 kHz. Although you are doubtless unaware of it, this is true of all the protons in your body as you read this. As we have seen, in connection with MRI, only certain orientations of the spins are allowed with respect to the magnetic field. For the spin one-half nuclei with which we shall be exclusively concerned, there are two. Irradiation with electromagnetic radiation at the Larmor frequency induces transitions between these energy states: this is the phenomenon of nuclear magnetic resonance. For practically attainable magnetic fields (up to 14 T or about

300,000 times the earth's field), the radiation is at the low-frequency end of the electromagnetic spectrum, typically in the radiofrequency region. Consequently, it is nonionizing. That is to say, there is no danger of ejecting an electron and thereby disrupting a molecular bond. This is one reason why NMR is attractive for *in vivo* biochemical studies—it will not damage samples and can be safely used for clinical diagnosis *in situ*. The low-energy nature of NMR represents a major disadvantage in another respect, however—the method has very low sensitivity compared with traditional analytical methods. Its use is therefore restricted to metabolites present at high intracellular concentrations (typically ≥ 10 μM).

In addition to the large differences in resonance frequency due to the different nuclear magnetogyric ratios, much smaller differences exist between nuclei of the same atomic species located in different molecular environments. These differences arise because it is the field at an individual nucleus which determines the resonance frequency:

$$B_{nucleus} = B_{applied}(1-\sigma)$$

where σ = the shielding constant.

This is the basis of the NMR spectrum. Nuclei in different functional groups are distinguished on the basis of their different electronic environment. These differences are known as chemical shifts. They are normally measured in parts per million from some arbitrarily chosen reference:

$$\delta = \frac{(f - f_{ref}) \times 10^6}{f_{ref}}$$

where δ =   the chemical shift
        f =   the observed frequency
        f_{ref} =   the reference frequency

For ^{31}P NMR, the normal choice of reference (for which δ is set to 0) is phosphocreatine, whereas for ^1H and ^{13}C NMR tetramethylsilane (TMS) is standard. Provided the spectra are recorded under fully relaxed conditions, the areas under the peaks correspond directly to the number of nuclei resonating at that frequency and can hence be used to determine concentrations. In the case of ^{31}P NMR spectra, it is normally possible to discern signals from the high-energy phosphates phosphocreatine and ATP, inorganic phosphate (see below), and various phosphomonoesters and phosphodiesters, generally believed to be intermediates in the synthesis and breakdown of lipids, respectively. Other key biochemical/physiological parameters can sometimes also be deduced, for example, intracellular pH, pH_i.

There are numerous examples of NMR resonances which titrate over the physiological range of pH and which, in principle, could be used to determine intracellular pH. The first example to be described in the literature was the use of ^{31}P NMR to monitor the shift of the inorganic phosphate, Pi, resonance in erythrocytes.[30] This method has survived the test of time and remains the most popular. Pi is subject to the following equilibria:

$$H_3PO_4 \leftrightarrow H^+ + H_2PO_4^- \qquad \text{pK } 2.0$$

$$H_2PO_4^- \leftrightarrow H^+ + HPO_4^{2-} \qquad \text{pK } 6.8$$

$$HPO_4^{2-} \leftrightarrow H^+ + PO_4^{3-} \qquad \text{pK } 12.0$$

Thus, under normal physiological conditions, inorganic phosphate exists primarily as $H_2PO_4^-$ and HPO_4^{2-}. These species have ^{31}P chemical shifts relative to phosphocreatine of 3.29 and 5.81 ppm, respectively. They are in rapid chemical exchange and so the pH can be determined from the following expression:

$$pH = 6.8 + \log\left[\frac{(3.29 - \delta)}{(\delta - 5.81)}\right]$$

where δ = the observed ^{31}P shift of the inorganic phosphate peak.

More commonly, an empirically determined titration curve is used to read off pH from the observed shift. It is important that this calibration be performed under intracellular conditions: a medium containing 150 mM K$^+$, 5 mM Na$^+$, and 1 mM Mg^{2+} is often used. In practice, the titration curve is little shifted, even by substantial changes in these concentrations. However, such effects contribute to an uncertainty in the absolute pH$_i$ of perhaps 0.1 units. Changes in pH can be measured to rather higher accuracy, normally better than 0.05 units.

The clinical application of localized NMR spectroscopy stems from small-scale studies conducted at roughly the same time as the demonstrative imaging experiments. The successful demonstration that high-resolution ^{31}P spectra could be recorded from isolated but intact skeletal muscle[31] led to the widespread use of this technique for monitoring tissue bioenergetics. Clinical studies were pioneered in Oxford by Professor Radda and were initially targeted towards the diagnosis of in-born errors of muscle metabolism for which purpose they proved extremely successful.[32] Other early successes include the monitoring of neonates suspected to have been exposed to an ischemic episode (birth asphyxia). Measurement by ^{31}P NMR of the ratio of the concentrations of phosphocreatine to inorganic phosphate in these children proved to be an accurate indicator of survival prospects and of possible brain damage.[33] The ^{31}P NMR spectrum is an excellent indicator of ischemia/hypoxia: it is therefore extremely attractive to use ^{31}P NMR to perform regional studies in adult brain and heart. Such studies require the use of rather more sophisticated localization techniques than were employed in the early studies on muscle and infantile brain.[34]

^{13}C NMR is well suited to the elucidation of metabolic pathways and the measurement of fluxes through them. Recently, human studies involving the incorporation of ^{13}C label from $1 - ^{13}$C glucose into the C1 of muscle glycogen have shown that muscle is responsible for the uptake of virtually all the excess glucose during hyperglycemia and that, in patients with non-insulin-dependent diabetes mellitus, it is a failure of glucose transport, rather than a defect in glycogen synthase, that is responsible for the reduced rate of glycogen synthesis compared to control subjects.[35] Attractive though ^{13}C studies are, they are both expensive and relatively insensitive. There is no inherent reason for the high cost, and as clinical ^{13}C NMR becomes more widely used we can expect to see a reduction by at least an order of magnitude in isotope costs from perhaps $1000 to $100 per investigation. However, the problem of low sensitivity will remain and much attention is, therefore, now also being focused on ^{1}H MRS.[36] This can be used directly, for example, as in the measurements of cerebral glucose in patients with insulin-dependent diabetes mellitus,[37] or as an indirect measure of attached ^{13}C-labeled metabolites.

Drug metabolism can be monitored *in situ* by NMR provided the drug accumulates to sufficient concentration and has an appropriate "NMR label". For example, the metabolism of 5-fluorouracil, a drug widely used in the treatment of disseminated tumors of the colon, breast, and ovary, has been monitored in animal models but can now be monitored directly in patients undergoing therapy. There is a good correlation between the presence of active metabolite, detected by ^{19}F NMR, and therapeutic response.[38]

The recording of high resolution spectral information from humans has proved to be a considerable challenge and the technology is still under active development.[39] As it matures, we can expect to see a dramatic shift in emphasis towards direct study of human disease.

16.5 Future Developments

16.5.1 Trends

The main drive in the development of technology for MRI and MRS has been clinical, principally for diagnostic purposes, but increasingly also for research purposes. This is especially true of MRS which thus far has relatively few major diagnostic applications.

Whereas the ability to perform such investigations in humans is certain to greatly reduce the need for (inappropriate) animal models, it is certain that some animal studies will continue to be necessary for the forseeable future. The same MRI/S techniques that have been developed primarily for clinical use can also be used in smaller-scale equipment for these tests. The main benefit is the noninvasive nature of the measurements. This means that serial studies are possible, greatly reducing the numbers of animals that must otherwise be used to generate statistically meaningful results. A very high proportion of animal experimentation is concerned with "safety" testing of new and existing compounds. There is enormous scope for reduction of animal experimentation here—nonanimal alternatives, harmonization of international safety legislation, examination of the need for constant development of new products, especially in the cosmetic industries, etc.

16.5.2 Technological Advances and Availability

The very high cost of superconducting magnets distinguishes MRI/S from other diagnostic modalities and restricts its application to relatively few of the more prestigous healthcare institutions. In order for the technology to become more accessible, and the evidence of its clinical efficacy strongly suggests that there is such a need, magnet costs must be substantially reduced. In the longer term, the development of high T_c superconducting materials could have a profound effect on the industry. In the shorter term, magnet manufacturers are looking for acceptable compromises in magnet bore, field strength, and homogeneity—the problem being that the NMR is an inherently insensitive technique (when compared to other branches of spectroscopy) and image quality is impaired if cheaper (lower-field) magnets are employed.

Permanent magnets are attracting increasing attention. Constructed from ferrite material, they can be made to generate a field of 0.2 T with a homogeneity of about 40 ppm over a spherical volume of diameter 36 cm, though with a substantially increased weight (8.5 t compared to the 3.5 t of a typical 0.5 T superconducting magnet). Such a system has recently been released in Japan by Siemens-Asahi. Over the period 1988 to 1990, about 100 similar sytems were installed in Japan by Hitachi. We can certainly anticipate substantial world growth in this area.

Apart from cost, another problem limits the wider application of MRI, namely siting difficulties. High-field magnets generate substantial peripheral fields which represent a potential hazard to patient and equipment (particularly devices employing cathode ray tubes) alike. Permanent magnets solve this problem by being self-shielding; manufacturers of other magnet systems seek to reduce the problem by employing passive[40] or, more recently, active shields.

Conventional MRI systems require the patient to be slid deep within the bore of a superconducting magnet. There is considerable risk of claustrophobia, and a relatively high patient-refusal rate results. This can be alleviated by sympathetic counseling in which the genuine noninvasiveness of the technique (compared, for example, to explorative surgery!) is emphasized. Oxford Magnet Technology has proposals for flatbed (one-sided) magnets which would greatly improve accessibility and reduce patient anxiety. Unfortunately, a high price would be paid in terms of peripheral field.

REFERENCES

1. Lauterbur, P. C. "Image Formation by Induced Local Interactions: Examples Employing Nuclear Magnetic Resonance," *Nature* 242(5394):190–191 (1973).
2. Mansfield, P. and P. K. Grannell. "NMR 'Diffraction' in Solids?," *J. Phys. C* 6(22):L422–L426 (1973).
3. Hounsfield, G. N. "Computerized Transverse Axial Scanning (Tomography): Part I. Description of System," *Brit. J. Radiol.* 46(552):1016–1022 (1973).
4. Mansfield, P. and A. A. Maudsley. "Medical Imaging By NMR," *Brit. J. Radiol.* 50(591):188–194 (1977).
5. Hinshaw, W. S., P. A. Bottomley, and G. N. Holland. "Radiographic Thin-Section Image of the Human Wrist by Nuclear Magnetic Resonance", *Nature* 270(5639):722–723 (1977).
6. Damadian, R., M. Goldsmith, and L. Minkoff. "NMR in Cancer: XVI. FONAR Image of the Live Human Body," *Physiol. Chem. Phys.* 9(1):97–100 (1977).
7. Mansfield, P., I. L. Pykett, P. G. Morris, and R. E. Coupland. "Human Whole Body Line-Scan Imaging by NMR," *Brit. J. Radiol.* 51(611):921–922 (1978).
8. Young, I. R., A. S. Hall, C. A. Pallis, N. J. Legg, G. M. Bydder, and R. E. Steiner. "Nuclear Magnetic Resonance Imaging of the Brain in Multiple Sclerosis," *Lancet* 2(8255):1063–1066 (1981).
9. Radon, J. "On the Determination of Functions from Their Integrals along Certain Manifolds," *Ber. Saechs. Akad. Wiss. Leipzig, Math. Phys. Kl* 69:262–277 (1917).
10. Bracewell, R. N. "Strip Integration in Radioastronomy," *Austr. J. Phys.* 9(1):198–217 (1956).
11. Morris, P. G. *Nuclear Magnetic Resonance Imaging in Medicine and Biology* (Oxford: Oxford University Press, 1986), chapter 4.
12. Ljunggren, S. "A Simple Graphical Representation of Fourier-Based Imaging Methods," *J. Magn. Reson.* 54(2):338–343 (1983).
13. Mansfield, P. "Multi-Planar Image Formation Using NMR Spin Echoes," *J. Phys. C* 10(3):L55–L58 (1977).
14. Hawksworth, D. "New Magnet Designs for MR," *Magn. Reson. Med.* 17(1):27–32 (1991).
15. Wedeen, V., R. Meuli, R. Edelman, S. Geller, L. Frank, T. Brady, and B. Rosen. "Projection Imaging of Pulsatile Flow with Magnetic Resonance," *Science* 230(4728):946–948 (1985).
16. Dumoulin, C., S. Souza, M. Walker, and W. Wagle. "Three-Dimensional Phase Contrast Angiography," *Magn. Reson. Med.* 9(1):139–149 (1989).
17. Van Dijk, P. "Direct Cardiac NMR Imaging of Heart Wall and Blood Flow Velocity," *J. Comput. Assist. Tomogr.* 8(3):429–436 (1984).
18. Nayler, G. L., D. N. Firmin, and D. B. Longmore. "Blood Flow Imaging by Cine Magnetic Resonance," *J. Comput. Assist. Tomogr.* 10(5):715–722 (1986).
19. Le Bihan, D. "Intravoxel Incoherent Motion Using Steady-State Free Precession," *Magn. Reson. Med.* 7(3):346–351 (1988).
20. Turner, R., D. Le Bihan, and A. S. Chesnick. "Echo-Planar Imaging of Diffusion and Perfusion," *Magn. Reson. Med.* 19(2):247–253 (1991).
21. Stehling, K., R. Turner, and P. Mansfield. "Echo-Planar Imaging: Magnetic Resonance Imaging in a Fraction of a Second," *Science* 254(5028):43–50 (1991).

22. Mansfield, P., A. M. Howseman, and R. J. Ordidge. "Volumar Imaging Using NMR Spin Echoes: Echo-Volumar Imaging (EVI) at 0.1T," *J. Phys. E* 22(5):324–30 (1989).

23. Belliveau, J. W., D. N. Kennedy, R. C. McKinstry, B. R. Buchbinder, R. M. Weisskoff, M. S. Cohen, J. M. Vevea, T. J. Brady and B. R. Rosen. "Functional Mapping of the Human Visual Cortex by Magnetic Resonance Imaging," *Science* 254(5032):716–719 (1991).

24. Fleischer, J., A. Takeishi, C. Drummond, M. Scheler, M. Grafe, M. Zornow, G. Shearman, and H. Shapiro. "MK-801, an Excitatory Amino Acid Antagonist Does Not Improve Neurologic Outcome Following Cardiac Arrest in Cats," *J. Cerebr. Blood Flow Metab.* 9(6):795–804 (1989).

25. Buchan, A., H. Li, and W. A. Pulsinelli. "The *N*-methyl-D-Aspartate Antagonist MK-801 Fails to Protect Against Neuronal Damage Caused by Transient Severe Forebrain Ischaemia in Rats," *J. Neurosci.* 11(4):1049–1056 (1991).

26. Park, C. K., D. G. Nehls, D. I. Graham, G. M. Teasdale, and J. McCulloch. "The Glutamate Antagonist MK-801 Reduces Focal Ischemic Brain Damage in the Rat," *Ann. Neurol.* 24(4):543–551 (1988).

27. Moseley, M. E., J. Kucharczyk, J. Mintorovitch, Y. Cohen, J. Kurhanewicz, N. Derugin, H. Asagari, and D. Norman. "Diffusion-Weighted MR Imaging of Acute Stroke: Correlation with T_2-Weighted and Magnetic Susceptibility Enhanced MR Imaging in Cats," *Am. J. Neurorad.* 11(3):423–29 (1990).

28. Moseley, M. E., Y. Cohen, J. Mintorovitch, L. Chileuitt, H. Shimizu, J. Kucharczyk, M. F. Wendland, and P. R. Weinstein. "Early Detection of Regional Cerebral Ischaemia in Cats: Comparison of Diffusion and T_2-Weighted MRI and Spectroscopy," *Magn. Reson. Med.* 14(2):330–346 (1990).

29. Cady, E. B. *Clinical Magnetic Resonance Spectroscopy* (New York: Plenum Press, 1990).

30. Moon, R. B. and J. H. Richards. "Determination of Intracellular pH by [31]P Magnetic Resonance," *J. Biol. Chem.* 248(20):7276–7278 (1973).

31. Hoult, D. I., S. J. W. Busby, D. G. Gadian, G. K, Radda, R. E. Richards, and P. J. Seeley. "Observation of Tissue Metabolites Using [31]P Nuclear Magnetic Resonance," *Nature* 252(5481):285–287 (1974).

32. Radda, G. K. "The Use of NMR Spectroscopy for the Understanding of Disease," *Science* 233(4764):640–645 1986.

33. Hope, P. L., A. M. Costello, E. B. Cady, P. A. Hamilton, A. M. De Costello, D. T. Delpy, A. Chu, E. O. Reynolds, and D. R. Wilkie. "Cerebral Energy Metabolism Studied with Phosphorus NMR Spectroscopy in Normal and Birth-Asphyxiated Infants," *Lancet* 2(8399):366–370 (1984).

34. Bottomley, P. A. and C. J. Hardy. "Strategies and Protocols for Clinical [31]P Research in the Heart and Brain," *Phil. Trans. R. Soc. Lond. A* 333(1632):531–544 (1990).

35. Shulman, G. I., D. L. Rothman, and R. G. Shulman. "^{13}C NMR Studies of Glucose Disposal in Normal and Non-Insulin-Dependent Diabetic Humans," *Phil. Trans. R. Soc. Lond. A* 333(1632):525–529 (1990).

36. Gadian, D. G. "Proton Studies of Brain Metabolism," *Phil. Trans. R. Soc. Lond. A* 333(1632):561–570 (1990).

37. Bruhn, H., T. Michaelis, K. D. Merboldt, W. Hanicke, M. L. Gyngell, and J. Frahm. "Monitoring Cerebral Glucose in Diabetics by Proton MRS," *Lancet* 337(8743):745–746 (1991).

38. Semmler, W., P. Bachert-Baumann, F. Guckel, F. Ermark, P. Schlag, W. J. Lorenz, and G. van Kaick. "Real-Time Follow-Up of 5-Fluorouracil Metabolism in the Liver of Tumor Patients by Means of F-19 MR Spectroscopy," *Radiology*, 174(1):141– 145 (1990).

39. Diehl, P., E. Fluck, H., Gunther, R. Kosfeld, and J. Seelig. Eds. *In-Vivo Magnetic Resonance Spectroscopy I: Probeheads and Radiofrequency Pulses, Spectrum Analysis* (Berlin/Heidelberg: Springer-Verlag, 1992).

40. Andrew, E. R. "Passive Magnetic Screening," *Magn. Reson. Med.* 17(1):22–26 (1991).

Index

A

Active Memory Technologies DAP, 154
Acute oral-toxicity testing, at Procter & Gamble, 28–29
Adaptive Resonance Theory (ART), 92–93
Adsorption, 218
Affinity chromatography, 218
Aging, 199
Agriculture/veterinary computation modeling, 131, 134
AIDS
    discovery of virus sequence in, 145
    epidemiologic studies of, 178–179
    human autopsies in study of, 199
    mathematical modeling of, 129
Alloparenting study, 107–109
α_2-adrenergic binding, 79
Alternative explanations, ruling out of, 176
Alternative testing methods
    at Procter & Gamble, 29–32
    validation of, 37–38
American Type Culture Collection, 50–51
Ames assays, 35
Ames Reverse Mutation Test, 16
Amino acid measurement, 151
Analysis problems, 120
Analytic epidemiology, 166–167
    case–control studies in, 167–169
    cohort studies in, 169–172
    cross-sectional studies in, 172
ANALYZE, 121
Animal
    alternatives to in preventive medicine, 191–193
    classification of, 190
    disease-control programs and, 189
    human health interconnections with, 189–190
    magnetic resonance and, 237–251
    public health and welfare of, 187–189
    venomous and dangerous, 190–191
    vermin, 191
Animal behavior studies
    ethological techniques of, 106–112
    goals of, 105–106
    history of, 103–105
Animal testing, 4
    replacement of, 20
    uses of, 11–12

Animalcules, 208
Anisotropic diffusion, 244
ANN, see Neural networks, artificial
Anopheline mosquito, 208
Antibiotic, first, 208
Antibody detection, 212
Antidepressants, action of, 78–79
Antigen detection, 213
Antipsychotic drugs, action of, 79–81
Aristotle, 103
Artificial intelligence, 89, see also Computer
Asepsis, 209
Aseptic surgical technique, 208–209
Association, measurement of, 176
Autopsies, 195–199
Avery, Oswald, 208
Avon Corporation, elimination of animal testing in, 20
AZT, 179

B

Bacteria, medically important, 209–210
Bacteriology, medical, 209
Beagles, in lung cancer study, 192
Behavior
    evolution of, 104
    goals of studies of, 105–106
Behavioral science
    early history of, 87–91
    neural networks and, 87–99
    nonanimal models of, 96
Behavioral variable studies, epidemiologic, 173
Behavioristic psychology, 105
β-adrenoceptor binding, 79
Biogenic amines, 76
Bioimplants design, 127
Biological data matrix, 134–135
Biological/medical systems
    cognitive and sensory processes in, 91–92
    computation modeling of, 115–135
Biological research
    physicochemical techniques in, 217–221
    in psychiatry, 73–81
Biology, human genome in, 148–149
Biomarkers, 181–182
Biomedical research, 195–199
Biophysical properties, 130
Biostatistics study, 129–130
Biotechnology databases, 146–147